OBJECTIVE CARDIOLOGY

AF655314

OBJECTIVE CARDIOLOGY

Mahesh Chandra
Chief, Intensive Care Unit
Department of Medicine
King George's Medical University
Lucknow–226003

PUBLISHING FOR ONE WORLD

NEW AGE INTERNATIONAL (P) LIMITED, PUBLISHERS
New Delhi • Bangalore • Chennai • Cochin • Guwahati • Hyderabad
Jalandhar • Kolkata • Lucknow • Mumbai • Ranchi
Visit us at www.newagepublishers.com

Copyright © 2009, New Age International (P) Ltd., Publishers
Published by New Age International (P) Ltd., Publishers
First Edition: 2009

All rights reserved.
No part of this book may be reproduced in any form, by photostat, microfilm, xerography, or any other means, or incorporated into any information retrieval system, electronic or mechanical, without the written permission of the copyright owner.

Branches:

- 36, Malikarjuna Temple Street, Opp. ICWA, Basavanagudi, **Bangalore**. ✆ (080) 26677815
- 26, Damodaran Street, T. Nagar, **Chennai**. ✆ (044) 24353401
- Hemsen Complex, Mohd. Shah Road, Paltan Bazar, Near Starline Hotel, **Guwahati**. ✆ (0361) 2543669
- No. 105, 1st Floor, Madhiray Kaveri Tower, 3-2-19, Azam Jahi Road, Nimboliadda, **Hyderabad**. ✆ (040) 24652456
- RDB Chambers (Formerly Lotus Cinema) 106A, Ist Floor, S.N. Banerjee Road, **Kolkata**. ✆ (033) 22275247
- 18, Madan Mohan Malviya Marg, **Lucknow**. ✆ (0522) 2209578
- 142C, Victor House, Ground Floor, N.M. Joshi Marg, Lower Parel, **Mumbai**. ✆ (022) 24927869
- 22, Golden House, Daryaganj, **New Delhi**. ✆ (011) 23262368, 23262370

ISBN: 978-81-224-2615-1

Rs. 200.00

C-09-03-3473

Printed in India at Mohan Lal Printers, Delhi.
Typeset at In-house

PUBLISHING FOR ONE WORLD

NEW AGE INTERNATIONAL (P) LIMITED, PUBLISHERS
4835/24, Ansari Road, Daryaganj, New Delhi-110002
Visit us at **www.newagepublishers.com**

To

My Wife

Mrs. Usha Agarwal

&

My Daughter

Dr. Swati Chandra

PREFACE

In this era of super-specialisation almost every postgraduate student has the zeal of acquiring training in a specialised way. One of the most fascinating branches for the students of Medicine is Cardiology. As the pattern of DM entrance examination is based on multiple choice questions and there is scarcity of such books, I took up this task and tried to fill the lacuna by writing a book containing MCQs for DM entrance exams and also supplementing it with updated version of recent advances. I have tried to cover each topic with appropriate stress upon often repeated facts.

The questions are authentic and the answer of each and every question has been checked from various textbooks.

Every effort is made to minimize grammatical errors and spelling mistakes. I hope that you would pardon me for any inadvertent error.

Mahesh Chandra

Acknowledgement

I owe this book first and foremost to my wife, Mrs. Usha Agarwal and my daughter, Dr. Swati Chandra who made all the resources available to me for the making of this book and making no demands on my time when I was writing this book. In fact, it is our dream vision which has taken a real shape.

This book would not have been so complete without the help of my students Dr. Lanlan Jha, Dr. Saurabh Srivastva and Dr. Rupali Khanna of SGPGI, Lucknow; Prof. Pankaj Kumar, Dr. Pradeep Kumar, Dr. Arun Prasath, Dr. Ritesh Sangari, Dr. Akshyaya Kumar Pradhan, Dr. Vivek Raj Singh, Dr. Gaurav Chaudhary, Dr. Abhishek Singh, Dr. Abhilash Chandra, Dr. Shiresh Mishra, Dr. Rakesh Kumar and Dr. Jahangeer Rashid Beg of KGMU and Mr. Vikas Roy, Area Manager of New Age International (P) Limited, Publishers, Lucknow Branch.

In fact, all the residents of Medicine have given me immense support throughout.

Mahesh Chandra

ABBREVIATIONS

ASD	=	Atrial Septal Defect
ASH	=	Asymmetrical Septal Hypertrophy
ATVL	=	Anterior Tricuspid Valve Leaflet
AV	=	Atrioventricular
AVA	=	Aortic Valve Area
AVR	=	Aortic Valve Replacement
CAD	=	Coronary Artery Disease
CO	=	Cardiac Output
CS	=	Coronary Sinus
CT	=	Computed Tomography
ECG	=	Electrocardiogram
Echo	=	Echocardiography
EF	=	Ejection Fraction
HCM	=	Hypertrophic Cardiomyopathy
HOCM	=	Hypertrophic Obstructive Cardiomyopathy
HR	=	Heart Rate
LA	=	Left Atrium
LAA	=	Left Atrial Appendage
LADCA	=	Left Anterior Descending Coronary Artery
LAE	=	Left Atrial Enlargement
LPA	=	Left Pulmonary Artery
LV	=	Left Ventricle
LVH	=	Left Ventricular Hypertrophy
LVE	=	Left Ventricular Enlargement

LVI = Left Ventricular Inflow
MI = Myocardial Infarction
MR = Mitral Regurgitation
MRI = Magnetic Resonance Imaging
MS = Mitral Stenosis
PA = Pulmonary Artery
PD = Pulsed Doppler
PDA = Patent Ductus Arteriosus
PDA = Posterior Descending Artery
PE = Pericardial Effusion
RA = Right Atrium
RAE = Right Atrial Enlargement
RCA = Right Coronary Artery
RCC = Right Coronary Cusp
RF = Regurgitant Fraction
SV = Stroke Volume or Sample Volume
SVC = Superior Vena Cava
TOF = Tetralogy of Fallot
TR = Tricuspid Regurgitation
TS = Tricuspid Stenosis
TSV = Total Stroke Volume
VAS = Ventriculo Atrial Septum
VSD = Ventricular Septal Defect
WPWS = Wolff-Parkinson-White Syndrome

Contents

SECTION–1

Clinical and Investigational Cardiology

1. Loud first heart sound is heard in

(a) Mitral stenosis
(b) Mitral regurgitation
(c) Mitral valve prolapse
(d) Calcified mitral stenosis

2. Commonest cause of pulsus paradoxus is

(a) Cardiac tamponade
(b) Adhesive pericarditis
(c) Constrictive pericarditis
(d) Chylopericardium

3. Roth's spots are seen in the

(a) Pharynx (b) Heart
(c) Fundus (d) Palms

4. Bisferiens pulse may be seen in all except

(a) Combined aortic stenosis + Aortic regurgitation
(b) Hypertrophic subaortic stenosis
(c) Normal individuals
(d) Chronic severe atrial regurgitation

5. Cannon 'a' waves are seen in

(a) Sinus bradycardia
(b) Complete heart block
(c) Pulmonary stenosis
(d) Atrial fibrillation

6. Anacrotic pulse is present in

(a) Aortic regurgitation
(b) Mitral regurgitation
(c) Mitral stenosis
(d) Aortic stenosis

7. Pulsus alternans is seen in
(a) Left ventricular failure
(b) Digitalis poisoning
(c) Aortic stenosis with aortic regurgitation
(d) Mitral stenosis with mitral regurgitation

8. Electrical alternans is pathognomic of
(a) Pericardial tamponade
(b) Pericardial effusion
(c) Left ventricular failure
(d) All of the above

9. Rib notching is seen in
(a) Patent ductus arteriosus
(b) Ventricular septal defect
(c) Coarctation of aorta
(d) Tetralogy of fallot

10. Mid diastolic rumble in the tricuspid region is found in which of the following.
(a) Atrial septal defect
(b) Ventricular septal defect
(c) Patent ductus arteriosus
(d) Mitral regurgitation

11. Graham steel murmur is heard in
(a) Aortic regurgitation
(b) Pulmonary hypertension
(c) Aortic stenosis
(d) Tricuspid stenosis

12. Which statement is true for left ventricular free wall thickness?
(a) Uniform
(b) Thickest toward apex
(c) Thickest toward base
(d) Thickest in mid segment

13. Papillary muscles are not found in
(a) Mitral valve
(b) Aortic valve
(c) Tricuspid valve
(d) All the above

14. Current technique of bed side assessment of jugular venous pressure was described by

(a) Pierre-carl potain (b) James mackenzie
(c) Claudius galen (d) Thomas lewis

15. Nobel prize in electrocardiography was given to

(a) Von kalliker (b) Augsentus walter
(c) William einthoven(d) None of the above

16. Which tricuspid leaflet is least mobile?

(a) Anterior (b) Posterior
(c) Septal (d) None of these

17. Which is the smallest tricuspid leaflet?

(a) Anterior (b) Posterior
(c) Septal (d) None of these

18. Coronary origin of angina was first appreciated by

(a) William heberden (b) Edward jenner
(c) John hunter (d) None of the above

19. Mean pulmonary arterial pressure is best estimated by

(a) Loud P2
(b) Narrow split S2
(c) Right ventricular heave
(d) Diameter of the right pulmonary artery at the widest point

20. P mitrale has all the following features except

(a) More than normal duration
(b) Best seen in L1
(c) Notched
(d) Flat top

21. ECG–RVH in mitral stenosis suggest all except.

(a) Bad prognosis without surgery
(b) More prone to right ventricular failure
(c) More prone to infective endocarditis
(d) None of the above

22. Most specific sign of pulmonary hypertension in mitral stenosis is

(a) P2 loud (b) P2 palpable
(c) ESM in PA
(d) Right ventricular heave

23. In mild mitral stenosis the diastolic murmur is confined to

(a) Middiastole
(b) Presystolic
(c) Both middiastolic and presystolic murmur with gap between two
(d) Holodiastolic

24. Non significant mitral regurgitation in presence of mitral stenosis is suggested by

(a) Presence of presystolic murmur
(b) Absence of loud S1
(c) Absence of opening snap
(d) None of the above

25. A patient having loud S1 with atrial fibrillation the most common diagnosis is

(a) Constrictive pericarditis
(b) Cor pulmonale
(c) Mitral stenosis
(d) Mitral regurgitation

26. What S2–OS duration means that mitral stenosis is critical?

(a) > 0.10 sec (b) 0.1 sec
(c) 0.09 sec (d) < 0.08 sec

27. Normal diastolic mitral valve flow is approximately

(a) 70 ml/sec (b) 100 ml/sec
(c) 150 ml/sec (d) 200 ml/sec

28. Boot shaped cardiac silhouette is characteristic of

(a) Aortic stenosis
(b) Mitral stenosis
(c) Aortic regurgitation
(d) Transposition of great arteries

29. All the following statements are incorrect regarding pulmonary regurgitation except

(a) Murmur increases with hand grip
(b) Comes after A2
(c) Murmur decreases with amyl nitrite
(d) Murmur begins just after P2

30. Austin flint murmur has all the features except

(a) S3 is present
(b) Opening snap is present
(c) Left ventricular enlargement is present
(d) Murmur decreases with amyl nitrite

31. Pulsus parvus occurs in

(a) Compensated aortic stenosis
(b) Aortic stenosis and aortic regurgitation
(c) Decompensated aortic stenosis
(d) All the above

32. All statements regarding cooing dove murmur are correct except

(a) Musical murmur of aortic stenosis
(b) Musical murmur of aortic regurgitation
(c) Due to perforation of aortic cusp
(d) Occurs in aortic valve infective endocarditis

33. Ascending aorta dilatation is usual in the all following except

(a) IHSS
(b) Congenital supravalvular aortic stenosis
(c) Congenital valvular aortic stenosis
(d) Congenital subvalvular aortic stenosis

34. Double apex beat is usually found in

(a) IHSS (b) Aortic stenosis
(c) Supravalvular aortic stenosis
(d) None of the above

35. Aortic ejection sound is most commonly found in

(a) Congenital valvular stenosis
(b) Acquired valvular aortic stenosis
(c) Congenital subvalvular stenosis
(d) Congenital supravalvular stenosis

36. Which of the following is a sail sound?

(a) Normal M1 (b) Normal T1
(c) Exaggerated T1 (d) Exaggerated M1

37. Reverse splitting of S1 is found in all except

(a) Right ventricular pacing
(b) Severe aortic stenosis
(c) Left atrial myxomia
(d) Right bundle branch block

38. All are high frequency heart sound except

(a) A2 (b) P2
(c) S4 (d) Non ejection sound

39. Summation fallop is a fusion of

(a) A2 and P2 (b) M1 and T1
(c) S3 and S4 (d) All of the above

40. Most common cause of kussmauls sign is

(a) Constrictive pericarditis
(b) Severe right side heart failure
(c) Right ventricle infarction
(d) Cardiac tamponade

41. Giant 'a' wave is most commonly present in

(a) PS
(b) PS with VSD
(c) PS with ASD
(d) PS with ASD and VSD

42. Bisferiens pulse is found in all of the following except

(a) Aortic regurgitation
(b) Aortic stenosis + Aortic regurgitation
(c) HCM
(d) Mitral regurgitation

43. Central venous pressure and wave forms are best appreciated in

(a) Right internal jugular vein
(b) Left internal jugular vein
(c) Right external jugular vein
(d) None of the above

44. Osler's node has all of the following features except

(a) Present on distal pad of fingers
(b) Are non tender
(c) Reddish purple
(d) Tender

45. Pulsatile liver is found in which condition?

(a) Mitral regurgitation
(b) Tricuspid regurgitation
(c) Aortic stenosis
(d) None of the above

46. Katz-Wachtel phenomenon in ECG occurs in

(a) Mitral regurgitation
(b) Ventricular septal defect
(c) Tricuspid regurgitation
(d) Aortic stenosis

47. In severe chronic mitral regurgitation all are commonly found except

(a) S1 soft (b) Wide split S2
(c) S3 (d) S4

48. All are contraindication to exercise testing in ischemic heart disease except

(a) Within 48hr of acute myocardial infraction
(b) High risk of unstable angina
(c) Sinus bradycardia with mild hypertension
(d) Symptomatic severe aortic stenosis

49. In presence of RBB block ST depression in which lead suggests presence of Ischemia?

(a) L1, aVL (b) V2, V3
(c) V1 (d) L2, L3, aVF

50. Tall T waves in patients of hyperkalemia are differentiated from tall T waves of myocardial infarction by

(a) Tall 'P' wave
(b) Short QT interval
(c) Prolonged QT interval
(d) None of the above

51. False positive exercise test is found in all except

(a) Hypertension (b) Aortic stenosis
(c) Recent food intake (d) 1° AV block

52. Myocardial dysfunction is best assessed by

(a) History
(b) Physical examination
(c) Chest X-ray
(d) ECG

53. Myocardial ischemia is best assessed by

(a) Physical examination
(b) Resting ECG
(c) Exercise ECG
(d) Holter monitoring

54. Functional capacity of heart disease is best assessed by

(a) History
(b) ECG (Resting)
(c) Exercise ECG
(d) Physical examination

55. Valvular function is best assessed by

(a) Chest X-ray (b) ECG exercise
(c) Echo (d) All of the above

56. When is pulsus paradoxus is absent in cardiac tamponade?

(a) Associated with left ventricular failure
(b) Regional tamponade
(c) When associated with ASD
(d) All of the above

57. Which of the following is best for diagnosis of constrictive pericarditis?

(a) Chest X-ray (b) CT
(c) Cine CT (d) MRI

58. Which ECG feature is pathognomic for cardiac tamponade?

(a) Low voltage QRS complex
(b) Generalized T wave inversion
(c) Abnormal Q waves
(d) Total electrical alternans

59. Which of the following is powerful predictor of cardiac temponade?

(a) Anteriorly echo free space of 5 mm
(b) Posteriorly echo free space of 10 mm
(c) Circumferential echo free space > 10 mm
(d) None of the above

60. Peak gradient on doppler ultrasound suggestive of high likelihood of severe aortic stenosis is

(a) 60 mmHg (b) 50 mmHg
(c) 70 mmHg (d) > 80 mmHg

61. Myocardial disarray is found in all except

(a) Hypertrophic cardiomyopathy
(b) Hypertension
(c) Aortic stenosis
(d) Aortic regurgitation

62. Probable largest organ of body is

(a) Lungs (b) Brain
(c) Endothelium (d) Liver

63. Left ventricular enlargement in presence of LBBB is suggested by all except

(a) Left atrial enlargement
(b) Left axis deviation
(c) V2 S + V5 R = 45 mm or more
(d) QRS duration > 0.14 S

64. Which statement is incorrect regarding still's murmur?

(a) Common in infancy
(b) Common after age 3 years
(c) Decreases towards adolescence
(d) Systolic vibratory murmur

65. Following ECG findings are strongly suggestive of acute corpulmonale except

(a) S1-Q3-T3 pattern with T wave inversion in V1-V3
(b) S1-Q3-T3 pattern with RBBB
(c) RBBB
(d) S1-T3 pattern

66. **All the following drugs causes false positive exercise test except**
   (a) Digitalis (b) Diuretics
   (c) Antidepressants (d) Calcium blockers

67. **All of the following drugs causes false negative exercise test except**
   (a) Nitrates (b) Aspirin
   (c) Propranolol (d) Verapamil

68. **Which arrhythmia is not indication for termination of exercise test?**
   (a) VT (b) AT
   (c) RBBB (d) Atrial fibrillation

69. **All the following findings are of clinical significance during exercise testing**
   (a) S3
   (b) S4
   (c) Systolic murmur at mitral area
   (d) loud S1

70. **All of the following are absolute contraindications to exercise test except**
   (a) Atrial fibrillation (b) CHB
   (c) Heart failure (d) 1° AV block

71. **Pseudo left axis deviaton is found in**
   (a) Diffuse myocardial disease
   (b) Diffuse pulmonary disease
   (c) Left ventricular enlargement
   (d) Left anterior fascicular block

72. **S1, S2 and S3 syndromes are found in all except**
   (a) Right ventricular enlargement
   (b) COPD
   (c) Myocardial infraction
   (d) RBBB

73. **Negative T wave is found in all except**
   (a) Coronary artery disease
   (b) Aortic regurgitation
   (c) Mitral regurgitation
   (d) Aortic stenosis

74. Tall T wave is found in all except

(a) Mitral stenosis
(b) Hyperkalemia
(c) Left ventricular enlargement
(d) Polycythemia

75. QT interval is prolonged in all except

(a) Left ventricular enlargement
(b) Acute myocardial infarction
(c) Mitral valve prolapse
(d) Digitalis

76. RSR' in V1 with prolonged QRS duration is found in

(a) RBBB
(b) RBBB with RV enlargement
(c) RBBB with left posterior hemiblock
(d) All of the above

77. Poor R wave progression is found in all of the following except

(a) COPD
(b) LBBB
(c) Anterior myocardial infarction
(d) PS

78. Fixed & wide split of S2 was first detected by

(a) Cardiac nurse (b) Cardiac technician
(c) Cardiac resident (d) Cardiac consultant

79. Snowman's heart on X-ray is found in

(a) Tetralogy of fallot
(b) Transposition of great vessels
(c) Total anomalous pulmonary venous drainage
(d) Pulmonary arteries-venous fistula

80. All are auscultatory features of cortriatriatum except

(a) Systolic murmur
(b) Early diastolic murmur at pulmonary area
(c) Loud P2
(d) Middiastolic murmur at mitral area

81. Narrow upper mediastinum with cardiomegaly is seen in

(a) Tetralogy of fallot
(b) Trilogy of fallot
(c) Complete transposition of great vessels
(d) None of the above

82. Right aortic arch is seen in all except

(a) TOF
(b) Pulmonary artesia with VSD
(c) Common arterial trank
(d) ASD (OS)

83. High volume pulse in premature baby is found in

(a) ASD
(b) VSD
(c) PDA
(d) Atrial regurgitation

84. P mitrale suggest

(a) Right atrial enlargement
(b) Left atrial enlargement
(c) Right ventricle enlargement
(d) None of the above

85. Abnormal LAD of 'P' wave is found in

(a) OP ASD (b) OS ASD
(c) SV ASD (d) PFD

86. Which is least common auscultatory finding in pulmonary hypertension?

(a) Graham steel murmur
(b) Right sided S3
(c) Right sided S4
(d) Tricuspid regurgitation

87. All are common ECG findings of RVH in CLD except

(a) Partial RBBB with RAD
(b) Complete RBBB with normal axis
(c) R/S ratio in V1 >1
(d) QR in V1

88. Pathologic LV S3 is found in all the following conditions except

(a) Left ventricular dysfunction
(b) Mitral regurgitation
(c) Restrictive cardiomyopathy
(d) Mitral stenosis

89. Pericardial knock has all following features except

(a) Occurs in constrictive pericarditis
(b) High pitched
(c) Best heard in expiration
(d) Best heard in inspiration

90. Paradoxic splitting of S2 has all the following features except

(a) Increases during inspiration
(b) Splitting maximum during expiration
(c) Found in LBBB
(d) Found in aortic stenosis

91. Early systolic murmur is found in all except

(a) TR with normal PAH
(b) TR with PAH
(c) Acute mitral regurgitation
(d) VSD

92. Apex beat is usually palpable in

(a) < 20% (b) < 40%
(c) About 50% (d) 70%

93. Most specific indicator of left ventricle enlargement is

(a) Lateral shift from left mid clavicular line
(b) Down & outward shift from left mid clavicular line
(c) > 10 cm shift from mid sternal line
(d) Apical diameter > 3 cm

94. Which is the most specific feature of dyspnea due to left ventricle dysfunction?

(a) Dyspnea on exertion
(b) Orthopnea
(c) Paroxysmal nocturnal dyspnea
(d) All of the above

95. All are common causes of non cardiac syncope except

(a) Vaso vagal
(b) Situational
(c) Orthostatic hypotension
(d) Cardiovascular

96. Idiopathic dilatation of pulmonary artery has all the following features except

(a) Systolic murmur in pulmonary area
(b) Right ventricular hypertrophy
(c) Pulmonary ejection sound
(d) Mid systolic murmur in pulmonary area

97. Which right heart event decreases during inspiration?

(a) Murmur (b) T1
(c) P2 (d) Ejection click

98. Left axis deviation of 'P' wave is found in which of the following?

(a) Ostium secondum ASD
(b) Ostium premium ASD
(c) Single atrium
(d) VSD

99. Complete A-V septal defect has all the features except

(a) Fixed split S2
(b) Left axis deviation
(c) Right ventricular hypertrophy
(d) Right axis deviation

100. All are modes of stress in stress echo except

(a) Dopamine (b) Adenosine
(c) Dipyrimadole (d) Isoprenaline

101. All following features regarding pulsus alternans are correct except

(a) Found in severe depression of left ventricular performance
(b) Better appreciated in carotid
(c) Confirmed by blood pressure Instruments
(d) Usually associated with left ventricular S3

102. Sustained pulsations in pulmonary area are found in all the following except

(a) Pulmonary hypertension
(b) Pulmonary stenosis
(c) Idiopathic dilatation of pulmonary artery
(d) ASD

103. Aortic ejection sound has all the features except

(a) Best heard on left sternal border
(b) Found in non calcific aortic stenosis
(c) Best heard in mitral area
(d) Best heard in 2nd intercostal space

104. Tall notched 'P' with is found in

(a) Emphysema
(b) Acute left ventricular failure
(c) Tachycardia
(d) Tricuspid atresia

105. Negative 'P' wave is found in all the following except

(a) True dextrocardia
(b) Left atrial rhythm
(c) Severe RA enlargement
(d) Low atrial rhythm

106. ECG finding in subarachnoid hemorrhage includes all except

(a) ST segment changes
(b) T wave inversion
(c) Short QT interval
(d) Isnacre

107. Which cardiac disease is not associated with sweating?

(a) Acute myocardial infarction
(b) Infective endocarditis
(c) Heart failure
(d) None of the above

108. Wide splitting S2 in constrictive pericarditis has following features except

(a) Abrupt and shut hand
(b) Occurs in expiration
(c) Occurs throughout inspiration
(d) Occurs in early insbiration

109. Pulsus paradoxus is best detected in

(a) Carotid (b) Brachial
(c) Radial (d) Femoral

110. ECG finding highly suggestive of TR is

(a) P pulmomale (b) Atrial fibrillation
(c) RBBB (d) QR in V1

111. All the following suggest severe mitral stenosis except

(a) Right ventricular hypertrophy
(b) S2-OS interval short
(c) Full length diastolic murmur
(d) Loud S1

112. Hilar dance on X-ray chest is feature of

(a) Mitral stenosis (b) VSD
(c) ASD (d) PDA

113. Mean right atrial pressure is

(a) 0.3 mm Hg (b) 2.7 mm Hg
(c) 1.5 mm Hg (d) 0.2 mm Hg

114. Large 'a' waves is seen in

(a) Tricuspid stenosis
(b) Right ventricular failure
(c) Pulmonary hypertension
(d) All of the above

115. Normal mean pulmonary artery pressure ranges between

(a) 19–29 mm Hg (b) 0–9 mm Hg
(c) 9–19 mm Hg (d) 9–29 mm Hg

116. In mild PAH the mean pulmonary artery pressure ranges between

(a) 9–19 mm Hg
(b) 20–29 mm Hg
(c) 39–49 mm Hg
(d) More than or equal to 50 mm Hg

117. PCWP may be greater than LA pressure in

(a) Veno occlusive disease of lungs
(b) Pulmonary venous thrombosis
(c) Pulmonary venous obstruction by a tumor mass
(d) All of the above
(e) None of the above

118. PCWP may be more than pulmonary artery diastolic pressure

(a) Acute VSD
(b) Acute miral regurgitation
(c) Chronic mitral regurgitation
(d) Severe mitral stenosis
(e) All except C

119. In severe PVH the PCWP is between

(a) 13–19 mm Hg
(b) 20–24 mm Hg
(c) More than or equal to 25 mm Hg
(d) None of the above

120. Mitral valve area calculation by pressure half-time method is affected by all of the following except

(a) Left ventricular compliance
(b) Aortic regurgitation
(c) Pulmonary hypertension
(d) Mitral regurgitation

121. Displaced heart with out cardio megaly is featured by

(a) Lateral and upward
(b) Downward & lateral
(c) Upward only
(d) Downward only

122. Pulsations in right 1st & 2nd intercostal space occur with

(a) Coarctation of aorta
(b) Aneurysm of ascending aorta
(c) Supra valvular aortic stenosis
(d) None of the above

123. Central chest bulge frequently associated with

(a) PDA (b) VSD Large
(c) TOF (d) All of the above

124. Left chest bulge is after seen in

(a) Large ASD (b) Large PDA
(c) PS (d) AS

125. Jugular venous pressure is raised in all the following except

(a) Right heart failure
(b) High out put state
(c) Constrictive pericarditis
(d) Chronic lax pericardial effusion

126. Prominent x descent is found in which of the following?

(a) TR
(b) Atrial fibrillation
(c) Constrictive pericarditis
(d) Acute pericarditis

127. Enlargement of main PA only with normal right & left pulmonary A. suggests

(a) PS
(b) Eissenmenger syndrome
(c) Primary PA
(d) Idiopathic dilatation of PA

128. Cardiac calcification is rarely found in which of the following?

(a) Valves (b) Pericardium
(c) Myocardium (d) Aorta

129. Which of the following valve is rarely calcified?

(a) Mitral (b) Aortic
(c) Pulmonary (d) Tricuspid

130. Most common cause of rib notching is

(a) Aortic stenosis
(b) Coarctation of aorta
(c) Cyanotic congenital heart disease when subclavian artery is used for palliative shunt
(d) Superior vena cava occlusion

131. Intermittent RBBB occurs in

(a) Acute myocardial infarction
(b) Myocarditis
(c) ASD
(d) During paroxysmal SVT

132. Most specific clinical sign for LV enlargement is

(a) Shift of apex beat from midclavicular line
(b) Shift of apex beat from midsternal line
(c) Size of apex beat
(d) Any one of the above

133. Presystolic accentuation of MDM not found in all except

(a) Mitral regurgitation
(b) VSD
(c) Anuthnia
(d) Austin flint murmur

134. At which valve the peak gradient is often used instead of valve orificearea?

(a) Pulmonary (b) Aortic
(c) Mitral (d) All of the above

135. Valvular regurgitant fraction indicating severe lesion is

(a) 20 – 40% (b) 50 %
(c) 55 % (d) 60 %

136. Sphygmomanometer is used either in diagnosis or treatment in all the following except

(a) Cardiogenic edema
(b) To bring out murmur of AR
(c) Pulsus alternans
(d) Mitral stenosis

137. Total ischemic burden on ambulatory monitoring is indicative of poor prognosis

(a) 15 mts (b) 30 mts
(c) 45 mts (d) >60 mts

146. Hoarseness of voice may occur in all except

(a) LA enlargement
(b) PA dilation
(c) Ascending aortic aneurysm
(d) Arch of aorta aneurysm

147. Einthovens triangle is constituted by all except

(a) Left arm – Right arm
(b) LL – RA
(c) LL – LA
(d) RL – LA

148. Splenomegaly is found in all except

(a) Severe heart failure
(b) Constrictive pericarditis
(c) Infective endocarditis
(d) Rheumatic fever

149. Continuous vascular murmur is heard when

(a) Obstruction is 40% of luminal diameter
(b) Obstruction is 50% of luminal diameter
(c) Obstruction is 60% of luminal diameter
(d) Obstruction is 80% of luminal diameter

150. Which investigation is best for determining cardiac chamber size?

(a) X-ray chest
(b) Echocardiography
(c) Radionuclide ventriculography
(d) Myocardial scintigraphy

151. Valvular stenosis/regurgitation are best shown by

(a) Echocardiography
(b) Cardiac catheterization
(c) Radionuclide ventriculography
(d) Clinical examination

152. Tissue characterisation is best done by

(a) X-ray chest
(b) Echo
(c) CC–expond
(d) Radionucleotide ventriculography

153. Ventricular diastolic function is best determined by

(a) Radionuclide ventriculography
(b) Echocardiography
(c) Clinical
(d) Myocardial scintigraphy

154. Coronary anatomy is best determined by

(a) Digital angiography
(b) MRI
(c) FCT expand
(d) Echocardiography

155. Investigation of choice in dilated cardiomyopathy

(a) X-ray
(b) Echocardiography
(c) Cardiac catheterisation
(d) Radionuclide study

156. Investigation of choice in infective endocarditis is

(a) Echocardiography (b) FCT–expond
(c) MRI (d) X-ray chest

157. Best investigation for pericardial disease is

(a) X-ray
(b) Echocardiography
(c) Cardiac catheterisation
(d) FCT–expond

158. Which function is least common in systolic heart failure?

(a) Cardiomegaly (b) S3
(c) S4
(d) Mitral regurgitation functional

159. Valvular function is best assessed by

(a) Echo (b) X-ray
(c) ECG (d) Holter

160. Which finding is least common in diastolic heart failure?

(a) Hypertension (b) S4
(c) Pulmonary congestion
(d) Soft heart sounds

161. Syncope occurring with arm exercise is found in

(a) Atrial myxoma
(b) Orthostatic hypotension
(c) Vasovagal syncope
(d) Subclavian steal

162. Important causes of neurological syncope are

(a) TIA
(b) Migraine
(c) Epilepsy
(d) Brain tumor

163. Non infarction Q wave are found in all except

(a) Hypertrophic cardiomyopathy
(b) Myocarditis
(c) Cardiac amyloidosis
(d) Acid base disturbances

164. All following drugs may cause T wave inversion except

(a) Digoxin
(b) Anti arrhythmics
(c) Lithium
(d) β-blockers

165. Which of the continous murmur is louder in diastole than systole?

(a) PDA
(b) Arterial constriction
(c) Mammary souffle
(d) Venous hum

166. Valsalva maneuver should not be performed in

(a) Mitral regurgitation
(b) Aortic stenosis
(c) IHSS
(d) Ischemic heart disease

167. Variable intensity of Ist heart sound is found in all except

(a) Atrial fibrillation
(b) Atrial flutter with fixed block
(c) Complete heart block
(d) Ventricular tachycardia

168. All of the following are causes of wide splitting of S1 except

(a) RBBB (b) ASD
(c) Ebsteins anamoly (d) VSD

169. Prominent 'a'wave in JVP in cyanotic congenital heart disease suggests all the following except

(a) Tricuspid atresia
(b) Pulmonary atresia with intact IVS
(c) TAPVD
(d) Single ventricle

170. JVP is elevated in VSD in all the following except

(a) Small VSD (b) Large VSD with HF
(c) A-V Canal VSD (d) Gerbode's defect

171. All are the finding of JVP in cardiac tamponade except

(a) JV pressure is elevated
(b) X descent is prominent
(c) Y descent is prominent
(d) A & V wave are equal

172. Systolic retraction of apex beat occurs in all the following except

(a) Constrictive pericarditis
(b) ASD
(c) TR (d) AS

173. Decreased pulmonary flow in congenital heart disease is determined by all the following except

(a) Usually no cardiac enlargement
(b) Left parasternal lift
(c) Systolic thrill in pulmonary area
(d) Palpable pulmonary artery

174. All are clinical features of increased pulmonary flow in congenital heart disease except

(a) Cardiac enlargement
(b) S3 with MDM in mitral area
(c) P2 Palpable
(d) Absence of heart failure

175. All are high frequency murmur except

(a) AR (b) PR
(c) MR (d) Organic TR

176. All are high frequency sounds except

(a) Ejection click (b) Pericardial knock
(c) Opening snap (d) S1

177. All are mixed frequency murmurs except

(a) AS (b) PS
(c) VSD (d) MR

178. Which is the commonest component of pericardial rub?

(a) Systolic whole (Halosystalic)
(b) Mid systolic
(c) Early diastolic (d) Late diastolic

179. Where the pericardial rub is best heard?

(a) Apex
(b) Pulmonary area
(c) Left sternal border at 3rd and 4th ICS
(d) Over whole precordium

180. Murmur of coronary artery stenosis has all the following features except

(a) Diastolic murmur
(b) Crescendo decrescendo
(c) High pitched
(d) Most easily heard in supine position

181. MDM at tricuspid valve occurs in all of the following except

(a) Rheumatic (b) Ebsteins anamoly
(c) ASD (d) VSD

182. Tricuspid flow diastolic murmur occurs in all the following except

(a) ASD (b) TAPVD
(c) PDA (d) TR

183. Nonpan systolic murmur in MR is found in all the following except

(a) MVP
(b) Papillary muscle dysfunction
(c) Acute mitral regurgitation
(d) Functional mitral regurgitation

184. Silent mitral regurgitation is found in all the following except

(a) Acute mitral regurgitation
(b) Para prosthetic mitral regurgitation
(c) Post BMV
(d) Moderate mitral regurgitation

185. Systolic thrill in mitral regurgitation is usually found in all the following except

(a) Chordal rupture
(b) Infective endocarditis
(c) Severe chronic mitral regurgitation
(d) Mitral regurgitation following episode of ischemia

186. All the following mitral regurgitation may produce unmusical murmur except

(a) Chordal rupture
(b) Vegetation of infective endocarditis
(c) MVP
(d) Traumatic mitral regurgitation

187. All are associated physical finding in TR except

(a) Pulsatile liver
(b) Prominent 'V' in jugular venous pulse
(c) RV S3
(d) High volume pulse

188. All are causes of diastolic murmur due to increased flow through tricuspid valve except

(a) ASD
(b) TAPVD
(c) Ruptured sinus of valsalva
(d) Ebstein's anomaly

189. Functional diastolic murmur of mitral regurgitation has all following features except

(a) Mid diastolic
(b) Preceded by S3
(c) Indicates severe mitral regurgitation
(d) Presystolic murmur is always present

190. All are causes of functional TR because of increased flow in cyanotic congenital heart disease except

(a) TAPVD
(b) Single RA
(c) Hypo plastic left heart syndromes
(d) Ebstein's anomaly

191. Austin flint murmur has all the features except

(a) Thrill rare
(b) decrease HS is not loud
(c) Opening snap is absent
(d) Pulmonary hypertension is usual

192. Sustained apical impulse is found in all except

(a) Aortic stenosis
(b) Hypertension
(c) Mitral regurgitation
(d) Left ventricular aneurysm

193. All are diagnostic criteria for RBBB except

(a) QRS duration ≥ 0.12 sec
(b) M pattern of QRS in V1 – V3
(c) Deep slurred S in L1, aVL, V4 – V6
(d) Secondary ST/T changes V1 – V6

194. All following are diagnostic criteria for LBBB except

(a) QRS ≥ 0.12 sec
(b) M pattern of QRS in L1, avL, V4 – V6
(c) No Q in L1, aVL, V4 – V6
(d) Secondary ST/T changes in V1 – V6

195. LBBB is rarely found in which of the following?

(a) Coronary artery disease
(b) Hypertensive heart disease
(c) Cardiomyopathy
(d) Rheumatic heart disease

196. Electrocardiography signs of sub endocardial Ischemia are all except

(a) Prolonged QT (b) Tall T wave
(c) Both 'a' & 'b' (d) T wave inversion

197. Systolic murmur at left sternal border with brisk carotid upstroke the possible cause for syncope is

(a) Aortic stenosis with aortic regurgitation
(b) Aortic stenosis
(c) HCM
(d) CHB

198. Early systolic murmur is found in all except

(a) Acute severe mitral regurgitation
(b) Chronic severe mitral regurgitation
(c) Small VSD
(d) Large VSD with PH

199. Regular cannon 'a' wave in jugular vein occurs in all the following except

(a) Junctional rhythm
(b) VT
(c) Isorhythmic AV dissociation
(d) Complete healt block

200. Brockenbrongh sign is found in all the following except

(a) HOCM
(b) Constrictive pericarditis
(c) Severe left ventricular dysfunction
(d) Mild aortic stenosis

201. In a normal person upright posture causes all the following except

(a) Tachycardia
(b) Bradycardia
(c) Decrease in systolic blood pressure < 5 mm Hg
(d) Increase in dystolic blood pressure < 5 mm Hg

202. Which physical sign is virtually diagnostic of constrictive pericarditis?

(a) Systolic retraction of apex
(b) Rapid deep 'y' descent
(c) Pericardial knock
(d) Prompt wide splitting of S2 for one beat only

203. Maximum blood volume is in

(a) Left heart (b) Right heart
(c) Arteries (d) Veins

204. Narrow fixed splitting of S2 is found in

(a) Eisenmenger complex
(b) Pulmonary hypertension
(c) ASD
(d) PDA

205. Wide and fixed splitting of S2 in MR is found in all the following except

(a) Severe mitral regurgitation with heart failure
(b) Associated ASD
(c) Mitral regurgitation as a part of AV canal defect
(d) Mitral regurgitation with RBBB

206. Loud A2 with aortic regurgitation is found in all the following except

(a) Syphilis
(b) Marfan's syndrome
(c) Aortic dissections
(d) Rheumatic

207. All the following usually cause soft or absent OS in MS except

(a) Calcification
(b) Fibrosis
(c) Aortic regurgitation
(d) Extremely low flow

208. Juvenile 'T' wave pattern is due to all except

(a) Positional change of subject
(b) Up ward displacement of diaphragm
(c) Anxiety
(d) Exposed to hot environment

209. Which ECG finding is not found in pericarditis?

(a) T wave inversion
(b) ST depression
(c) Low voltage of QRS
(d) Abnormal Q wave

210. Commonest ECG finding in single vertricle is

(a) RVH (b) LVH
(c) BVH (d) RAD

211. Which of the following is associated with reversed splitting of S2?

(a) Congenital aortic stenosis
(b) Subvalvular aortic stenosis
(c) Supravalvular aortic stenosis
(d) HOCM

212. Aortic ejection sound is commonly found in

(a) Congenital non calcific aortic stenosis
(b) Subvalvular aortic stenosis
(c) Supravalvular aortic stenosis
(d) HOCM

213. All following left ventricular outflow tract obstruction are associated with slow rising pulse except

(a) Congenital valvular aortic stenosis
(b) Subvalvular aortic stenosis
(c) Aquired valvular aortic stenosis
(d) HOCM

214. S3 with short diastolic rumble indicates

(a) Significant mitral stenosis
(b) Mild mitral stenosis
(c) Carrey coomb's murmur
(d) Left atrial myxoma

215. Most common ECG finding in ostium secundum ASD is

(a) Incomplete RBBB
(b) Complete RBBB
(c) RAD
(d) RVH

216. All can cause slow 'y' descent except

(a) Tricuspid stenosis
(b) Cardiac tamponade
(c) Tension pneumothorax
(d) Constrictive pericarditis

217. All following are the cause of shock with out 3rd HS except

(a) Hypovolemia
(b) Septic shock
(c) Tension pneumothorax
(d) Cardiogenic shock

218. All following are the causes of pathological S4 except

(a) LVH
(b) Coronary artery disease
(c) Acute regurgitant lesions
(d) Short PR interval

219. Ejection click in LVOT obstruction has all following features except

(a) Widely audible
(b) Indicates valvular obstruction
(c) Indicates valvular pliability
(d) Indicates severity of aortic stenosis

220. Roths spots are found in all the following except

(a) Infective endocarditis
(b) Severe anemia
(c) Collagen vascular diseases
(d) Rheumatic fever

221. All of the following are causes of chest pain except

(a) Esophageal spasm
(b) Esophageal reflux
(c) Esophageal rupture
(d) Hepatitis

222. Hypokinetic pulse is found in all the following except

(a) Mitral stenosis
(b) Constrictive pericarditis
(c) LVF
(d) Hypervolemia

223. Mid systolic murmur occurs in all the following except

(a) Aortic stenosis
(b) Mitral regurgitation due to papillary muscle dysfunction
(c) PS
(d) Rheumatic mitral regurgitation

224. ECG is more reliable for diagnosis of RVH in which of in following

(a) Sleep apnoea
(b) Obstructive airway disease
(c) Parenchymal lung disease
(d) All the above

225. ECG changes may be non diagnostic in following situations except

(a) Presence of old infarct marking the new infarct
(b) Apical infarct
(c) LBBB preexisting
(d) Anteroseptal myocardial infarction

226. Inverted 'P' wave in L1 occurs in all except

(a) Dextrocardia
(b) Left atrial rhythm
(c) Anterolateral infarction
(d) Technical dextrocardia

227. Negative 'U' wave is found in all except

(a) Hypertension
(b) Aortic regurgitation
(c) Mitral regurgitation
(d) Dilated cardiomyopathy

228. 'P' pulmonale is found in all the following except

(a) Right atrial enlargement
(b) Emphysema
(c) Coronary artery disease
(d) Acute rheumatic fever

229. Left atrial enlargement pattern is found in all except

(a) Pulmonary embolism
(b) Mitral valve disease
(c) Hypertension
(d) Constrictive pericarditis

230. Pulsus alternans in heart failure may occurs in all the following but particularly occurs in which condition

(a) Heart failure in aortic stenosis
(b) Heart failure in ischemic heart disease
(c) Heart failure in cardiomyopathy
(d) Heart failure in mitral regurgitation

231. All of the following causes localized edema except

(a) Cellulitis
(b) Filariarsis
(c) Deep venous thrombosis
(d) Heart failure

232. Duplex scanning is most useful for

(a) Aorta (b) Iliac
(c) Common femoral (d) Popliteal

233. Increase jugular venous pressure occurs in all the following except

(a) RHF (b) TS
(c) IVC obstruction (d) SVC obstruction

234. Hypoperfusion is suggested by all except

(a) Narrow pulse pressure
(b) Decreased renal function
(c) Hypernatremia
(d) Mental obtundation

235. Which auscultatory sign is not found in significant mitral stenosis?

(a) M1 Increase loud S1
(b) S3
(c) MDM
(d) OS

236. Most sensitive indicator of right ventricular hypertrophy in COPD is

(a) R/S ratio > 1 in V1
(b) Right axis deviation
(c) P. pulmonale
(d) Poor 'r' wave progression in precordial leads

237. Commonly considered specific ECG finding in acute pulmonary embolism is

(a) T wave inversion
(b) ST and T abnormality
(c) Right axis deviation
(d) S1 q3 T3 pattern

238. Clubbing is a feature of all the following except

(a) Cyanotic congenital heart disease
(b) Rheumatic fever
(c) Pulmonary arteriovenous fistula
(d) Infective endocarditis

239. Cardiac chamber is best measured by

(a) X-ray
(b) Echo
(c) Radionuclide ventriculography
(d) None of the above

240. Myocardial mass is best known by

(a) X-ray
(b) ECG
(c) Echo
(d) Radionuclide ventriculography

241. Intra cardiac masses are best detected by

(a) X-ray
(b) Echo
(c) Myocardial scintigraphy
(d) Radionuclide ventriculography

242. Pericardial disease is best detected by

(a) Clinical (b) X-ray
(c) ECG (d) Echo

243. Valvular heart disease is best detected by

(a) Clinical (b) X-ray
(c) ECG (d) Echo

244. Coronary anatomy is best detected by

(a) Echo
(b) Coronary angiography
(c) EBCT
(d) All the above

245. Ventricular systolic function is best known by

(a) Clinical (b) X-ray
(c) Echo (d) ECG

246. Ventricular diastolic function is best known by

(a) Clinical
(b) X-ray
(c) Cardiac catheterization
(d) Echo

247. Myocardial tissue characterization is best known by

(a) Cardiac catheterization
(b) Radionuclide ventriculorgraphy
(c) Echo
(d) Radionuclide ventriculography

248. Myocardial blood flow is best known by

(a) Myocardial angiography
(b) Clinical
(c) Echo
(d) Cardiac catheterization

249. Myocardial metabolism is best known by

(a) Myocardial scintigraphy
(b) Clinical
(c) ECG
(d) All of the above

250. Post PVC increase the murmur of

(a) TR (b) VSD
(c) MVP (d) MOCM

251. Presystolic increase of MDM is not found in all except

(a) Mitral regurgitation
(b) VSD
(c) Arrthymia
(d) Austin flint murmur

252. Austin flint murmur has all following feature except

(a) Frequently found in syphilitic AR
(b) MDM with presystolic Increase
(c) M1 may be loud
(d) No OS

253. The term diastolic shock on palpation of precardium is used for

(a) Palpable M1 (b) Palpable A2
(c) Palpable S3 (d) Palpable P2

254. Murmur of organic TS has all feature except

(a) Radiates to cardiac apex
(b) Louder during inspiration
(c) High frequency
(d) Low frequency

255. Venous pulsations have all the feature except

(a) Laterally derated and superficial
(b) Multiple
(c) Better palpable than seen
(d) Alters with respiration

256. Mammary shuffle has all following features except

(a) Due to inceased blood flow to breast
(b) Continuous with late systolic accentuation
(c) Usually no thick
(d) Charge with respiration

257. Pathological venous hum is found in all the following except

(a) Anemia (b) Thyrotoxicosis
(c) A–V Frstula (d) Myxedema

258. Which physical sign of pulmonary hypertension indicates the pressure in PA is equal to suprasystemic pressure

(a) Loud P2
(b) Grahm steel murmur
(c) Ejection click
(d) Pulmonary ejection systolic murmur

259. Excimer laser angiography is indicated in all except

(a) Differs disease (b) Lang lesion
(c) Ostial stenosis (d) Refracting restorer

260. Absence of EC in aortic stenosis suggest gradient to be

(a) < 30 mmHg (b) 30–35 mmHg
(c) 35–50 mmHg (d) > 50 mmHg

261. Split S2 is best heart in right side of stenosis except

(a) Dextrocardia
(b) Persistent tancescerterosis PDA
(c) TGA
(d) ASD

262. Which of the following suggest the pulmonary hypertension is primary?

(a) P2 Loud and palpable
(b) Grahm steel murmur
(c) Pulmonary ejection click
(d) Vibratory S1

263. Nonparadoxical reversed splitting is found in

(a) Aortic stenosis with heart failure
(b) Aortic stenosis with aortic regurgitation
(c) LBBB with AWMI
(d) LBBB with normal heart

264. All are causes of late OS except

(a) Mild mitral stenosis
(b) Mitral stenosis with myocardial dysfunction
(c) Mitral stenosis with aortic regurgitation
(d) Mitral stenosis with tachycardia

265. Soft or absent OS in significant mitral stenosis is found in all the following except

(a) Calcification
(b) Associated mitral regurgitation
(c) Extremely low flow through MV
(d) Thick chest wall

266. Peripheral cyanosis seen of all following places except

(a) Nail beds (b) Earlobeg
(c) Nose (d) Inner surface of lips

267. Aortic ejection click is found in all the following except

(a) Aortic stenosis
(b) Hypertension
(c) Bicuspid aortic valve with out stenosis
(d) IHSS

268. Widest reversed splitting of S2 occurs is

(a) Left bundle brunch block
(b) Aortic stenosis
(c) Large PDA
(d) Acute ventricular dysfunction

269. Reversed splitting of S2 in aortic stenosis indicates gradient to be

(a) < 30mmHg (b) 30–40 mmHg
(c) 40–50 mmHg (d) Around 60 mmHg

270. RV S3 has all following features except

(a) Heard over RV area (lower sternal area)
(b) Louder in inspiration
(c) Usually associated with RV failure
(d) Usually associated with prominent 'a' wave

271. Bifid notched 'P' wave are seen in all the following except

(a) Mitral stenosis
(b) Constrictive pericarditis
(c) IHSS
(d) PS

272. Ear lobe crease more frequently in which cardiovascular disease

(a) Hypertension
(b) Aortic stenosis congenital
(c) Coronary artery disease
(d) Restrictive CMP

273. All haemodynamic finding occur during sudden squatting position except

(a) Increase venous return
(b) Decrease PVR
(c) Increase SVR
(d) Increase arterial pressure

274. All the following murmur become louder during squatting except

(a) Aortic stenosis (b) PS
(c) Mitral stenosis (d) TR

275. Abnormal Q wave in L1 is found in all except

(a) Ant lat myocardial infarction
(b) Superior myocardial infarction
(c) Dextrocardia
(d) Levocardia

276. All following are haemodynamic feature of dicrotic pulse except

(a) Decrease cardiac output
(b) Decrease SV
(c) Increase PUR
(d) Normal LV and diastolic pressure

277. Abnormal pulsatron in strno clavocular area are found in all except

(a) Aortic dissection
(b) Anurysm of aorta
(c) Follots tetralogy
(d) Mild aortic regurgitation

278. Pedal edema is not reoyted with which Ca-blocker

(a) Nifidipine (b) Verapamil
(c) Nimodipine (d) Bepridil

279. Headache may occur with all the Ca-channel blockers except

(a) Nifedipine
(b) Verapamed –Verapamil
(c) Diltiazem (d) Bepridil

280. Soil sound is

(a) Exaggerated T1 (b) Loud M1
(c) Normal oral P2 (d) RVS3

281. Calcium itucouale is effective in reversing all in following Ca-blocker and used complication except

(a) Hypertension (b) LV dysfunction
(c) Suns burly cardia (d) A–V nodal block

282. Abnormal LAD is found in all except

(a) LAHB
(b) Diffuse myocardial disease
(c) Ostium primum defect
(d) Left ventricular ectopic rhythm

283. Negative 'V' waves are found in all except

(a) Coronary artrey disease
(b) Hypertension
(c) Aortic regurgitation
(d) Mitral stenosis

284. Tall 'V' waves are found in all except

(a) CHB (b) Hypokalemia
(c) Hypocalcaemia (d) Hypomagnesaemia

285. QT prolongation is found in all except

(a) Hypercalcaemia
(b) Acute myocardial infarction
(c) Subarachnoid hemorrtiage
(d) Quinidine

286. Prolonged QRS interval is found in all except

(a) BBB (b) Quinidine
(c) Procainamide (d) RVH

287. RSQ in V1 with normal QRS is found in all except

(a) S1, S2, S3 syndromes
(b) LAHB
(c) Post myocardial infarction
(d) Complete RBBB

288. Poor 'r' wave progression in V1-V3 is found in all except

(a) Anterior septal myocardial infarction
(b) LBBB
(c) LAHB (d) 'P' RBB

289. Narrow pulse pressure is found in all except

(a) Aortic stenosis
(b) Cardiac temponade
(c) AVNRT
(d) Mitral stenosis with mild PH

290. Incomplete RBBB may be produced by all the following except

(a) Variable conduction through main trunk
(b) Delayed activation of crista supra ventriculars
(c) Conduction delay because of elongated right bundle
(d) Localized delay in purkinje-myocardial area

291. All are heart rate indications of recpradings except

(a) Differentiation of supraventricular from ventricular rhythm
(b) Evaluation of wide QRS tachycardia is with pre excitation
(c) Evaluation of syncope with uncertain origin
(d) 1 Degree AV block

292. Following murmur may be heard by patients except

(a) VSD
(b) Aortic regurgitation due to retro version of aortic cusp
(c) Mitral regurgitation due to rupture of CT
(d) ASD

293. PND is found in all the following except

(a) LVF
(b) Pulmonary embolism
(c) Hyperventilation
(d) Neurogenic pulmonary edema

294. For cardiac diagnosis maximum information is obtained by

(a) Medical history
(b) Physical examination
(c) Investigation
(d) All similar

295. What strategy should be applied regarding β-blocker for stress ECG

(a) Abrupt withdrawl
(b) Should be continued
(c) Withdraw in 48 hrs.
(d) Gradual withdrawal

296. All are contraindications to exercise testing except

(a) Acute myocardial infarction < 48 hours
(b) Severe symptomatic aortic stenosis
(c) Symptomatic heart failure
(d) AF with controlled VR

297. All are indications for stopping exercise testing in IHD except

(a) A drop of SBP > 10 mmHg from base line
(b) Mod – severe angina
(c) ST elevation
(d) Ventricular ectopics

298. Tall R wave in V1 is found in all the following except

(a) Post myocardial infarction
(b) RVH
(c) Constrictive pericarditis
(d) Acute pericarditis

299. P2 is loud in all following except

(a) TPVR (b) Truncus arteriosus
(c) C – TGA (d) Ebstein anamoly

300. P2 decrease in all the following except

(a) TOF (b) Common atrium
(c) Tricuspid atresia (d) Ebsteins disease

301. CT ratio is normal in all the following except

(a) TOF
(b) Tricuspidatresia
(c) Eissenmenger syndrome
(d) TAPVC

302. MPA is concave in all the following except

(a) C – TGA
(b) TOF
(c) Tricuspidatresia
(d) Eissenmenger syndrome

303. Earliest ECG change in hyperkalemia is

(a) Tall tented T
(b) Decrease P wave
(c) PR
(d) Widening elevation of QRS

304. Pseudo infarction pattern or ECG is found in all except

(a) HCM
(b) LBBB
(c) WPW syndrome
(d) Cerebral thrombosis

305. Most common cause of aortic systolic murmur in elderly is

(a) Aortic stenosis (b) Aortic sclerosis
(c) Anemia (d) Hypertension

306. Regular cannon 'a' waves are found is

(a) CHB (b) SVT
(c) VT (d) AF

307. Sinequa non of cardiac tamponade is

(a) Cardiomegaly
(b) Pericaricardial knock
(c) Pulsus paradoxus
(d) Absent Y

308. Most common type of normal continuous murmur

(a) Venous hum
(b) Mammary soufflé
(c) Cephalic continuous murmur
(d) All the above

309. RVH is not the feature of which PH

(a) Acute cor pulmonale (Embolic)
(b) Passive PH
(c) Primary pulm. HTN
(d) PH in CHD

310. Ischemic ST depression is found in all the following except

(a) Prinzmetal angina
(b) Ventricular aneurysm
(c) Acute myocardial infarction (Tranusmural)
(d) Acute myocardial infarction (Sub endocardial)

311. Osborn wave is associated with all except

(a) Hypothermia
(b) ST elevation
(c) Ventricular arrhythmia
(d) Hyperthermia

312. Pulsus paradoxus may be absent in cardiac tamponade in all the following except

(a) LV dysfunction
(b) ASD
(c) Positive pressure breathing
(d) Malignant etiology

313. Diagnostic method of choice for pericardial effusion is

(a) MRI (b) CT
(c) Echo (d) Clinical

314. Which auscultatary sign in mitral stenosis is not palpable

(a) Opening snap
(b) Myocardial infarction
(c) P2
(d) Murmur

315. All the following conditions are associated with left parasternal heave except

(a) PS
(b) PH
(c) Eissenmenger's syndrome
(d) Fallots tetralogy

316. Graham steell murmur has all the following features except

(a) Early diastolic murmur
(b) Low pitched
(c) Ejection click
(d) In pulmonary hypertension

317. Austin flint murmur has all the following feature except

(a) S3 is present
(b) LV enlargement
(c) Murmur decrease by amylnitrile
(d) S1 is loud

318. Musical aortic regurgitation murmur is found in all the following except

(a) IE
(b) Syphilis
(c) Rheumatic fever
(d) Ankylosing spondylitis

319. Hemoptysis may occur in all following cardiac lesion except

(a) Pulmonary venous hypertension
(b) Pulmonary infarction
(c) Eissenmengers physiology
(d) Aortic stenosis uncomplication

320. Jaundice may occur in all following cardiac complications except

(a) Hepatic congestion due to heart failure
(b) Prosthetic valve
(c) Severe aortic stenosis
(d) Fallot's tetralogy

321. Dynamic exercise causes all the following change except

(a) O_2 uptake is increased
(b) Cardiac out put is increased
(c) Peripheral vascular resistance is decreased
(d) Blood pressure is increased

322. Static exercise cause all the following hemodynamic change except

(a) O_2 uptake least increase
(b) Co least increase
(c) Peripheral resistance is least decrease
(d) Blood pressure is decreased

323. Superior axis on ECG usually occurs in except

(a) Endocardial cashion defects
(b) Single ventricle
(c) DORV with PS
(d) Truncus arteriosus

324. Egg on side appearance of heart on X-ray is found in

(a) TGA (b) Fallot's
(c) Tricuspid atresia (d) TAPVS

325. Functional TR usually develops with RVSP (Right Ventricular Systolic Pressure) of

(a) 15 mm Hg (b) 30 mm Hg
(c) 40 mm Hg (d) > 55 mm Hg

326. The TS should be suspected in patients of mitral stenosis by all the following except

(a) Prominent 'a' wave with out pulmonary hypertension
(b) Rapid Y descent
(c) MDM in TA increase with inspiration
(d) Ascles tricuspidanea

327. RVH is asceles consistently found at which RVSP

(a) 50 mm Hg (b) 70 mm Hg
(c) 90 mm Hg (d) > 100 mm Hg

328. Kereley A lines are indicate mitral stenosis to be

(a) Minimal (b) Mild
(c) Moderate (d) Severe

329. Thrill of aortic stenosis is best appreciated in which posture

(a) Sitting (b) Leaning forward
(c) In held expiration (d) Standing

330. In which aortic stenosis A2 may be increase?

(a) Congenital bicuspid valve pliable
(b) Rheumatic aortic stenosis pliable
(c) Degenerative aortic stenosis
(d) None of the above

331. Paradoxic splitting of S2 in aortic stenosis signifies

(a) A – V gradient –50 mm Hg
(b) A – V gradient –60 mm Hg
(c) A – V gradient –70 mm Hg
(d) A – V gradient –75 mm Hg

332. All the following may be heard in pregnancy except

(a) Systolic murmur (b) Mammary soufflé
(c) Diastolic murmur (d) Loud S1

333. Negative V wave occurs in all except

(a) LVH
(b) LVH with dilation
(c) Myocardial ischemia/infarction
(d) Dilated CMP

334. Coronary angiography may cause

(a) Myocardial infarction
(b) Arrhythmia
(c) Coronary dissection
(d) All the above

335. All following abnormal Q/R ratio act as evidence of Pathological Q except

(a) > 25% in L1, L2, L3 are F
(b) > 50% in Are
(c) > 15% in V4 – V6
(d) > 10% in V2 – V3

336. Himalayan 'P' waves are found in

(a) Eissenmengers disease
(b) Fallot's tetralogy
(c) TGA
(d) Ebseins anomaly

337. Most specific ECG finding of RVH is

(a) RAD (b) R/S V1 >1
(c) RS V6 < 1 (d) S1 S2 S3

338. Splenomegaly occurs in all the following except

(a) Tricuspid valve disease
(b) Infective endocarditis
(c) Constrictive pericarditis
(d) Left ventricular failure

339. Non cardioganic pulmonary edema has all following features except

(a) High flow state (b) S3 per cent
(c) JVP normal (d) Dry crepts

340. All following arrhythmia have abnormal splitting of S2 except

(a) RBBB (b) CHB
(c) VT (d) 1° AV block

341. Globular cardio megaly on X-ray is found in all except

(a) Dilated CMP
(b) Pericardial effusion
(c) Ebsteins disease
(d) ASD

342. Absence of 'P' in ECG occurs in all the following except

(a) Chronic progressive cardiac disease in old age
(b) Chronic neuromuscular disease in young patients
(c) Hyperkalemia
(d) Acidosis

343. Pulsus alternans can occur in normal heart in which situation?

(a) During bradycardia
(b) During tachycardia
(c) With sinus arrhythmia
(d) All the above

344. Pulses alternans particularity occurs in LVF of which etiology?

(a) Myocardial infarction
(b) Cardiomyopathy
(c) Aortic stenosis
(d) Hypertension

345. Cyanosis leads to clubbing after which time period?

(a) Immediately (b) At one month
(c) At two months (d) After three months

346. Up right exercise does not cause the following changes in blood pressure except

(a) Systolic blood pressure falls
(b) Diastolic pressure falls
(c) Both systolic and diastolic blood pressure falls
(d) All of the above

347. Inverted is v in ECG suggest all except

(a) HT
(b) Coronary artery disease
(c) LVH
(d) On exercise ECG suggest no significant CAD

348. Most specific ECG evidence of RVH is

(a) R/S, V1 >1 (b) RAD
(c) S1, S2, S3 (d) R/S, V6 <1

349. Prediction of significant PH by ECG is best done by

(a) RAD
(b) R/S, V1 >1
(c) R in, V1 > 12 mm
(d) None of the above

350. Prediction of reduced cardiac index is best done by

(a) RAD
(b) RAD + R/S, V6 < 2
(c) R/S, V1 >1
(d) S1 S2 S3

351. Which murmur is named after Gibson's

(a) Aortic regurgitation
(b) Coronary arteris – venous fistula
(c) PDA
(d) VSD

352. All are causes of continuous murmur except

(a) Large PDA
(b) Long namone murmur PDA
(c) Infant with PDA
(d) All of the above

353. First description of angina was given by

(a) William Henerder
(b) Edward Jenner
(c) Johan Hunter
(d) Samuel Block

354. Which variety of shock is associated with pathologic S3?

(a) Hypovolemic shock
(b) Septic shock
(c) Cardiac tamponade
(d) Cardiogenic shock

355. Which heart failure cause is associated with pathologic S3?

(a) Cardiac tamponade
(b) Acute myocardial infarction with LVF
(c) Mitral stenosis with heart failure
(d) Aortic stenosis with heart failure

356. S4 may be heard in mild LVOT obstruction in all the following situations except

(a) HOCM
(b) Aortic stenosis mild
(c) Mild aortic stenosis with CAD
(d) Mild aortic stenosis with HT

357. Dilated IVC and hepatic veins indicates the estimated RAP to be

(a) 5–10 mm Hg (b) 10–15 mmHg
(c) 15–20 mmHg (d) > 20 mmHg

358. All are the echo findings in old myocardial infarction except

(a) Infarct area decreases
(b) Increased echogenicity of infarct area
(c) Decrease motion
(d) Systolic thickening preserved

359. All are indications of contrast echocardiography except

(a) Detection of ASD
(b) Detection of VSD
(c) Detection of PFO
(d) Myocardial perfusion

360. All are false positive causes of ST depression during EST except

(a) Digitalis
(b) Hypokalemia
(c) Recent food intake
(d) Palycythemia

361. All the following are cardiac causes of false positive EST except

(a) Aortic stenosis
(b) MVP
(c) WPW
(d) Rheumatic mitral valve disease

362. Myocardial function is best evaluated by

(a) History
(b) Physical examination
(c) X-ray chest
(d) ECG

363. Myocardial ischemia is best evaluated by

(a) History
(b) Physical examination
(c) X-ray
(d) ECG

364. Functional capacity best evaluated by

(a) Physical examination
(b) History
(c) Examination ECG
(d) Chest X-ray

365. In which location of acute myocardial infarction the ventricular septal defect occurs?

(a) Antero septal (b) Apical
(c) Post intact (d) Anterolateral

366. The late systolic murmur in MVP is

(a) Crescendo – Decrescendo
(b) Decrescendo
(c) Crescendo (d) Same necessity

367. In which valve lesion the systolic murmur may radiate to top of head?

(a) MVP chordal rupture mitral regurgitation
(b) Aortic stenosis
(c) PS (d) TR

368. Changing intensity of apical systolic murmur occurs in all the following except

(a) Rheumatic fewer
(b) Bacterial endocarditis
(c) Papillary muscle dysfunction
(d) HOCM

369. Collapsing pulse in cyanotic congenital heart disease is found in all the following except

(a) Fallots with bronchopulmonary collaterals
(b) Truncus arteriosus
(c) Pulmonary atresia
(d) Ebstein anomaly

370. All the following are causes of chest pain with collaping pulse except

(a) Aortic regurgitation severe
(b) RSOV

(c) Aortic dissection with aortic regurgitation
(d) PDA

371. Chest pain with bisferiens pulse is found in all except

(a) HOCM
(b) Aortic regurgitation
(c) Aortic stenosis + Aortic regurgitation
(d) RSOV

372. Verrucae exhibit all the following feature except

(a) Most often observed on dorsal line of mitral and aortic value
(b) Location on atrial surface AV of valves
(c) Location on ventricular surface of similunar valves
(d) Found in infective endocarditis

373. In all the following situations S1 is decrease in aortic regurgitation except

(a) Severe aortic regurgitation
(b) Increase PR interval
(c) Decrease PR interval
(d) Sinus brachycardia

374. Which is characteristic change on fundus examination?

(a) Micro infarction (b) Micro aneurysm
(c) Arterio venous anustomosis around disc
(d) Hemorrhage

375. Early RVH in myocardial infarction is suggested by

(a) Deep S in L1 (b) RAD
(c) S in V6
(d) Non descriptive QRS in V1 with marked diminution in amplitude of S wave

376. Dock's murmur has all following features except

(a) Early diastolic murmur
(b) Significant stenosis of proximal LAD
(c) Best head 2nd 3rd left intercostals space lateral to sternal border
(d) Mid diastolic murmur

377. Least amount of fluid detectable by echocardiography is

(a) 5 ml (b) 10 ml
(c) 15 ml (d) 20 ml

378. Presence of both anterior and posterior pericardial effusion in supine position indicates what amount of fluid

(a) 100 ml (b) 200 ml
(c) 300 ml (d) > 300 ml

379. Paradoxical pulse occurs in all the following except

(a) Cardiac tamponade
(b) Acute cor pulmonale
(c) Hypovolemic shock
(d) Lax pericardial effusion

380. Most characteristic X-ray finding in constrictive pericarditis is

(a) Decrease or absent cardiac pulsations on fluoroscopy
(b) Distension of superior vena cava and calcification of azygous vein
(c) Pericardial calcification
(d) Cardiac shadow often not enlarged

381. All the following signs are unusual in cardiac tamponade except

(a) Pulsus paradoxus
(b) Kussmaul's sign
(c) Liver enlargement
(d) Ascites

382. Electrical alternans most commonly develop in which etiology of cardiac tamponade?

(a) Tuberculosis (b) Uremia
(c) Viral (d) Malignant

383. Single diagnostic feature of pericardial pain is

(a) Substernal location
(b) Stabbing
(c) Variation with position
(d) Radiates to neck

384. Pericardial rub has all following features except

(a) Scratchy
(b) Leather like series of sounds
(c) Low pitched
(d) Has 3 components

385. Following low frequency phenomenon are best left by heal of palm except

(a) Mid diastolic murmur of mitral stenosis
(b) Right ventricular lift
(c) LV Lift
(d) 3rd and 4th heart sound

386. Most common cause of liver enlargement in cardiac disease is

(a) Increase RAP (b) Increase LAP
(c) Increase LVSP (d) Increase RVSP

387. Best tool for imaging pericardium is

(a) X-ray chest (b) Echocardiography
(c) CT (d) MRI

388. S1 Q3 T3 pattern is found in which pulmonary hypertension?

(a) Primary pulmonary hypertension
(b) Passive pulmonary hypertension
(c) Reactive pulmonary hypertension
(d) Pulmonary embolism

389. In which of following causes of pulmonary hypertension LVH is found in ECG?

(a) Mitral stenosis (b) Aortic disease
(c) COPD (d) PPH

390. ECG shows LAD + LVH in all the following valvular heart disease except

(a) Mitral stenosis
(b) Mitral regurgitation
(c) Aortic stenosis
(d) Aortic regurgitation

391. Extreme pulmonary hypertension with RVH without heart failure occurs in which of the following

(a) Lung disease
(b) Primary pulmonary hypertension
(c) Persons living at high altitude (> 10,000 ft)
(d) Mitral stenosis

392. Foremost symptom of myocardial ischemia is

(a) Chest pain (b) Dyspnea
(c) Syncope (d) Palpitation

393. Most common precipitating factor for angina is

(a) Exertion (b) Emotional distress
(c) Cold weather (d) Eating

394. Hypokinetic pulse is found in all except

(a) Hypovolemia
(b) Left ventricular failure
(c) Mitral stenosis
(d) Mitral regurgitation

395. Dicrotic pulse is found in

(a) Mitral stenosis
(b) Aortic stenosis
(c) Dilated cardiomyopathy
(d) Hypertrophic cardiomyopathy

396. Which neck vein is best for accurate measurement of central venous pressure?

(a) Left external jugular vein
(b) Right internal jugular vein
(c) Left internal jugular vein
(d) Right external jugular vein

397. Most common cause of Kussmaul's sign is

(a) Constrictive pericarditis
(b) Severe right sided failure
(c) RV infarction
(d) All of the above

398. In acute pericarditis ST segment is elevated in

(a) V1 – V6
(b) L2, L3, aVF
(c) All Leads
(d) All Leads except AVR & V1

399. Most common alteration of PR segment in acute pericarditis is

(a) Elevated
(b) Isoelectric
(c) Depressed
(d) Any of the above

400. Which changes don't occur in ECG in acute pericarditis?

(a) PR elevation
(b) Reciprocal changes of ST elevation
(c) Abnormal Q wave
(d) All of the above

401. Pure ST segment alternans is a sign of

(a) Sub endocardial ischemia
(b) Severe transmural myocardial ischemia
(c) Pericardial effusion
(d) Myocarditis

402. U-wave alternans is found in

(a) Idiopathic QT prolongation
(b) Ischemic heart disease
(c) Drug induced
(d) Myocarditis

403. QRS alternans is usually found in

(a) Rapid SVT with concealed bypass tract
(b) Myocarditis
(c) Cardiac tamponade
(d) Drug induced

404. On ECG presence of RA enlargement left axis deviation and LVH indicates which disorder?

(a) Single ventricle
(b) Truncus arteriosus
(c) Fallot's tetralogy
(d) Tricuspid artesia

405. Which up thrust is found in atrial fibrillation in neck veins?

(a) a-wave
(b) c-wave
(c) v-wave
(d) cv-wave

406. Pulmonary venous hypertension is best known by

(a) Clinical
(b) ECG
(c) Radiology
(d) Echocardiography

407. Broad QRS tachycardia associated with coronary artery disease is likely to be VT in which % of cases

(a) 50% (b) 70%
(c) 95% (d) 100%

408. All are ECG criteria of AV dissociation except

(a) Independent 'P' wave at slower rate than VR
(b) Captured beats
(c) Fusion beats (d) LBBB

409. Kussmaul's sign is found in all except

(a) Constrictive pericarditis
(b) RV infarction
(c) Pulmonary embolism
(d) Cardiac tamponade

410. Rapid 'x' descent is found in

(a) Atrial fibrillation
(b) Atrial paralysis
(c) Cardiac tamponade
(d) AVNRT

411. Marked delay in T1 occurs in

(a) TS (b) TR
(c) Ebstein's disease (d) None of the above

412. Causes of palpable presystolic impulse at apex are all the following except.

(a) Aortic stenosis (b) IHSS
(c) SH
(d) Restrictive cardiomyopathy

413. All the following are causes of BP differences in arms and legs except

(a) Dissection of aorta
(b) Coarctation of aorta
(c) Supravalvular aortic stenosis
(d) Aneurysm of ascending aorta

414. Pulmonary artery pulsation are found in pulmonary area in all the following except

(a) ASD (b) PS
(c) PH (d) VSD

415. Commonest symptom of pulmonary hypertension is

(a) Dyspnea (b) Fatigue
(c) Chest pain (d) Syncope

416. Which is the commonest murmur found in pulmonary hypertension?

(a) TR (b) PR
(c) Pulmonary systolic murmur
(d) All the above with same frequency

417. Commonest X-ray finding in thoracic aortic dissection is

(a) Abnormality in the region of aortic knob
(b) Mediastinal widening
(c) Indistinct aortic margins
(d) No definite finding

418. Oslers nodes have all the following features except

(a) Small (b) Vascular
(c) Due to infected micro emboli
(d) Purplish

419. Fundus examination is useful in all except

(a) Valvular heart disease with atrial fibrillation
(b) Hypertension
(c) Infective endocarditis
(d) Congenital acyanotic heart disease

420. Ear lobe crease is often found in

(a) Hypertension
(b) Coronary artery disease
(c) Diabetes mellitus
(d) Hyperlipoproteinemia

421. Tallest precordial T is found in which leads?

(a) V1 – V2 (b) V3 – V4
(c) V5 – V6 (d) V3 – V6

422. Massive hemoptysis occurs in all the following except

(a) Acute pulmonary edema
(b) Rupture of pulmonary artery aneurysm
(c) Thoracic aortic aneurysm
(d) Arteriovenous malformations

423. Following are the causes of fatigue in cardiac disease except

(a) Severe pulmonary hypertension with heart failure
(b) α-Methyldopa
(c) β-blockers
(d) ACE inhibitors

424. All the following features of bisferiens pulse are correct except

(a) Best felt in femoral artery
(b) Found in HOCM
(c) Found in aortic stenosis with aortic regurgitation
(d) Found in pure aortic regurgitation

425. Pulses alternans is characterized by all the following except

(a) Best felt in carotids
(b) Found in LV dysfunction
(c) Found in cardiac tamponade
(d) The systolic blood pressure difference in two beats is ≥ 20 mm Hg

426. Examination of apex beat provide information about

(a) Cardiomegaly (b) LV size
(c) LV function (d) All of the above

427. In what percentage apex beat is palpable in normal persons?

(a) 70% (b) 80%
(c) 50% (d) 100%

428. Peri bronchial cuffing is best visualized at which location?

(a) Superior portion of pulmonary hilum
(b) Apex of lung
(c) Base of lung
(d) Peripheral part of lung

429. All are features of ischemic T wave except

(a) Deep (b) Symmetrical
(c) Arrow head (d) Shallow

430. Earliest radiological sign in mitral stenosis is

(a) Left atrium enlargement
(b) Right atrium enlargement
(c) RV enlargement
(d) Kerley's B lines

431. All the following valve lesions have left atrium and left ventricular enlargement except

(a) Mitral stenosis
(b) Mitral regurgitation
(c) Aortic stenosis
(d) Aortic regurgitation

432. Hemoptysis is found in which valve lesion?

(a) Mitral stenosis
(b) Mitral regurgitation
(c) Aortic stenosis
(d) Aortic regurgitation

433. Acute mitral regurgitation has all the following except

(a) Normal apical impulse
(b) S3
(c) Pansystalic murmur
(d) Mod – Severe heart failure

434. Most common cause of cardiac enlargement

(a) CHF
(b) Attelete heart
(c) Pericardial effusion
(d) Absence of pericardium

435. All are causes of narrow pulse pressure except

(a) Heart failure
(b) Shock
(c) Cardiac temponade
(d) Use of vasodilators

436. Systolic thrill in AV disease in found in all following except

(a) Severe aortic stenosis
(b) Severs aortic regurgitation with mild aortic stenosis
(c) Moderate aortic regurgitation with moderate aortic stenosis
(d) Mild aortic stenosis

437. Long fields on X-ray in cardiac temponade are frequently

(a) Normal (b) Hyperaemic
(c) Oligenic (d) All the above

438. Which is the most sensitive method for delection atrial thrombosis?

(a) Trans thoracic echo
(b) Trans esophageal echo
(c) Ultra fast CT (d) All the above

439. Inadequate rise of blood pressure during exercise < 120mm Hg systolic indicate

(a) Double vessel disease
(b) Presence of LBBB
(c) LV dysfunction
(d) Autonomic dysfunction

440. ST segment elevation during exercise testing indicates all the following except

(a) Elevation occurring in levels with Q indicates severs Prox CAD
(b) Indicates spams
(c) With prior Q indicates deepberetic area
(d) Indicates low ejection fraction

441. Which is commonest finding in primary pulmonary hypertension?

(a) Dysphasia (b) Fatigue
(c) Loud P2 (d) EDM of PR

442. Which is commonest finding in thrombo-embolic PH?

(a) Dysper (b) Loud P2
(c) EDM of PR (d) RVH

443. Kerley's A line are not due to which of the following?

(a) Fluid in inter lobular septal
(b) Perivascular cutting
(c) Peribronctrial cutting
(d) All of the above

444. S3 Gallop has all following feature except

(a) Heard best at apex
(b) Heard best during expiration

(c) Positions of patients should be lasts interval
(d) After persist after heart best of heart failure

445. Most common cause of cannon a waves in jugular is

(a) Complete heart block
(b) Junctional tachycardia
(c) Ventricular fibrillation
(d) Pacemaker syndrome

446. Most common cause of cyclic ischemic chest pain at rest is

(a) Stable angina (b) Unstable angina
(c) Variant angina (d) All of the above

447. Small cardiac chambers on echocardiography is found in

(a) Acromegaly (b) Myxoedema
(c) Addison's disease (d) Diabetes mellitus

448. Which is most uncommon cause of S4?

(a) Aortic stenosis (b) Athletes heart
(c) Hypertension
(d) Hypertrophic cardiomyopathy

449. Most common cause of cyanosis is

(a) Cor pulmonale (b) Tetralogy of fallot
(c) Tricuspid atresia (d) Ebstein's anomaly

450. All are common causes of ejection click except

(a) Aortic stenosis (b) Bicuspid valve
(c) Mitral valve prolapse
(d) Pulmonary stenosis

451. Most common site for pericardial rub in acute pericarditis is

(a) Aortic area (b) Mitral area
(c) Pulmonary area (d) Left sternal border

452. Sustained apex beat is found in all the following except

(a) Mitral regurgitation with left ventricular failure
(b) Aortic stenosis
(c) HCM
(d) VSD

453. Most sensitive ECG marker of tricyclic antidepressant cardiac toxicity is

(a) QT prolongation
(b) QRS prolongation
(c) Terminal R wave in AVR
(d) Ventricular arrhythmia

454. RA enlargement without RVH is found in

(a) Mitral stenosis (b) ASD
(c) TS (d) All of the above

455. RA enlargement with LVH and oligemic lung fields is found in

(a) Ebstein's anomaly (b) Fallots tetralogy
(c) TGA (d) Tricuspid atresia

456. First indication of cor pulmonale usually is

(a) Increase JVP (b) Liver enlargement
(c) Edema (d) All of the above

457. All are clinical signs of hypercapnia except

(a) High volume pulse
(b) Flapping tremors
(c) Papillodema
(d) None of the above

458. Most sensitive indicator of RVH in Cor pulmonale is

(a) RAD (b) P pulmonale
(c) R/S in V1 >1 (d) R/S ratio V6 < 1

459. S3 /knock is found in all except

(a) Constrictive pericarditis
(b) Endomyocardial fibrosis
(c) Amyloid heart disease
(d) Primary restrictive cardiomyopathy

460. Step ladder 'P' waves are found in

(a) Restrictive cardiomyopathy
(b) Constrictive pericarditis
(c) Dilated cardiomyopathy
(d) None of the above

461. Gold standard test for diagnosis of pulmonary hypertension is

(a) Echocardiography
(b) Lung scan
(c) Lung biopsy
(d) Right heart catheterization

462. Lung scan is of most value in which etiological type of pulmonary hypertension
(a) Mitral stenosis
(b) Left ventricular failure
(c) Thrombo embolic
(d) Left–Right shunt

463. Which is best technique to know the vulnerablity of plaque?
(a) Angioscopy
(b) Intravascular ultrasound
(c) Optical coherence topography
(d) None of the above

464. All the following indicate moderately severe LA hypertension except
(a) Orthopnea
(b) Short S2 - OS
(c) Long mid diastolic murmur
(d) RVF

465. Most specific criteria for LVH is
(a) Sokolow lyon criteria
(b) Romhilt - estes score
(c) Cornell criterion
(d) Talbot criterion

466. Apical mid diastolic murmur of mitral stenosis is masked in which of the following?
(a) Calcification
(b) Atrial fibrillation
(c) Right ventricle enlargement
(d) Mitral regurgitation

467. Dicrotic pulse is characterized by all following haemodynamic features except
(a) Peripheral resistance is low
(b) Blood pressure is low
(c) Cardiac out put probably low
(d) Arterial tree increase tone

468. Unilateral clubbing is found in

(a) Aneurysm of ascending aorta
(b) Aneurysm of arch of aorta
(c) Reversed PDA
(d) Aneurysm of subclavian artery

469. All the following cardiac diseases are not associated with prominent 'a' wave except

(a) Tricuspid regurgitation
(b) Constrictive pericarditis
(c) Fallot's tetralogy
(d) Pulmonary stenosis

470. P2 in pulmonary stenosis has all the features except

(a) Delayed (b) Diminished
(c) High Pitch (d) Low Pitch

471. Murmur of TR has all the following features except

(a) Usually holosystolic
(b) Increases with inspiration
(c) TR & RHF the murmur does not increase with inspiration
(d) Usually associated with thrill

472. TS murmur has all the following features except

(a) Low pitched
(b) Increases with inspiration
(c) Loudest at lower left sternal border
(d) High pitched

473. Pulsatile liver is found in which of the following lesion

(a) Mitral regurgitation (b) VSD
(c) TR (d) Aortic stenosis

474. Murmur with thrill is usually present in which of the following lesion?

(a) Mitral regurgitation (b) TR
(c) VSD (d) ASD

475. S2 in acute mitral regurgitation is

(a) Normal split (b) Wide split
(c) Single S2 (d) All the above

476. All the following events are best felt in left lateral position except

(a) S3 (b) S4
(c) Size of apex beat (d) S2

477. Type B lesion on coronary angiography has all the following features except

(a) Tubular 10–20 mm length
(b) Concentric
(c) Moderate angulation 45 – 90° angle
(d) Moderate to heavy calcification

478. Type c lesion an coronary angiography has all the following features except

(a) Diffuse 20 mm in length
(b) Extreme angulation > 90°
(c) Total occlusion < 3 months
(d) Excessive torturusity of proximal segment

479. Type A lesion on coronary angiography has all the following features except

(a) Discrete < 10 mm
(b) Eccentric
(c) Non angulated < 45° angle
(d) Smooth contour

480. Single best physical sign for severity of aortic valve stenosis is

(a) Pulsus parvus et tardus
(b) Decrease A2
(c) S4
(d) Ejection click

481. Which of the following is correct for apex beat of aortic stenosis?

(a) Forceful only
(b) Sustained only
(c) Shifted from normal position
(d) Forceful and sustained

482. Palpable S1 in mitral stenosis indicates

(a) AML pliable
(b) PML pliable
(c) Both are pliable
(d) None of the above

483. All the following method increase intensity of korotokoff sound in case they are less loud except

(a) Rapidly inflating bladder
(b) By raising the arm for few seconds before taking blood pressure
(c) Hand closing and opening ten times before taking blood pressure
(d) Taking the blood pressure in standing position

484. Murmur of papillary dysfunction is decreased in the following situations except

(a) Post PVC (b) Valsalva
(c) Standing (d) Squatting

485. Murmur of aortic stenosis is decreased in all the following situations except

(a) Post PVC (b) Valsalva
(c) Handgrip (d) Standing

486. MVP murmur is decreased in all the following except

(a) Post PVC (b) Handgrip
(c) Squatting (d) Standing

487. Calcification of proximal pulmonary artery occurs in

(a) Severe long standing pulmonary hypertension
(b) PS
(c) PR
(d) All the above

488. Abnormal convexity of right border of heart on X-ray is found in all except

(a) RA Enlargement (b) LA Enlargement
(c) LV Enlargement (d) RV Enlargement

489. Aortic valve calcification occurs most commonly in

(a) Bicuspid valve
(b) Rheumatic endocarditis
(c) Senile degenerating
(d) Ankylosing spendylitis

490. Reduced HR variability in myocardial infarction is indicative of all except

(a) Severe coronary artery disease
(b) Coronary artery disease with LV dysfunction
(c) Propensity to arrhythmia
(d) Strony predictor of mortality

491. All following CNS neurotrans mittor are Involved in HR variability except

(a) Acetyl Choline (b) Norepinephrine
(c) Serotonin (d) Dobutamine

492. LA Hypertrophy is better known by

(a) Abnormal 'P' terminal force in V1
(b) Abnormal P duration L2
(c) Both of the above
(d) All of the above

493. LA Dilatation is best known by

(a) Abnormal 'P' terminal force in V1
(b) Abnormal duration
(c) Both of the above
(d) None of these

494. In collapsing paluse carllapse related to

(a) Back flow in to the rentide
(b) Reflex vasodillation
(c) Both of the above
(d) None of the above

495. All following are physiological cause of sinus bradycardia except

(a) Athletes (b) During sleep
(c) Neorutes (d) Pregnancy

496. All following drugs causes sinus bradycardia except

(a) Lithium (b) Clonidium
(c) Amiodarone (d) ACE inhibitcrs

497. Jugular venous pulse in cardiac tamponade result in all the following except

(a) Pressure is increased
(b) Y is absent
(c) X is prominent
(d) a wave larger than V-wave

498. Reduced pulse pressure is found in all except

(a) Aortic stenosis
(b) Heart failure
(c) Cardiac tamponade
(d) Renal failure

499. Which of the following sign is always associated with severe aortic stenosis?

(a) S4
(b) Pulsus parvus et tardus
(c) Late peaking murmur
(d) Reverse splitting of S2 in absence of LBBB

500. Sustained PA pulsation in PA are felt in

(a) Post stenotic dilation of PA
(b) PH
(c) Both of the above
(d) None of the above

501. Pulsation s in supraclavicular area are seen in all the following except

(a) Aortic stenosis
(b) Aortic regurgitation
(c) Aneurysm of aorta
(d) Dissection of aorta

502. Which murmur is heard in extensive venous embolism?

(a) Systolic
(b) Diastolic
(c) To and fro
(d) Churning continuous

503. Upright T wave in V1 after Ist week of life suggests which diagnosis

(a) Tricuspid atresia
(b) Pulmonary atresia with hypoplastic RV
(c) Ebstein's disease
(d) Fallot's tetralogy

504. Pulses alternans is amplified by all the following except

(a) Aortic regurgitation
(b) Hypotension
(c) Nitroglycerine administration
(d) Lying down position

505. Most common causes of cannon 'a' waves in neck veins

(a) Complete heartblock
(b) Non-paroxysmal junctional tachycardia
(c) Pacemaker syndrome
(d) Ventricular tachycardia

506. Most common cause of continuous murmur is

(a) Patent ductus arteriosus
(b) Ventricular septal defect with aortic regurgitation
(c) Aortopulmonary window
(d) Fallots tetralogy

507. Most common cause of central cyanosis

(a) Corpulmonale
(b) Eisenmengers syndrome
(c) Fallots tetralogy
(d) Tricuspid atresia

508. Most common cause of pedal edema

(a) Heart failure
(b) Hypothyroidism
(c) Constrictive pericarditis
(d) Lymph edema

509. Most common cause of systolic ejection sound

(a) Bicuspid aortic valve
(b) Pulmonary hypertension
(c) Pulmonary stenosis
(d) None of the above

510. Most common cause of elevated jugular venous pressure is

(a) Heart Failure (Right)
(b) Restrictive cardiomyopathy
(c) Right ventricular infarction
(d) Superior vena caval syndrome

511. Most common cause of cardiogenic cerebral dysfunction is

(a) Cardiogenic shock
(b) Digitalis toxicity
(c) Infective endocarditis
(d) Mitral stenosis

512. Reversed opening snap is found in

(a) Mitral stenosis
(b) Tricuspid stenosis
(c) Pulmonary stenosis
(d) Bicuspid valve

513. Reversed opening snap is

(a) Aortic ejection click
(b) Pulmonary ejection click
(c) Mitral opening snap
(d) Non ejection click

514. Aneurysm of sinus of valsalva commonly involves which cusp?

(a) Right aortic cusp (b) Posterior cusp
(c) Left cusp (d) All the above

515. Cannon 'a' wave most commonly found

(a) Atrioventricular nodalhis block
(b) Nonparoxysmal junctional tachycardia
(c) Pacemaker syndrome
(d) Ventricular tachycardia

516. Systolic murmur in axilla represents which lesion

(a) PDA
(b) Pulmonary valve stenosis
(c) Peripheral pulmonary stenosis
(d) Venous hum

517. Which sound is absent in atrial fibrillation?

(a) S1 (b) S2
(c) S3 (d) S4

518. Anacrotic notch in aortic stenosis is best felt in

(a) Brachial artery (b) Carotid artery
(c) Radial artery (d) Femoral artery

519. Who auscultated the heart first?

(a) Lennec (b) Nectar
(c) Austinflint (d) Nicolas corvisart

520. How the auscultation of heart was carried first?

(a) Ear applied to chest
(b) Cylinder of paper on the chest

(c) Roll of pasted card board
(d) Wooden cylinder

521. Who invented spectral phonocardiogram?

(a) Alfredo luisade (b) Aubrey leathen
(c) Victor mekusick (d) MB rappaport

522. Most anterosuperior part of heart is

(a) Aortic valve (b) Pulmonary valve
(c) Left atrium (d) Right atrium

523. Pulses paradoxus is best detected in

(a) Carotid artery (b) Femoral artery
(c) Brachial artery (d) Radial artery

524. Which finding is diagnostic of constrictive pericarditis?

(a) Raised JVP (b) Hepatomegaly
(c) Ascites
(d) Wide splitting of S2 for one beat only

525. The murmur of pulmonary arteriovenous fistula is heard at all following sites except

(a) Right lower lobe (b) Left lower lobe
(c) Right middle lobe (d) Left middle lobe

526. All following are features of pulmonary arteriovenous fistula except

(a) Cyanosis (b) Clubbing
(c) Murmur (d) Abnormal ECG

527. Mitral opening snap is best heard at

(a) Between left sternal border and apex
(b) Pulmonary area
(c) Mitral area (d) Aortic area

528. Infants have typically which axis?

(a) Right axis deviation
(b) Left axis deviation
(c) Extreme right axis deviation
(d) Normal axis

529. L1 shows upward QRS and lead aVF downward QRS which axis is that

(a) Right axis deviation
(b) Left axis deviation
(c) Extreme right axis deviation
(d) Normal axis

530. All are the non cardiac causes severe left axis deviation

(a) Ascites (b) Pregnancy
(c) Aging (d) Infants

531. If L1 and aVF show downward QRS which axis is that?

(a) Left axis deviation
(b) Right axis deviation
(c) Normal axis
(d) Extreme right axis deviation

532. It lead I has downward QRS complex and lead aVF upward QRS complex which axis deviation is it?

(a) Left axis deviation
(b) Right axis deviation
(c) Normal axis
(d) Extremer right axis deviation

533. If L1 and aVF show up right QRS which electrical axis is the?

(a) Right axis deviation
(b) Normal axis
(c) Left axis deviation
(d) Extremer right axis deviation

534. Which electrolyte disorder produces RBBB?

(a) Hypokalemia (b) Hyperkalemia
(c) Hypocalcaemia (d) Hyponatremia

535. Which is the best lead to monitor VT?

(a) V1 (b) L11
(c) L111 (d) V4

536. On predischarge exercise ECG in acute myocardial infarction which parameter has highest positive predictive valve

(a) ST Depression
(b) Impaired systolic blood pressure
(c) Excercise duration
(d) Angina

537. After 6 hours of chest pain which of the following marker is most specific in acute myocardial infarction?

(a) Total CK.MB activity
(b) Total CK.MB mass
(c) Troponin-I
(d) Trrponin-T

538. All following can cause situational syncope except

(a) Swallowing (b) Defecation
(c) Micturition (d) Sneezing

539. All are causes of paradoxical splitting of size except

(a) Aortic stenosis (b) LBBB
(c) LVF (d) RBBB

540. Early systolic ejection sound is found in all the following except

(a) Aortic regurgitation
(b) Aortic stenosis
(c) PS (d) Ebsteins Anomaly

541. P Mitrale is suggestive of

(a) Left atrial enlargement
(b) LV hypertrophy
(c) RV hypertrophy
(d) RA enlargement

542. Extremely tall P wave is seen in

(a) Pulmonary hypertension due to mitral stenosis
(b) Pulmonary hypertension due to cor-pulmonale
(c) Pulmonary hypertension due to eisseum-enger's syndrome
(d) Ebsteins anomaly

543. Variable intersity of S1 occurs in all except

(a) CHB (b) AVNRT
(c) VT (d) Atrial fibrillation

544. Paradoxical splitting of S2 due to mechanical delay of A2 occurs in all the following except

(a) Aortic valve stenosis
(b) HCM
(c) Aortic regurgitation
(d) Mitral regurgitation

545. All following features regarding pericardial knock are correct except

(a) 1st Recognized by bottom
(b) Found in cous
(c) Low pitched sound
(d) It can be palpated

546. Continuous murmur may be found in all the following except

(a) Small ASD
(b) Anomalous left coronary artery
(c) High VSD
(d) Pulmonary artery branch stenosis

547. All following sounds can be palpable except

(a) Loud P2 (b) Loud M1
(c) Ejection click (d) Tumour plop

548. Carotid arterial pulse in chronic AR has all following features except

(a) Rapidrise (b) Bifid
(c) Short curation
(d) Reduced dicrotic notch

549. Friction rubs over liver suggest

(a) Viral hepatitis
(b) Serum hepatitis
(c) Amoebic liver abscess
(d) Gonococcal endocarditis

550. Outward lift over precardium occurs in all the following except

(a) RV enlargement
(b) LV enlargement
(c) Left atrium
(d) Dilated ascending aorta

551. Which ECG finding best correlate with LVEF?

(a) Q wave in precordial leads
(b) LVH
(c) RBBB
(d) Low voltages

552. Cabrera's sign in ECG is found in

(a) LBBB with RV pacing and extension anterior myocardial infarction

(b) Extension inferior myocardial infarction
(c) RV pacing with LBBB
(d) RV pacing with diffuse myocardial disease

553. Which of the following ECG is most important in diagnosis of MI in presence of LBBB?

(a) ST elevation of 1 mm or more with concordant QRS
(b) ST depression of ≥ 1 mm V1 – V3
(c) ST elevation of ≥ 5 mm with discordant QRS
(d) All of the above

554. Which is most sensitive method for predicting cardiac failure after myocardial infarction?

(a) Exercise ejection fraction
(b) Rest ejection fraction
(c) Killips class
(d) Position exercise test

555. Which complication does not occurs during exercise testing?

(a) SVT (b) VT
(c) BBB (d) CHB

556. Right anterior oblique view is useful in detection of all the following except

(a) Right atrial enlargement
(b) Left atrial enlargement
(c) RV enlargement
(d) Left ventricular enlargement

557. PA is used as injection site during angiocardiograpy in which lesion?

(a) PS
(b) Fallots tetralogy
(c) Atrial septal defect
(d) LA myxoma

558. In OSASD which site is used of injection during angiocardiography?

(a) RA
(b) RV
(c) LA
(d) Right upper lobe pulmonary view

559. Most specific and sensitive method for predicting cardiac events after myocardial infarction

(a) Exercise EF
(b) Exercise EF
(c) Positive exercise test
(d) Killip class

560. LV is used as injection site during angiocardiography in all the following except

(a) Mitral stenosis
(b) Aortic stenosis
(c) Atrial regurgitation
(d) Mitral regurgitation

561. Hand grip test integrity which part of autonomic nervous system

(a) α-sympathetic (b) β-sympathetic
(c) Parasympathetic (d) Baroceptor

562. Orthostatic test does not show integrity of which part of ANS?

(a) β-sympathetic (b) β-sympathetic
(c) Parasympathetic (d) Baroreceptor

563. Isoprenaline test show integrity of which part of ANS?

(a) β-sympathetic (b) β-sympathetic
(c) Parasympathetic (d) Baroreceptor

564. Broken brough's sign is found in

(a) HOCM
(b) Aortic stenosis
(c) Mitral regurgitation
(d) PS

565. ECG findings in common atrium include all the following except

(a) RA hypertrophy
(b) RV hypertrophy
(c) Prolonged PR interval
(d) Left axis deviation

566. All are ECG changes in trained athletes except

(a) Sinus bradycardia
(b) 1 Degree AV block

(c) QRS voltages of LVH
(d) ST segment elevation

567. Wide splitting of S1 is found in all except
(a) Ebsteins disease
(b) RBBB
(c) Preexcitation syndrome (LV connection)
(d) Sinus tachycardia

568. Clubbing occurs first in which part of the hand?
(a) Index finger (b) Little finger
(c) Thumb (d) Other two finger

569. Mammary souffle has all following feature except
(a) Continuous murmur
(b) Arterial origin
(c) Venous origin
(d) Louder in systole

570. Gallop de block term is applied for
(a) 3rd HS
(b) 4th HS
(c) 2nd HS (A2)
(d) None of the above

571. Echocardiogram confirms the diagnosis of
(a) Coarctation of aorta
(b) Reno vascular disease
(c) Hypothyroidism
(d) Phaeochromocytoma

572. Left parasternal lift in severe mitral regurgitation has all following features except
(a) Occurs later then LV apex
(b) Synchronous with 'v' wave of LA pressure curve
(c) Due to RV
(d) Due to enlarged expanding LA

573. RV lift occur best at which site
(a) Upper left parasternal area
(b) Middle left parasternal area
(c) Lower left parasternal area
(d) Whole left parasternal area

574. Diastolic mitral regurgitation occurs

(a) Mitral stenosis
(b) Chronic aortic regurgitation
(c) Acute aortic regurgitation
(d) None of the above

575. All following cardiac signs may be found during pregnancy with normal heart except

(a) Pedal edema (b) Basilar rales
(c) Systolic murmur (d) Diastolic murmur

576. Following changes may occurs in ECG in subarcheroid haemorrhage except

(a) Short PR interval
(b) Long QT interval
(c) Inverted T wave
(d) Depressed ST segment

577. Procedure of choice for diagnosis of pericardial effusion

(a) X-ray chest (b) ECG
(c) Clinical (d) Echo

578. What happens to S3 gallop with the treatment of heart failure?

(a) Often persist (b) Often disappear
(c) Always persist (d) Always disappears

579. All following are correct regarding aortic ejection sound except

(a) High pitched
(b) Usually best heard at apex
(c) Usually best heard at aortic area
(d) Disappears with calcification of aortic valve

580. Which of the following is associated with most marked bisferiens pulse?

(a) Pure severe aortic regurgitation
(b) Mild aortic stenosis + Moderate aortic regurgitation
(c) Moderate aortic stenosis + Severe aortic regurgitation
(d) Severe aortic stenosis with moderate aortic regurgitation

581. Which type of aortic stenosis produces bisferiens pulse?
(a) Severe aortic valve stenosis
(b) Supravalvular aortic stenosis
(c) HOCM (d) All the above

582. Dicrotic wave is palpable in all the following except
(a) Tamponade (b) Severe heart failure
(c) Low output states (d) Mitral stenosis

583. Bisferiens pulse found in
(a) Mild aortic regurgitation
(b) Moderate aortic regurgitation
(c) Severe aortic regurgitation
(d) All the above

584. Very rapid rising pulse with more pulse pressure is found in all the following except
(a) Mitral regurgitation
(b) VSD
(c) Idiopathic hypertrophic subaortic stenosis
(d) PDA

585. Dyspnea and ascites precedes edema likely diagnosis is
(a) Cirrosis of liver
(b) Constrictive pericarditis
(c) CHF
(d) None of the above

586. Dyspnoea occurring with anginal discomfort is how frequent
(a) 10% (b) 20%
(c) 33% (d) 50%

587. Facial flushing is seen in which all following cardiac condition except?
(a) Carcinoid heart disease
(b) Post stokes adam's attack
(c) Cushing's syndrome
(d) All the above

588. Which location of edema tends to rule out cardiac origin?
(a) Pedal (b) Sacral
(c) Abdominal (d) Hand

589. Mosque sign in ECG is found in

(a) Congenital hypothyroidism
(b) Congenital hyperthyroidism
(c) Marfan's syndrome
(d) All the above

590. Systolic retraction of apex beat is found in

(a) Mitral stenosis
(b) Tricuspid regurgitation
(c) PS
(d) Constrictive pericarditis

591. Audible splitting of S1 in normal subject is heard in

(a) 20% (b) 40%
(c) 60% (d) 85%

592. Which is in correct regarding ejection sound heard in pulmonary hypertension?

(a) Better heard lower down in the chest
(b) Decrease with Inspiration
(c) Usually not changed by respiration
(d) All of the above

593. Most common cause of abnormal left axis deviation

(a) Left anterior hemiblock
(b) Normal
(c) Inferior myocardial infarction
(d) Chronic diffuse pulmonary disease

594. Supraclavicular systolic murmurs have all the following features except

(a) In children and young adults
(b) Can reach to grade 4/6
(c) Crescendo – Decrescendo
(d) Louder on Left Side

595. Most common form of innocent murmurs in adults is

(a) Still's murmur
(b) Supraclavicular murmur
(c) Systolic mammary soufflé
(d) Aortic systolic murmur

596. Vibratory systolic murmur has all the following features except

(a) Twanging sound
(b) In children between 2–6 years
(c) Intensity 1–3/6
(d) High frequency

597. Innocent pulmonary systolic murmur has all the following features except

(a) Maximal in 2nd left intercostals space
(b) Crescendo – Decrescendo
(c) 2/6 intensity
(d) Best heard on standing

598. Exercise induced ischemia causes all the following except

(a) Increase end diastolic size of LV
(b) Increase end systolic size of LV
(c) Increase end diastolic filling rate
(d) Ejection fraction increased

599. ST elevation of acute pericarditis has all the following features except

(a) Concavity upward
(b) Not > 5 mm
(c) Lead avR is spared
(d) Lead avL is spared

600. Mammary soufflé has all following features except

(a) Changes with respiration
(b) Heard over breasts
(c) During advanced pregnancy/lactation
(d) Due to increased blood flow to the breast

601. All are pathological causes of vinous heart except

(a) Anaemia
(b) Thyrotoxicosis
(c) Intracranial AV Fistula
(d) Pregnancy

602. Most specific sign of severe PAH

(a) Loud palpable P2
(b) Ejection systolic murmur in PA
(c) Ejection click
(d) Graham steel murmur

603. Loud A2 in ASD suggest all the following except

(a) Associated coarctation of aorta
(b) TGA with VSD
(c) Systemic hypertension
(d) Associated ASD (OS)

604. P2 is absent in all the following except

(a) TOF
(b) TGA
(c) Pulmonary artesia
(d) Eissenmenger syndrome

605. All causes loud S1 except

(a) Mitral stenosis (b) ASD
(c) Tachycardia (d) Bradycardia

606. High frequency murmur have all following features except

(a) Soft (b) Blowing
(c) Musical (d) Rumbling

607. All are high frequency sound except

(a) Ejection clicks
(b) Non ejection clicks
(c) Pericardial knock
(d) 4th HS

608. All are low frequency murmur except

(a) MDM
(b) Austin flint murmur
(c) PR with normal PA pressure
(d) PR with pulmonary hypertension

609. Aortic ejection click of aortic stenosis has all the following features except

(a) Usually best heard in aortic area
(b) Does not vary with respiration
(c) Indicate severity of aortic stenosis
(d) Disappears with calcified valve

610. All following are cause of shock without S3 except

(a) Hypovolemic shock
(b) Cardiogenic shock following anterior MI
(c) Cardiac tamponade
(d) Septic shock

611. All following points regarding LV S3 are correct except

(a) Best head at apex (b) Widely audible
(c) Low pitched (d) Palpable

612. All following points regarding split of S2 are correct except

(a) Best heard in PA (b) Localized
(c) High pitched
(d) Better heard in expiration

613. All following are causes of aortic valvular click except

(a) Aortic stenosis
(b) Aortic regurgitation
(c) Systemic hypertension
(d) Fallots tetralogy

614. All following are causes pulmonary valvular clicks except

(a) Left-Right shunts
(b) Pulmonary hypertension
(c) Idiopathic dilatation of pulmonary artery
(d) Pulmonary stenosis

615. Diastolic murmur has following features except

(a) Nearly always organic
(b) Graded by intensity
(c) Graded by duration
(d) Presence/absence of thrill is noted

616. Murmur of mitral stenosis increase by all except

(a) Standing
(b) Amylnitrite inhalation
(c) Isotonic exercise
(d) During expiration

617. Opening snap may not be heard in mitral stenosis in all following situations except

(a) Mitral regurgitation
(b) Aortic regurgitation
(c) LVF
(d) PAH

618. Musical early diastolic murmurs of aortic regurgitation occurs in all the following except

(a) Infective endocarditis
(b) Syphilis
(c) Congenital
(d) All of these

619. Austin flint murmur has all the following features except

(a) Thrill is common
(b) Opening snap is absent
(c) LV S3 may occurs
(d) Significant pulmonary hypertension is unlikely

620. Which block causes flow mid diastolic murmur in mitral area?

(a) 1° AV block
(b) LBBB
(c) Complete AV block
(d) None of the above

621. Which is the most reliable sign for severity of mitral stenosis?

(a) Loud 1st heart sound
(b) Length of diastolic murmur
(c) Presence of opening snap
(d) Presence of pulmonary hypertension

622. Functional mid diastolic murmur have all following except

(a) Begin in mid diastole
(b) Preceding 3rd heart sound
(c) Presence of presystolic accentuation
(d) Usually without thrill

623. All following ECG finding are found in subarachnoid hemorrhage except

(a) Diffuse inverted broad T
(b) QT prolongation
(c) ST elevation
(d) Short PR interval

624. Giant a wave in jugular pulse is found in which lesion?

(a) TS (b) TR
(c) MR (d) AS

625. Large 'V' wave in jugular pulse is found in

(a) TS (b) TR
(c) AR (d) MS

626. Tall 'P' wave with normal axis is found in

(a) TR (b) TS
(c) MS (d) AR

627. Bulge in lower sternal area occurs in

(a) PDA (b) ASD
(c) VSD (d) MS

628. Bulge and pulsation of upper right sternum is found in

(a) Aneurysm of arch of aorta
(b) Aneurysm of ascending aorta
(c) Aortic regurgitation
(d) All the above

629. Oslers node in infective endocarditis are all except

(a) Tender
(b) Red
(c) Occasionally found
(d) Commonly found

630. Jaundice is found in all following cardiac disorder except

(a) Prosthetic valves
(b) Constrictive pericarditis
(c) CHF
(d) Severe rheumatic fever

631. Ischamic T wave has all the features except

(a) Deep
(b) Symmetrical
(c) Peak like arrow head
(d) Peak rounded

632. All following are physiological causes of hyperkinetic state except

(a) After hot bath (b) Vigorous excercise
(c) Pregnancy (d) In children

633. Most common ECG abnormality in stroke patients is

(a) QT prolongation (b) Ischaemic changes
(c) 'V' wave (d) ST elevation

634. Which of the situs is not associated with TOF?

(a) Situs solitarus (b) Situs MV wave
(c) Situs ambiguces (d) All of the above

635. Which finding is unusual in TOF in ECG?

(a) RAD
(b) Abnormal atrial rhythm
(c) RVH
(d) None of these

636. Most specific test to diagnose LV thrombus

(a) Echo TTE
(b) MRI
(c) Radionuclide angiography
(d) Indium III platelet scintigraphy

637. Most sensitive method to detect LV thrombus

(a) Echo TTE
(b) Radionuclide angiography
(c) CT
(d) Indium III platelet scintigraphy

638. Most sensitive and specific test to detect LA thrombus

(a) Echo TTE (b) Echo TEE
(c) CT (d) Angiography

639. Small quite heart with raised JVP the likely diagnosis is

(a) Constrictive pericarditis
(b) MS with CHF
(c) Restrictive cardiomyopathy
(d) All the above

640. Pulsus paradoxus is found in all following conditions except

(a) Cardiac tamponade
(b) Pneumothorax
(c) Massive pulmonary embolism
(d) Pleural effusion

641. Bruit over an artery is not heard with which degree of obstruction

(a) 60% (b) 70%
(c) 80% (d) 90–100%

642. All are causes of nocturnal angina except

(a) Left main disease
(b) Vasospastic angina
(c) Angina in aortic regurgitation
(d) Angina in aortic stenosis

643. Normal cardiac output is

(a) 2 L/m (b) 3 L/m
(c) 4–8 L/m (d) > 8 L/m

644. Paradoxical splitting in aortic stenosis indicates the gradient occurs the aortic valve is

(a) 30–40 mmHg (b) 40–50 mmHg
(c) 50–60 mmHg (d) > 70 mmHg

645. All following features are correct regarding innocent murmurs except

(a) Occurs in children and young adults
(b) Mid systolic
(c) Originate is out-flow tracts
(d) Originate at aortic or pulmonary valve

646. All are causes of mid systolic murmur except

(a) Functional mitral regurgitation
(b) Functional TR
(c) Aortic stenosis
(d) Moderate VSD

647. Which is the most reliable funding in excluding the severe aortic stenosis?

(a) S4
(b) Normal split S2
(c) Soft S1
(d) Ejection systolic murmur

648. Supra sternal notch pulsation occurs in all following except?

(a) Hypertension
(b) Coarctation of aorta
(c) Aortic regurgitation
(d) Aortic stenosis

649. Enlarged lymph nodes in neck may indicate

(a) Infective endocarditis
(b) Rheumatic fever
(c) Viral pericarditis
(d) Cardiomyopathy due to hodgkins disease

650. In bisferiens pulse all the following are correct except

(a) Found in combined AS and AR
(b) If amplitude of 'P' is more + AS is dominant
(c) If amplitude of T is greater than P AR is dominant
(d) If amplitude of T is greater than P AS is dominant

651. Least reliable sign of RHF is

(a) Increase JVP (b) Hepatomeguly
(c) Pedal edema (d) None of the above

652. Ascites appears early than edema in all the conditions except

(a) CHF
(b) TS
(c) Constrictive pericarditis
(d) All of the above

653. Pulses parvus et tardus is found in all the following except

(a) Aortic stenosis
(b) Supravalvular aortic stenosis
(c) Subvalvular AS by fibrous diaphragm
(d) HOCM

654. The gradient in HCM is increased by all except

(a) Hypovolemia (b) Hypotension
(c) Nitrates (d) β-Blockers

655. Which is commonest adverse effect of dipyridamall thallium scintigraphy?

(a) Chest pain
(b) Myocardial infarction
(c) Hypertension
(d) Death

656. All are cardiac causes of collapsing pulse except

(a) Arterio – Venous fistula
(b) Pagets disease
(c) Pregnancy
(d) Hepatic disease

657. In moderate – severe PH which of the following statement is correct?
(a) P2 and A2 equally loud
(b) P2 more moud than A2
(c) P2 less loud than A2
(d) All the above

658. Commonest cause of cardiac syncope
(a) Tachyarrhythmias
(b) Bradyarrhythmia
(c) Carotid sinus syncope
(d) Aortic stenosis

659. Enlarged heart is less common in all except
(a) Acute myocardial infarction
(b) ASD
(c) Eissenmenger's syndrome
(d) Aortic regurgitation chronic

660. S4 is more common in all the following except
(a) Aortic stenosis
(b) Hypertension
(c) Myocardial infarction
(d) Restrictive cardiomyopathy

661. Most common cause of crescendo decrescendo murmur
(a) Aortic stenosis
(b) Mitral regurgitation
(c) Thyrotoxicosis
(d) HCM

662. Kerley's lines have all the following features except
(a) Less common B lines in PVH
(b) Are longer than B lines
(c) Radiate from hilum of lung to midzone
(d) Radiate from hilum of lung in to lower zone

663. Which is most sensitive parameter for RVH in COPD?

(a) RAD
(b) R/S ratio > 1 in V1
(c) R/S ratio < 1 in V6
(d) T decrease in right pericardial leads

664. In constrictive pericarditis all are found except

(a) Pulses paradoxus (b) Kusmaul's sign
(c) Pericardial knock (d) Murmurs

665. Most common direction of T waves in adults V1 is

(a) Upright (b) Flat
(c) Inserted (d) All the above

666. Earliest change in RVH in ECG is

(a) RAD (b) R/S $\geq$ 1 in V1
(c) R/S $\leq$ 1 in V6 (d) All the above

667. All following are usual causes of tricuspid murmur except

(a) ASD
(b) TR
(c) Anomalous pulmonary venous drainage
(d) Hyperkinetic cuculation

668. Inverted P in L1 is found in all following condition except

(a) Dextrocardia (b) Left atrial rhythm
(c) Low atrial rhythm (d) Dextroversion

669. Prominent aortic knob indicates

(a) PDA
(b) VSD
(c) ASD
(d) None of the above

670. All are non cardiac conditions associated with abnormal Q except

(a) Pepes excavatum (b) Emphysema
(c) Pneumothorax (d) Pleuritis

671. Pulmonary ejection sound is heard in all the following except

(a) PS
(b) PH
(c) ASD without PH
(d) Idiopathic dilatation of PA

672. Respiratory variation of pulmonary ejection click occurs in which position

(a) Standing
(b) Sitting
(c) Lying supine
(d) Lying in lateral position

673. All following are causes of non ejection click except

(a) Atrial septal aneurysm
(b) Ventricular septal aneurysm
(c) Mitral valve prolapse
(d) None of these

674. Short QT syndrome has all following features except

(a) QRS is wide
(b) ST segment is absent
(c) T narrow, tall and symmetrical
(d) Recurrent syncope

675. ST increase occurs in which of the following

(a) Acute myocarditis
(b) Chronic myocarditis
(c) Inflammatory cardiomyopathy
(d) All the above

676. All are causes of acute right bundle branch block except

(a) Myocardial infarction
(b) Repair of VSD
(c) Myocarditis
(d) Corpulmonale

677. All are causes of chronic right bundle branch block except

(a) Fibrosis
(b) Ebsteins anomaly
(c) Cardiomyopathy
(d) Cardiac catheterization

678. All are causes of acute left bundle branch block except

(a) Myocardial infarction
(b) Septal myomectomy
(c) Myocarditis
(d) Aortic stenosis

679. Nuclear cardiology is not useful in which cardiac disease?

(a) IHD
(b) CMP
(c) Valvular heart disease
(d) Pericardial disease

680. In which globular cardiomegaly the cardiophrenic angle is obtuse?

(a) Dilated cardiomyopathy
(b) Multivalvular disease
(c) Ebstein's anomaly
(d) Pericardial effusion

681. No jugular veins are visible in which of the following condition?

(a) SVC obstruction
(b) Tricuspid stenosis
(c) Pulmonary hypertension
(d) Constrictive pericarditis

682. Narrow pulse pressure is found in all except

(a) Shock
(b) Severe heart failure
(c) Hypovolemia
(d) Hypothyroidism

683. All are cardiac causes of haemoptysis except

(a) Left ventricular failure
(b) Eissenmengers syndrome
(c) Mitral stenosis
(d) Pulmonary stenosis

684. Presystolic murmur of TS is

(a) Crescendo
(b) Decrescendo
(c) Crescendo – Decrescendo
(d) All the above

685. Left parasternal lift of severe mitral regurgitation has all following features except

(a) Produced by enlarged LA
(b) Occurs later then apical impulse
(c) Synchronous with V wave of left atrial pressure curve
(d) Due to anterior displacement of RV by enlarged LA

686. RV left is felt best at which location?

(a) Upper left parasternal
(b) Mid left parasternal
(c) Lower left parasternal
(d) Whole of peft parasternal region

687. Thrill is most commonly associated with

(a) Aortic stenosis
(b) Mitral regurgitation
(c) VSD
(d) Aortic regurgitation

688. All following medium pitched murmurs except

(a) Aortic stenosis
(b) Mitral regurgitation
(c) TR
(d) Aortic regurgitation

689. Which is the least common change in ECG in myxedema?

(a) Flattening or inversion of T wave
(b) Low P wave
(c) Low voltage of QRS
(d) Tachyarrhythmias

690. Ascites precsx is a features of

(a) Contrictive pericarditis
(b) Corpulmonale
(c) Advanced heart failure
(d) All the above

691. In all following condition diaphoresis may occur except

(a) Acute myocardial infarction
(b) Severe aortic regurgitation
(c) Heart failure in infant
(d) Bradyarrhythmias

692. Dysphagia may occur in all the following

(a) Aortic arch anomaly
(b) Extremely long LA
(c) Ventricular aneurysm
(d) None of these

693. Hiccups occurs in which cardiac condition?

(a) Stable angina
(b) Unstable angina
(c) Acute myocardial infarction
(d) Heart failure

694. Arterial pulsation over right sternoclavicular joint are due

(a) Aneurysm of aorta
(b) Dissection of aorta
(c) Aortic regurgitation
(d) Aortic stenosis

695. Arterial pulsation in right sternoclavocular joint with chest pain is caused by

(a) Aortic regurgitation
(b) Aneurysm
(c) Dissection of aorta
(d) Right sided aortic arch

696. Sustained double apical impulse is found in

(a) Cong valvular aortic stenosis
(b) Acquired valvular aortic stenosis
(c) Congenital subvalvular aortic stenosis
(d) Hypertrophic obstructive cardiomyopathy

697. Split S2 is normal in all the following except

(a) Congenital aortic stenosis valvular
(b) Acquired valvular aortic stenosis
(c) Supravalvular aortic stenosis
(d) Subvalvular aortic stenosis

698. ST increase right precordial leads occurs in all the following except

(a) LVH
(b) Long QT syndrome type 3
(c) Acute pulmonary embolism
(d) Right ventricular hypertrophy

699. Innocent murmurs have all following features except

(a) Soft
(b) Mid systolic
(c) Left sternal border
(d) Radiation is present

700. All haemodynamic changes of respiration are correct except (during inspiration)

(a) JV pulse decrease
(b) Heart rate decrease
(c) Blood pressure decrease
(d) S2 Splits

701. During expiration all following haemodynamic changes occurs except

(a) JV Pulse increase
(b) Blood pressure increases
(c) Heart rate increases
(d) S2 split fuses

702. Myocardial ischemic pain has which characteristic?

(a) Sharp (b) Standing
(c) Knifelike (d) Burning

703. Cheyne stokes respiration is found in

(a) Acute left ventricular failure
(b) Constrictive pericarditis
(c) Hypertrophic cardiomyopathy
(d) Pulmonary hypertension

704. Bulge along the left cardiac border with retrosternal double density is diagnostic of

(a) Biventricular hypertrophy
(b) Left ventricular hypertrophy
(c) Right ventricular hypertrophy
(d) LV aneurysm

705. All are complications of right heart catheterization except

(a) Hemothrorax
(b) Tracheal perforation
(c) RV perforation
(d) Left bundle branch block

706. All are cause of diastolic flow murmur at tricuspid valve except

(a) ASD (OS)
(b) Total anomalous pulmonary venous drainage
(c) TR
(d) Hyperkinetic curculation

707. Symmetrical T elevation in acute pericarditis is due to

(a) Subendocardial ischemia
(b) Epicardial ischemia
(c) Non specific
(d) Pericardial inflammation

708. Finger palpation of pulse is done when

(a) High volume pulse
(b) Biaferiesis pulse
(c) Small volume pulse
(d) All of the above

709. Bisferiens pulse may be felt in severe aortic regurgitation in how many patient?

(a) 30 %
(b) 50 %
(c) 75 %
(d) 100%

710. In which position of patient the apex beat should be felt usually?

(a) Sitting position with feet on bed
(b) Supine position
(c) Left lateral
(d) Any of the above

711. In which condition sustained displaced LV impulse is felt without LVH?

(a) Thin person
(b) Mitral regurgitation
(c) Anaemia
(d) Congenital absence of pericardium

712. Most common cause of chronic increased stiffness of left ventricle

(a) Hypertension
(b) Coronary artery disease
(c) Aortic stenosis
(d) L – R shunt

713. When does LV expand rapidly?

(a) Early diastole (b) Mid diastole
(c) Late diastole (d) Holo diastole

714. Post PVC pulse pressure in IHSS is never

(a) Wide (b) Narrow
(c) Same (d) All of the above

715. All following signs in severe aortic regurgitation picked up by auscultation except

(a) Pistal shot sounds over femoral artery
(b) Duroziez murmur
(c) Wide pulse pressure
(d) Bisferiens pulse

716. All are the causes of capillary pulsation except

(a) Severe aortic regurgitation
(b) Systolic hypertension
(c) Sinus bradycardia
(d) HOCM

717. In which phase of respiration the apex beat best felt?

(a) Fully held expiration
(b) Fully held inspiration
(c) Middle of inspiration or expiration
(d) Any of the above

718. Normally while measuring blood pressure, what should be used to hear the sounds?

(a) Bell of stethoscope
(b) Diaphragm of stethoscope
(c) Either of the two
(d) All of the above

719. Doppler probe is used to measure blood pressure in all the following except

(a) Infants
(b) Shock state
(c) During cardio pulmonary resuscitation to know the effective ness of blood flow
(d) For measuring both systolic and diastolic blood pressure

720. All are causes of non aortic non pulmonary ejection sounds except

(a) Persistent truncus arteriosus
(b) Mitral valve prolapse
(c) Membranous ventricular septal defect
(d) Ventricular aneurysm

721. Exaggerated left pure sternal movement occurs in all the following except

(a) TAPVD
(b) Aortic regurgitation
(c) Mitral stenosis
(d) ASD

722. All are causes of aortic ejection sound except

(a) Hypertension
(b) Aortic stenosis
(c) Bicuspid aortic valve
(d) Aortic regurgitation

723. Tissue doppler is particularly useful in all the following except

(a) LV function both systolic and diastolic
(b) Quantitative measurement of RWMA
(c) Evaluation of intracardiac masses
(d) Valvular stenosis density

724. Patients with pacemaker should avoid which of the following?

(a) Microwave (b) Electric brush
(c) CT Scan (d) MRI

725. Most common cause of raised JVP is

(a) CHF
(b) SVC obstruction
(c) Constrictive pericarditis
(d) Cardiac temponade

726. All are causes of low JVP except

(a) Hypovolemia
(b) Shock
(c) Addission's disease
(d) Myxedema

727. Absent 'y' descent is found in

(a) Constrictive pericarditis
(b) Cardiac temponade
(c) TS
(d) TR

728. 'V' wave is prominent in neck waves in

(a) TS (b) TR
(c) CHB (d) Tricuspid atresia

729. Positive hepatojugular reflux is found in

(a) RHF (b) LHF
(c) TR
(d) Budd-chiari syndrome

730. All are causes of reverse paradosus except

(a) HOCM
(b) Intermittent positive pressure
(c) A – V dissociation
(d) 1 Degree AV block

731. All are causes of dicrotic pulse except

(a) Typhoid fever
(b) Dehydration
(c) Cardiac tamponade
(d) Constrictive pericarditis

732. All are cardiac causes of low voltage ECG except

(a) Pericardial effusion
(b) Amyloid heart disease
(c) Cardiomyopathy
(d) Segmental myocardial ischemia

733. All are causes of changing murmur except

(a) Left atrial myxoma
(b) Infective endocarditis
(c) Cortriatriatum
(d) Atrial thrombosis

734. Wide and fixed splitting of S2 occurs in all except

(a) ASD (OS)
(b) Partial anomalous pulmonary venous damage
(c) Massive acute pulmonary embolism
(d) Sinus venosus ASD

735. All are common causes of kussmaul signs except

(a) Constrictive pericarditis
(b) Cardiac temponade
(c) RV infarction
(d) Severe right ventricular failure

736. All following skeletal abnormalities occurs in cardiac disease except

(a) Pectus excavatum (b) Arachnodactyly
(c) Absent radius (d) Absent ulna

737. Postural hypotension does not occurs with all following antihypertensives except

(a) Labetalol (b) α-Blockers
(c) Clonidine (d) Methyldopa

738. What is levine test?

(a) Disappearance of angina by clinched fist
(b) Nocturnal angina
(c) Linked angina
(d) Decrease in intensity of angina by carotid sinus massage

739. All are anginal equivalents except

(a) Palpitation (b) Fatigue
(c) Dyspnoea (d) Diaphoresis

740. All following are causes of platypnaea except

(a) Left atrial myxomia
(b) Left atrial thrombosis
(c) Pulmonary arteriovenous fistula
(d) LVF

741. Pulmonary ejection sound is found in

(a) Dome shaped pulmonary valve stenosis
(b) Dysplastic pulmonary valve stenosis
(c) Discrete subvalvular PS
(d) Pulmonary artery branch stenosis

742. Normal ECG is found in all the following except

(a) Innocent murmur
(b) Physiological murmur
(c) Idiopathic dilatation of pulmonary arteries
(d) Severe aortic stenosis

743. 1st HS in mitral stenosis has all features except

(a) Loud (b) Sharp
(c) Palpable (d) Split

744. Collapsing pulse is best appreciated by palmar aspect of four finger with in which artery

(a) Carotid (b) Axillary
(c) Brachial (d) Radial

745. Tapping apex beat in mitral stenosis suggest

(a) Normal sinus rhythm
(b) Anterior mitral leaflet is pliable
(c) Posterior mitral leaflet is pliable
(d) Both leaflet are pliable

746. All following sounds and murmurs are heard in supine position except

(a) Opening snap
(b) HS (S1-S2-S3-S4)
(c) Systolic murmur
(d) Aortic diastolic murmur

747. Which ECG change is found in hypoglycemia?

(a) Tall T (b) J wave
(c) ST increase (d) 1° AV block

748. Abnormal 'P' terminal force in V1 is found in all except

(a) Normal middle aged males
(b) Diffuse pulmonary disease
(c) Left atrial abnormality
(d) RV enlargement

749. V1-T wave > V6-T wave always indicates myocardial dysfunction due

(a) Hypertension
(b) Coronary artery disease
(c) Valvular heart disease
(d) May be found in normal

750. QS complexes in V1 and V2 are found in all except

(a) Emphysema
(b) Anteroseptal myocardial infarction
(c) LVH
(d) Cardiomyopathy

751. Notching with two collages QR in L1 decrease L2 is found in

(a) Myocardial infarction
(b) LVH
(c) Amyloidosis
(d) Myocardial fibrosis

752. False +ve exercise test occurs in all the following except

(a) MVP (b) HOCM
(c) WPW syndrome (d) Mitral stenosis

753. All following occurs in neck veins in TR

(a) Increase JVP (b) Early 'v' wave
(c) Rapid y descent (d) Prominent 'a' wave

754. Which is the least common change in ECG in athletes?

(a) ST decrease (b) ST increase
(c) RVH (d) RBBB

755. Pulses paradoxus may be absent in cardiac tamponade in all following situations except

(a) ASD (b) VSD
(c) AR (d) Hypotension

756. All following occurs in neck veins in TR

(a) Increase JVP (b) Early 'v' wave
(c) Rapid y descent (d) Prominent 'a' wave

757. Which is best method for assessment of myocardial ischemia?

(a) Histroy
(b) Physical examination
(c) X-ray chest
(d) ECG

758. Functional capacity is best assessed by

(a) Excercise test (b) Echo
(c) ECG (d) X-ray chest PA

ANSWERS

1. (*a*) 2. (*a*) 3. (*c*) 4. (*c*) 5. (*b*)
6. (*d*) 7. (*a*) 8. (*a*) 9. (*c*) 10. (*a*)
11. (*b*) 12. (*c*) 13. (*b*) 14. (*d*) 15. (*c*)
16. (*c*) 17. (*b*) 18. (*b*) 19. (*d*) 20. (*b*)
21. (*b*) 22. (*d*) 23. (*a*) 24. (*a*) 25. (*c*)
26. (*d*) 27. (*c*) 28. (*c*) 29. (*d*) 30. (*b*)
31. (*c*) 32. (*a*) 33. (*c*) 34. (*a*) 35. (*a*)
36. (*c*) 37. (*d*) 38. (*c*) 39. (*c*) 40. (*b*)
41. (*a*) 42. (*d*) 43. (*a*) 44. (*b*) 45. (*b*)
46. (*b*) 47. (*d*) 48. (*c*) 49. (*d*) 50. (*c*)
51. (*d*) 52. (*a*) 53. (*c*) 54. (*c*) 55. (*c*)
56. (*d*) 57. (*c*) 58. (*d*) 59. (*d*) 60. (*d*)
61. (*d*) 62. (*c*) 63. (*b*) 64. (*a*) 65. (*c*)
66. (*d*) 67. (*b*) 68. (*c*) 69. (*d*) 70. (*d*)
71. (*b*) 72. (*d*) 73. (*d*) 74. (*d*) 75. (*d*)
76. (*d*) 77. (*d*) 78. (*b*) 79. (*c*) 80. (*d*)
81. (*c*) 82. (*d*) 83. (*c*) 84. (*c*) 85. (*c*)
86. (*a*) 87. (*b*) 88. (*d*) 89. (*d*) 90. (*a*)
91. (*b*) 92. (*c*) 93. (*d*) 94. (*c*) 95. (*d*)
96. (*b*) 97. (*d*) 98. (*c*) 99. (*d*) 100. (*d*)
101. (*b*) 102. (*d*) 103. (*a*) 104. (*d*) 105. (*d*)
106. (*c*) 107. (*d*) 108. (*d*) 109. (*d*) 110. (*d*)
111. (*d*) 112. (*c*) 113. (*c*) 114. (*d*) 115. (*c*)
116. (*b*) 117. (*d*) 118. (*e*) 119. (*c*) 120. (*c*)
121. (*b*) 122. (*b*) 123. (*b*) 124. (*a*) 125. (*d*)
126. (*c*) 127. (*d*) 128. (*c*) 129. (*d*) 130. (*b*)
131. (*d*) 132. (*c*) 133. (*d*) 134. (*a*) 135. (*d*)
136. (*d*) 137. (*d*) 138. (*d*) 139. (*c*) 140. (*d*)
141. (*d*) 142. (*d*) 143. (*d*) 144. (*c*) 145. (*c*)
146. (*c*) 147. (*d*) 148. (*d*) 149. (*d*) 150. (*b*)
151. (*b*) 152. (*b*) 153. (*b*) 154. (*a*) 155. (*b*)
156. (*a*) 157. (*d*) 158. (*c*) 159. (*c*) 160. (*d*)

161. (*d*)	162. (*d*)	163. (*d*)	164. (*d*)	165. (*d*)
166. (*d*)	167. (*b*)	168. (*d*)	169. (*d*)	170. (*a*)
171. (*c*)	172. (*d*)	173. (*d*)	174. (*b*)	175. (*d*)
176. (*d*)	177. (*d*)	178. (*a*)	179. (*a*)	180. (*d*)
181. (*d*)	182. (*c*)	183. (*d*)	184. (*d*)	185. (*d*)
186. (*d*)	187. (*d*)	188. (*d*)	189. (*d*)	190. (*d*)
191. (*d*)	192. (*c*)	193. (*d*)	194. (*d*)	195. (*d*)
196. (*d*)	197. (*c*)	198. (*c*)	199. (*d*)	200. (*d*)
201. (*b*)	202. (*d*)	203. (*d*)	204. (*a*)	205. (*d*)
206. (*d*)	207. (*b*)	208. (*d*)	209. (*d*)	210. (*d*)
211. (*d*)	212. (*a*)	213. (*d*)	214. (*c*)	215. (*a*)
216. (*d*)	217. (*d*)	218. (*d*)	219. (*d*)	220. (*d*)
221. (*d*)	222. (*d*)	223. (*d*)	224. (*a*)	225. (*d*)
226. (*c*)	227. (*d*)	228. (*d*)	229. (*a*)	230. (*a*)
231. (*d*)	232. (*a*)	233. (*c*)	234. (*c*)	235. (*b*)
236. (*b*)	237. (*d*)	238. (*b*)	239. (*b*)	240. (*c*)
241. (*b*)	242. (*d*)	243. (*d*)	244. (*b*)	245. (*c*)
246. (*c*)	247. (*c*)	248. (*a*)	249. (*a*)	250. (*d*)
251. (*d*)	252. (*d*)	253. (*d*)	254. (*c*)	255. (*c*)
256. (*d*)	257. (*a*)	258. (*b*)	259. (*d*)	260. (*d*)
261. (*d*)	262. (*d*)	263. (*c*)	264. (*d*)	265. (*d*)
266. (*d*)	267. (*d*)	268. (*a*)	269. (*d*)	270. (*d*)
271. (*d*)	272. (*c*)	273. (*a*)	274. (*d*)	275. (*d*)
276. (*d*)	277. (*d*)	278. (*d*)	279. (*d*)	280. (*a*)
281. (*d*)	282. (*d*)	283. (*d*)	284. (*d*)	285. (*a*)
286. (*d*)	287. (*d*)	288. (*d*)	289. (*d*)	290. (*d*)
291. (*d*)	292. (*d*)	293. (*d*)	294. (*a*)	295. (*d*)
296. (*d*)	297. (*d*)	298. (*d*)	299. (*d*)	300. (*b*)
301. (*d*)	302. (*d*)	303. (*a*)	304. (*d*)	305. (*b*)
306. (*c*)	307. (*d*)	308. (*a*)	309. (*a*)	310. (*d*)
311. (*d*)	312. (*d*)	313. (*c*)	314. (*a*)	315. (*d*)
316. (*b*)	317. (*d*)	318. (*d*)	319. (*d*)	320. (*d*)
321. (*d*)	322. (*d*)	323. (*d*)	324. (*a*)	325. (*d*)
326. (*b*)	327. (*d*)	328. (*d*)	329. (*d*)	330. (*a*)
331. (*d*)	332. (*c*)	333. (*d*)	334. (*d*)	335. (*d*)
336. (*d*)	337. (*d*)	338. (*d*)	339. (*b*)	340. (*d*)

341. (*d*)	342. (*d*)	343. (*b*)	344. (*c*)	345. (*d*)
346. (*b*)	347. (*d*)	348. (*a*)	349. (*c*)	350. (*b*)
351. (*c*)	352. (*d*)	353. (*a*)	354. (*d*)	355. (*d*)
356. (*b*)	357. (*d*)	358. (*d*)	359. (*b*)	360. (*d*)
361. (*d*)	362. (*a*)	363. (*a*)	364. (*c*)	365. (*a*)
366. (*c*)	367. (*a*)	368. (*d*)	369. (*d*)	370. (*d*)
371. (*d*)	372. (*d*)	373. (*c*)	374. (*c*)	375. (*d*)
376. (*a*)	377. (*c*)	378. (*d*)	379. (*d*)	380. (*c*)
381. (*a*)	382. (*d*)	383. (*c*)	384. (*c*)	385. (*a*)
386. (*a*)	387. (*d*)	388. (*d*)	389. (*b*)	390. (*a*)
391. (*c*)	392. (*a*)	393. (*a*)	394. (*d*)	395. (*c*)
396. (*b*)	397. (*b*)	398. (*d*)	399. (*c*)	400. (*d*)
401. (*b*)	402. (*a*)	403. (*a*)	404. (*d*)	405. (*d*)
406. (*c*)	407. (*c*)	408. (*d*)	409. (*d*)	410. (*c*)
411. (*c*)	412. (*d*)	413. (*d*)	414. (*d*)	415. (*a*)
416. (*a*)	417. (*a*)	418. (*b*)	419. (*d*)	420. (*b*)
421. (*b*)	422. (*a*)	423. (*d*)	424. (*a*)	425. (*a*)
426. (*d*)	427. (*c*)	428. (*a*)	429. (*d*)	330. (*a*)
431. (*a*)	432. (*a*)	433. (*c*)	434. (*a*)	435. (*d*)
436. (*d*)	437. (*c*)	438. (*c*)	439. (*c*)	440. (*d*)
441. (*c*)	442. (*a*)	443. (*a*)	444. (*d*)	445. (*a*)
446. (*c*)	447. (*c*)	448. (*b*)	449. (*a*)	450. (*d*)
451. (*d*)	452. (*d*)	453. (*c*)	454. (*c*)	455. (*d*)
456. (*c*)	457. (*d*)	458. (*a*)	459. (*c*)	460. (*b*)
461. (*d*)	462. (*c*)	463. (*d*)	464. (*d*)	465. (*c*)
466. (*c*)	467. (*d*)	468. (*d*)	469. (*a*)	470. (*d*)
471. (*d*)	472. (*a*)	473. (*c*)	474. (*c*)	475. (*b*)
476. (*d*)	477. (*b*)	478. (*c*)	479. (*b*)	480. (*a*)
481. (*d*)	482. (*a*)	483. (*d*)	484. (*d*)	485. (*a*)
486. (*d*)	487. (*a*)	488. (*c*)	489. (*a*)	490. (*d*)
491. (*d*)	492. (*a*)	493. (*b*)	494. (*c*)	495. (*d*)
496. (*d*)	497. (*d*)	498. (*d*)	499. (*d*)	500. (*c*)
501. (*a*)	502. (*d*)	503. (*d*)	504. (*d*)	505. (*a*)
506. (*a*)	507. (*a*)	508. (*a*)	509. (*a*)	510. (*a*)
511. (*a*)	512. (*d*)	513. (*a*)	514. (*a*)	515. (*a*)
516. (*c*)	517. (*d*)	518. (*b*)	519. (*d*)	520. (*a*)

521. (*c*)	522. (*b*)	523. (*b*)	524. (*d*)	525. (*d*)
526. (*d*)	527. (*a*)	528. (*a*)	529. (*b*)	530. (*d*)
531. (*d*)	532. (*b*)	533. (*b*)	534. (*a*)	535. (*a*)
536. (*b*)	537. (*d*)	538. (*d*)	539. (*d*)	540. (*a*)
541. (*c*)	542. (*d*)	543. (*b*)	544. (*d*)	545. (*c*)
546. (*c*)	547. (*c*)	548. (*c*)	549. (*d*)	550. (*d*)
551. (*a*)	552. (*a*)	553. (*a*)	554. (*a*)	555. (*d*)
556. (*d*)	557. (*d*)	558. (*d*)	559. (*a*)	560. (*c*)
561. (*a*)	562. (*b*)	563. (*b*)	564. (*a*)	565. (*c*)
566. (*d*)	567. (*d*)	568. (*c*)	569. (*c*)	570. (*b*)
571. (*a*)	572. (*d*)	573. (*c*)	574. (*c*)	575. (*d*)
576. (*a*)	577. (*d*)	578. (*b*)	579. (*c*)	580. (*c*)
581. (*c*)	582. (*d*)	583. (*c*)	584. (*d*)	585. (*b*)
586. (*c*)	587. (*c*)	588. (*d*)	589. (*a*)	590. (*d*)
591. (*d*)	592. (*b*)	593. (*a*)	594. (*d*)	595. (*d*)
596. (*d*)	597. (*d*)	598. (*d*)	599. (*d*)	600. (*a*)
601. (*d*)	602. (*a*)	603. (*d*)	604. (*d*)	605. (*d*)
606. (*d*)	607. (*d*)	608. (*d*)	609. (*c*)	610. (*b*)
611. (*b*)	612. (*d*)	613. (*a*)	614. (*d*)	615. (*b*)
616. (*a*)	617. (*d*)	618. (*c*)	619. (*a*)	620. (*c*)
621. (*b*)	622. (*c*)	623. (*d*)	624. (*a*)	625. (*b*)
626. (*b*)	627. (*c*)	628. (*b*)	629. (*c*)	630. (*d*)
631. (*d*)	632. (*d*)	633. (*a*)	634. (*c*)	635. (*b*)
636. (*d*)	637. (*a*)	638. (*b*)	639. (*a*)	640. (*d*)
641. (*d*)	642. (*d*)	643. (*c*)	644. (*d*)	645. (*d*)
646. (*d*)	647. (*b*)	648. (*d*)	649. (*d*)	650. (*d*)
651. (*c*)	652. (*a*)	653. (*d*)	654. (*d*)	655. (*a*)
656. (*d*)	657. (*b*)	658. (*a*)	659. (*d*)	660. (*d*)
661. (*a*)	662. (*a*)	663. (*a*)	664. (*d*)	665. (*a*)
666. (*a*)	667. (*d*)	668. (*d*)	669. (*a*)	670. (*d*)
671. (*c*)	672. (*b*)	673. (*a*)	674. (*a*)	675. (*a*)
676. (*d*)	677. (*d*)	678. (*d*)	679. (*d*)	680. (*a*)
681. (*a*)	682. (*d*)	683. (*d*)	684. (*c*)	685. (*a*)
686. (*c*)	687. (*a*)	688. (*d*)	689. (*d*)	690. (*a*)
691. (*d*)	692. (*c*)	693. (*c*)	694. (*d*)	695. (*b*)
696. (*d*)	697. (*b*)	698. (*d*)	699. (*d*)	700. (*b*)

701. (*c*)	702. (*d*)	703. (*a*)	704. (*d*)	705. (*d*)
706. (*d*)	707. (*b*)	708. (*c*)	709. (*a*)	710. (*a*)
711. (*d*)	712. (*a*)	713. (*a*)	714. (*a*)	715. (*d*)
716. (*d*)	717. (*d*)	718. (*b*)	719. (*d*)	720. (*d*)
721. (*c*)	722. (*d*)	723. (*d*)	724. (*d*)	725. (*a*)
726. (*d*)	727. (*b*)	728. (*b*)	729. (*d*)	730. (*d*)
731. (*d*)	732. (*d*)	733. (*c*)	734. (*d*)	735. (*b*)
736. (*d*)	737. (*c*)	738. (*d*)	739. (*d*)	740. (*d*)
741. (*a*)	742. (*d*)	743. (*d*)	744. (*b*)	745. (*c*)
746. (*d*)	747. (*b*)	748. (*d*)	749. (*b*)	750. (*d*)
751. (*d*)	752. (*d*)	753. (*d*)	754. (*a*)	755. (*b*)
756. (*d*)	757. (*a*)	758. (*a*)		

SECTION–2

HEART FAILURE AND CARDIOMYOPATHY

1. Which is not a cause of chronic cor pulmonale?

(a) Chronic obstructive pulmonary disease
(b) Recurrent pulmonary emboli
(c) Mitral stenosis
(d) Kyphoscoliosis

2. Commonest cause of right ventricular failure is

(a) Corpulmonale
(b) Pulmonary involvement
(c) Endmyocardial fibrosis
(d) Left ventricular failure

3. Which of the following is false regarding hypertrophic obstructive cardiomyopathy?

(a) Digoxin is used
(b) Asymmetric septal hypertrophy
(c) Forward flow obstruction
(d) Anterior motion of mitral valve

4. All are true about hypertrophic obstructive cardiomyopathy except

(a) Asymmetric hypertrophy of septum
(b) Systolic motion of anterior leaflet of mitral valve
(c) Left ventricle outflow obstruction
(d) Beta blockers are not effective

5. Cardiac resynchronizing therapy does all except

(a) Improves LVEF
(b) Improves excercise tolerance
(c) Improves quality of life
(d) Decreases mortality

6. Least commonly encountered physical sign in pulmonary arterial hypertension is

(a) Loud P2
(b) Tricuspid regurgitation
(c) Right sided S4
(d) Graham steell murmur

7. Which atrial arrhythmia is most common the in heart failure?

(a) Atrial tachycardia
(b) AVN reentrant tachycardia
(c) Atrial flutter
(d) Atrial fibrillation

8. Drug of choice in case of betablocker overdose is

(a) Atropine (b) Glucagon
(c) Amrinone (d) Dobutamine

9. β-blockers are contraindicated in all of the following conditions except

(a) Severe heart failure
(b) Sick sinus syndrome
(c) High grade AV block
(d) 1degree AV block

10. Which position is best in pregnancy with heart failure?

(a) Right lateral (b) Left lateral
(c) Supine (d) Sitting

11. Which of the following drug is contraindicated in heart failure during pregnancy?

(a) Digoxin (b) Diuretics
(c) Hydralazine (d) ACE inhibitors

12. Commonest cause of heart failure is

(a) IHD
(b) Valvuler heart disease
(c) Hypertension
(d) Diluted CMP

13. Which beta-blocker is most cardioselective?

(a) Acebutalol (b) Carvedilol
(c) Propranolol (d) Bisoprolol

14. Which is not found in restrictive cardiomyopathy?

(a) Regurgitant (A-V) murmur
(b) Pericardial calcification
(c) Increased wall thickness
(d) Enlarged atrium

15. What extent of disarray is characteristic of hypertrophic cardiomyopathy?

(a) 1% of total myocardium
(b) 2% of total myocardium
(c) 2.4% of total myocardium
(d) > 5% of total myocardium

16. LVH in hypertrophic cardiomyopathy typically occurs

(a) During first years of life
(b) During adolescence
(c) Early twenties
(d) After 25 years

17. Abnormal Q in HCM is found in which leads

(a) Septal leads (V1-V3)
(b) V1-V6
(c) L1& aVL
(d) Inferolateral leads

18. All statement regarding secondary mitral regurgitation in heart failure are correct except

(a) Due to annular dilation
(b) Due to poor contraction of papillary muscle
(c) Mitral regurgitation regurgitant volume decreases by carvedilol
(d) Digoxin decreases mitral regurgitation in heart failure

19. All are haemodynamic findings in HOCM except

(a) Increased left ventricular inflow pressure
(b) Late peak systolic gradient
(c) Spike dome aortic flow
(d) Early peak systolic gradient

20. Potassium sparing diuretics acts at

(a) Distal tubule
(b) Loop of henle
(c) Cortical diluting segment
(d) All of the above

21. During of choice for HCM with obstruction at rest is

(a) Verapamil (b) Diltiazem
(c) Disopyrrmide (d) β-blocker

22. Drug of choice the latent obstructive HCM is

(a) β-blocker (b) Diltiazem
(c) Verapamil (d) Disopyramide

23. Drug of choice for nonobstructive HCM

(a) Calcium antagonist
(b) β-blocker
(c) Disopyramide
(d) Combined β-blocker & disopyramide

24. Atrial fibrillation in HCM is most commonly related to

(a) Extent of hypertrophy
(b) Presence of obstruction
(c) Absence of obstruction
(d) Left atrial enlargement

25. In which type of HOCM ST segment is usually elevated?

(a) When RV is involved
(b) Apical HCM
(c) Mid ventricular obstruction
(d) Sub aortic obstruction

26. Which inotropic agent has no effect on blood pressure?

(a) Dopamine (b) Dobutamine
(c) Adrenaline (d) Noradenaline

27. Which of the following inotropic agent increases SVR?

(a) Norepinephrine (b) Epinephrine
(c) Amrinone (d) Milrinone

28. Most common presenting symptom in pulmonary hypertension is

(a) Dyspnea (b) Fatigue
(c) Chest pain (d) Syncope

29. All of the following about carvedilol are correct except

(a) Antioxidant
(b) Both β-1 & β-2 blocker
(c) No direct smooth (vascular) muscle cell relaxation
(d) Does not act on 'α' receptors

30. Metoprolol has all the following features except

(a) β-1 blocker
(b) α-1 blocker
(c) No effect on β-2
(d) No antioxidant effect

31. All are possible mechanism of action of beta-blockers in improvement of heart failure except

(a) Upregulation of β-receptors
(b) Decreases heart rate so better myocardial perfusion
(c) Antiapoptosis effect
(d) Increases ventricular muscle hyper trophy

32. Which drug is indicated in asymptomatic left ventricular dysfunction?

(a) Digoxin
(b) Diuretics
(c) Hydralazine + Nitrate
(d) ACE inhibitors

33. All except inchoation of fab fraction antidigoxin antibody

(a) Hemodynamically unstable ventricular arrhythmia
(b) Ingestion of more than 10 mg of digoxia is adult
(c) Advanced AV blocker responsive to atropine
(d) 1 degree AV block

34. Low central venous pressure reflects

(a) Low blood volume
(b) Low right atrial pressure
(c) Low RVEDP
(d) All of the above
(E) None of the above

35. A 60 years aged female presents with acute breathlessness her haemodynamic parameters were as follows.

1. RA (mean) 12 mm Hg
2. RV systolic 50 mm Hg
3. PA systolic 50 mm Hg
4. PCWP 10 mm Hg

The likely diagnosis is

(a) Cardiac tamponade
(b) Right ventricular myocardial infarction
(c) Acute VSD
(d) Massive pulmonary embolism

36. Hypertrophic obstructive cardiomyopathy (HOCM) is characterized by all the following features except

(a) LVOT gradient (b) Septal hypertrophy
(c) Aortic stenosis (d) A small LV cavity

37. Patients of HOCM will have all the following symptoms except

(a) Syncope (b) Dyspnoea
(c) Nocturnal cough (d) Chest pain

38. The characteristic radial pulse in HOCM is

(a) Pulsus bisfierens (b) Collapsing pulse
(c) Jerky pulse (d) Anacrotic pulse

39. Characteristic apex beat in the classical HOCM is

(a) Well sustained and heaving
(b) Bifid apex
(c) Tapping
(d) Hyper dynamic

40. Diagnosis of HCM is confirmed by

(a) ECG (b) X-ray chest
(c) Echocardiography (d) Angiography

41. Following are the characteristic of HCM on doppler except

(a) Increased LVOT flow
(b) LV Diastolic dysfunction
(c) Mitral regurgitation
(d) Aortic regurgitation

42. Drugs used in the treatment of HOCM include all of following except

(a) Quinidine (b) Verapamil
(c) Amiodarone (d) Disopyramide

43. Apical cardiomyopathy is most frequent in one of the following countries

(a) India (b) USA
(c) Japan (d) UK

44. Surgical treatment is indicated in the following form of HCM except

(a) Concentric LVH
(b) Apical HCM
(c) Septal HCM
(d) Midventricular HCM

45. The type of pacemaker used in the HOCM is

(a) VVI pacemaker (b) DDD pacemaker
(c) AAI pacemaker (d) VDD pacemaker

46. All the following agents are used in β-blockers over dose except

(a) Isoprenaline (b) Dobutamine
(c) Glucagon (d) Atropine

47. All are clinical signs of abrupt β-blocker with drawl except

(a) Angina
(b) Myocardial infarction
(c) Sudden cardiac death
(d) Hypotension

48. β-blocker in acute Q wave myocardial infarction are beneficial in all except

(a) Reduce recurrent non fatal myocardial infarction
(b) Reduce sudden cardiac death
(c) Reduce total mortality
(d) Reduces LV dysfunction

49. Most common arrhythmia in heart failure is

(a) Atrial tachycardia
(b) Atrio ventricular node recentry tachycardia
(c) AVN tachycardia
(d) Atrial fibrillation

50. Which of the following condition produces both relaxation and restrictive diastolic dysfunction?

(a) Hypertrophy (b) Fibrosis
(c) Abnormal loading (d) Ischemia

51. Which is correct statement for mechanism of paroxysmal nocturnal dyspnea?

(a) Expansion of thoracic blood volume
(b) Elevation of diaphragm
(c) Reduced adrenergic drive
(d) All the above

52. Which mechanism of dyspnea in heart failure is incorrect?

(a) Decreased pulmonary compliance
(b) Hypoxemia
(c) Increased CO_2 production
(d) Metabolic alkalosis

53. Ascites in heart failure is due to all except

(a) Hepatic vein hypertension
(b) Peritoneal vein hypertension
(c) Lymphatic obstruction
(d) Protein losing enteropathy

54. Non cardiogenic pulmonary edema has all following features except

(a) No S3
(b) Bounding pulse
(c) ECG is usually normal
(d) PCWP > 18 mm Hg

55. Hypoperfusion is suspected from all except

(a) Wide pulse pressure
(b) Cool extremities
(c) Decreased urine output
(d) Mental obtundation

56. Which statement is incorrect for target dose of ACE inhibitors in heart failure?

(a) Ramipril 10 mg orally daily
(b) Lisinopril 10 mg orally daily
(c) Captopril 150 mg daily
(d) Enalapril 40 mg daily

57. Which Ca-blocker maximally increases digoxin levels?

(a) Nifedipine (b) Amlodipine
(c) Diltiazem (d) Verapamil

58. Which ECG finding strongly favours diagnosis congestive cardiomyopathy?

(a) Non specific ST/T changes
(b) Sinus tachycardia
(c) Right bundle branch block
(d) Left bundle branch block

59. Restrictive cardiomyopathy has all the following feature except

(a) AV valve regurgitant murmur
(b) Atrial fibrillation is common
(c) Conduction defects uncommon
(d) Pseudo infarct pattern is common

60. Which drug is contraindicated in hypertrophic cardiomyopathy?

(a) β-blockers (b) Verapamil
(c) Disopyramide (d) ACE inhibitors

61. Surgical interception is indicated in all the following in hypertrophic cardiomyopathy except

(a) Medical failure
(b) Out flow gradient < 30 mm Hg on rest
(c) Severe mitral regurgitation
(d) Very thick inter ventricular septum

62. Apical hypertrophic cardiomyopathy has all the following features except

(a) Low risk of sudden cardiac death
(b) Giant T wave inversion with high precordial QRS voltage
(c) Gradient at out flow tract
(d) Syncope uncommon

63. The risk features for development of doxorubicin cardiomyopathy are except

(a) Age > 70 years
(b) Prior cardiac disease
(c) Hypertension
(d) Dyslipidemia

64. Normal and deep Q wave is commonly encountered in

(a) IHSS (b) VSD
(c) Pectus excavatum (d) All the above

65. All are non heart failure cause of pathological S3 except

(a) Mitral regurgitation
(b) Aortic regurgitation
(c) Left to right shunt
(d) Hypovolemia

66. All following associated with pathological S3 in heart failure except

(a) Dilated left ventricular
(b) LVEF < 45 %
(c) LVEDP > 25 mm Hg
(d) Cardiac index > 2L /min / m^2

67. In hypertensive acute heart failure drug of choice is

(a) Nitroprusside (b) Hydralazine
(c) Beta-blocker (d) Nifedipine

68. RVF in secondary pulmonary hypertension is ineffable?

(a) Mild rise in PAP
(b) Moderate rise in PAP
(c) RVP is equal or more to systemic pressure
(d) None of the above

69. Gold standard method for diagnosis of pulmonary hypertension is

(a) Clinical
(b) Radiological
(c) ECG
(d) Cardiac catheterization

70. Pulmonary thromboembolic disease best diagnosed by

(a) X-ray chest
(b) ECG
(c) Ventilation / Perfusion scan
(d) Clinical

71. Most common cause of secondary pulmonary hypertension is

(a) Left ventricular failure
(b) MR without LVF
(c) Left-right shunt (Small)
(d) AV disease without LV dysfunction

72. Most effective therapy for long term use of PPH is

(a) Nitric oxide
(b) Ca-channel blockers
(c) I1oprost (Stable prostacyclin analogue)
(d) All of the above

73. All are indication of resynchronization therapy except

(a) True refractory heart failure
(b) EF < 35 %
(c) LBBB with QRS duration > 0.15 sec.
(d) Sinus node dysfunction

74. Nitrates are contraindicated in all the following except

(a) Heart failure
(b) Glaucoma
(c) Hypovolemia
(d) Right ventricular infarction

75. β-blockers are not contraindicated in which cardiac disorder

(a) Severe left ventricle failure
(b) Systolic blood pressure < 90 mm Hg
(c) All degrees of AVB
(d) LBBB

76. Digoxin is indicated in heart failure in all the following situations except

(a) Heart failure with atrial fibrillation
(b) Heart failure with S3
(c) Heart failure in NYHA III / IV
(d) All cases of heart failure

77. Commonest cause of death in cardiac transplant is

(a) Infarction
(b) Rejection
(c) Coronary artery disease
(d) Heart failure

78. All are risk features for sudden cardiac death in HCM except

(a) Angina
(b) Prior cardiac arrest
(c) Recurrent syncope
(d) Hypertension on exercise

79. Which β-blockers has partial sympathetic agonistic activity?

(a) Atenolol (b) Metaprolol
(c) Labetalol (d) Oxprenol

80. All the following statement are correct regarding ACE inhibitos induced cough except

(a) Due to inhibition of metabolism of Brodykinin
(b) Respiratory diseased patient are not at increased risk
(c) Appear after weeks or months after therapy
(d) Switaling to deferent ACE inhibitor is usually effective

81. All are goals of treatment of diastolic heart failure except

(a) Decrease HR
(b) Correct ischemia
(c) Use inotropic agents
(d) Reduce venous pressure

82. All are good after load reductors in heart failure except

(a) Hydrolazine (b) Nicorandil
(c) Nifedipine (d) Isosorbide nitrate

83. All are agent preload and after loud reductors in heart failure except

(a) Ramipril (b) Losartan
(c) Phantoprazol (d) Carvidulol

84. All are indication of cardiac transplantation except

(a) End stage ischemic CMD
(b) End stage idiopathic cardiomyopathy
(c) End stage valvular heart disease
(d) Markedly inceased PVR > 8 wood units

85. All following statements regarding peripartum CMP are correct except

(a) Presents only with RVF
(b) Immunologically based disease
(c) Develops during last month of pregnancy and 3–6 M post patients
(d) Strong case can be mode for treatment by immune suppression

86. All β-blockers removed by hemodialysis except

(a) Atenolol (b) Nadalol
(c) Sotalol (d) Propranotol

87. Ventricular tachycardia is usually not found in HCM in which age group VT in HOCM is rare in which age group

(a) < 15 Years (b) 16–30 Years
(c) 30–50 Years (d) None of these

88. Dopamine acts on all receptor except

(a) α1 (b) B1
(c) B2 (d) Dopaminengic

89. Epinephrine acts on all receptors except

(a) B1 (b) B2
(c) α (d) Dopaminengic

90. Maximum arterial dilatation occurs with

(a) Epinephine (b) Nitroprusside
(c) Nitroglycerine (d) Dopamine

91. Maximum isotropic effect is obtained by

(a) Dobutamine (b) Dopamine
(c) Epinephrine (d) Norepirephine

92. Mortality is highest in which age group of HCM?

(a) Children (b) Adult
(c) Adolescents (d) Elderly

93. Which arrhythmia carries highest mortality in HCM?

(a) Survivors of cardiac arrest
(b) Atrial fibrillation
(c) LBBB
(d) Runs of VT

94. Which echocardiographic finding carries very poor prognosis in HCM?

(a) Marked LVH
(b) Apical type
(c) Mid ventricular selection
(d) Thinning of LV walls with cavity dilatation

95. Which one is vasodilatory beta-blocker?

(a) Metaprolol (b) Bisopuolol
(c) Labetalol (d) Atenolol

96. Maximum tissue ACE affinity is with which ACE inhibitor

(a) Captopril (b) Enalapril
(c) Ramipril (d) Perindopril

97. Which of the following markedly increases murmur in HOCM?

(a) Valsalva (b) Amynitute
(c) Standing (d) Exercise

98. Common ECG changes is alcoholic CMP is

(a) ST depression (b) T wave inversion
(c) Peaked T wave (d) Abnormal Q wave

99. Which β-blocker has membrane stabilizing property?

(a) Atenolol (b) Propranolol
(c) Metaprolol (d) Nadolol

100. Dilated cardiomyopathy occurs as on adverse effect by all following drugs except

(a) Interferon alpha (b) Zidovudine
(c) Amphatericin B (d) Interleskin 2

101. Rales trail all are correct except

(a) Done in heart failure
(b) To evaluate efficacy of adding aldactone to ACE inhibitors

(c) Adding aldactone reduced the mortality rate
(d) Hospitalization was not reduced

102. Atlas study concluded all the following except
(a) High dose lisinopril more effective than Low dose in treatment of heart failure
(b) High dose reduces hospitalization rate
(c) High dose reduced all cause mortality
(d) High dose causes no change in cardiac mortality.

103. Which of the following auscultatory signs in primary pulmonary hypertension is always present?
(a) Mid systolic murmur in PA
(b) Early diastolic murmur in PA
(c) Pan systolic murmur in TA
(d) Loud P2

104. Most common symptom of primary pulmonary hypertension is
(a) Chest pain (b) Haemoptysis
(c) Breathlessness (d) Syncope

105. The initial pathologic finding in PPH is
(a) Medial hyperplasia of small pulmonary arteries
(b) Intimal hyperplasia
(c) Plexiform lesion
(d) Occlusion of pulmonary vasculature

106. Angina with HCM the choice of antianginal is
(a) β-blockers
(b) Dihydropyridne Ca-blockers
(c) Nitrates
(d) Metabolic modulator

107. Which cardiac disorder does not produce heart failure?
(a) Pericarditis
(b) Myocarditis
(c) Cardiomyopathy
(d) Valvular heart disease

108. All are hemodynamic goals of therapy of heart failure except

(a) PCWP 15 – 18 mm Hg
(b) RAP 5 to 8 mm Hg
(c) Cardiac index < 2.2 L/min/m^2
(d) Ventricular rate < 100/min

109. CRT improves all the following except

(a) EF
(b) NYHA functional class
(c) Hospitalization for worsening heart failure
(d) Prognosis

110. In CRT the electrode lead is placed in all the following sites except

(a) RA (b) RV
(c) Cardiac veins (d) LA

111. Which hormone is shown to be of therapeutic value in IDC?

(a) Thyroxin (b) Growth harmons
(c) Parathormone (d) None of the above

112. β-blockers in HCM Causes all the following except

(a) Decrease symptoms
(b) Decrease exercise gradient
(c) Decrease sudden cardiac death
(d) Decrease IE

113. Verapamil in HCM cause all the following except

(a) Decreases symptoms
(b) Decreases resting gradient
(c) Decreases exercise gradient
(d) SCR'S are unaffected

114. All the following clinical criteria suggest bad prognosis in heart failure except

(a) Coronary artery disease etiology of heart failure
(b) S3 Gallop
(c) Low pulse pressure
(d) Cardiomegaly

115. All the following biochemical alteration in heart failure relates to prognosis in heart failure except

(a) Increase norepinephrine
(b) Hyponatremia
(c) Hypernatremia
(d) Increase plasma renin

116. All are features of beriberi heart disease except

(a) Edema
(b) 3RD HS with MDM (Mid Diastolic Murmur)
(c) Enlarged heart
(d) Pansystolic murmur in mitralarea

117. All are good preload reducing agent in heart failure except

(a) Hydralazine
(b) Prazosin
(c) Nitroprosside
(d) Isosorbide dinitrate

118. All are clinical features of acute massive pulmonary embolism except

(a) Hypotension
(b) Increase J-V pressure
(c) RV S3
(d) Narrow split S2

119. Which of the following is not the feature of fat embolism?

(a) Acute right ventricular failure
(b) Non cardiogenic pulmonary edema
(c) Reduced cardiac out put
(d) Occurs after 2 weeks of major trauma to bones of legs and pelvis

120. Which clinical finding is present in non obstructive cardiomyopathy?

(a) Sustained apex beat
(b) Ejection SM
(c) Pan systolic murmur
(d) Jerky arterial pulse

121. All the following drugs reduce mortality in heart failure except

(a) ACE inhibitors (b) β-blockers
(c) Spironolactone (d) Inotropic drugs

122. All are non thrombotic causes of pulmonary embolism except

(a) Hydatid cyst (b) Fat
(c) Amniotic fluid (d) Calcium

123. All are causes of septic pulmonary embolism except

(a) Tran venous pacing electrodes
(b) Infective endocarditis of right heart
(c) Infection of head and neck
(d) Pyogenic liver abscess

124. In ACE inhibitor induced cough all following are correct except

(a) Dose independent
(b) May be related to bradylcinin
(c) May be related to substance 'P'
(d) May need cessation of therapy

125. Sulthydryl group related side effects of ACE inhibitors are all except

(a) Neutropenia (b) Rash
(c) Protinuria (d) Hyperkalemia

126. Which trial showed that sudden deaths are prevented by ACE inhibitors in heart failure?

(a) Consensus (b) V – heft II
(c) Solved – P (d) Solved – T

127. Which of the following has no vasoconstriction effect?

(a) Isoprenaline (b) Epinephrine
(c) Norepincphrine (d) Dopamine

128. Which of the following inotropic agent has maximum arrhythmogenic effect?

(a) Epinephrine (b) Norepinephrine
(c) Dobutamine (d) Dopamine

129. Maximum chronotropic effect is found in

(a) Inoprenaline (b) Norepinephrine
(c) Dopamine (d) Dobutamine

130. Most common cause of diuretic resistance is

(a) Increase salt intake
(b) Renal perfusion pressure
(c) Glomermular perfusion pressure
(d) Renal dysfunction

131. Women with heart failure exhibit all following except as complimed with more

(a) Less depressed EF
(b) Better prognosis
(c) More liberty to have underlying valvular heart disease as a cause of HF
(d) ACE inhibitors are more effective then men

132. Which genetic mutation is found with dilated CMP?

(a) Actin (b) Myosin
(c) Fibrilline (d) All the above

133. Commonest gene mutation in HCM is

(a) Beta-myosin heavy chain
(b) Actin
(c) Fibrillin
(d) Elastin

134. Genotyping is of prognostic importance in which of the following

(a) CAD
(b) HCM
(c) Marfan's syndrome
(d) None of the above

135. ACE inhibitor are superior to ARBS in hypertension in all following situation except

(a) Post myocardial infarction
(b) High coronary disease risk
(c) Recurrent stroke prevention
(d) Heart failure

136. Myocyte apoptosis is mediated by which adrenergic except?

(a) B1 (b) B2
(c) $\alpha 1$ (d) None of them

137. Anticoagulation is indicated in heart failure in all the following except

(a) DHF
(b) Heart failure with atrial flutter
(c) Heart failure with dilated LV
(d) Heart failure with LF < 35%

138. All following metal poisoning cause heart failure except

(a) Iron (b) Lead
(c) Phosphorous (d) Sclenim

139. Commonest non cardiac manitestation of digoxin intoxication is

(a) Vision disturbance (b) Nausea
(c) Vomiting (d) Gynecomastia

140. Which diuretic acts are proximal tubule?

(a) Loop diuretic (b) Thiazide
(c) K sparing diuretic (d) Acetazolamide

141. All are indicators of adequate divresis in heart failure except

(a) Normal lugular pressure
(b) No liver enlargement
(c) No edema
(d) Postural hypotension

142. Morphine in cardiogenic pulmonary edema causes all the following except

(a) Decrease after load
(b) Decrease preload
(c) Causes pharmacology phlebotomy
(d) Inotropic

143. All following cardiomyopathics produce sudden cardiac death except

(a) Arrhythmogenic RV dysplasia
(b) HCM
(c) Amyloid CMP
(d) EMF

144. Commonest cause of heart failure (Chronic) is CAD is

(a) Dilated CMP
(b) Mitral regurgitation

(c) VSD
(d) LV aneurysm

145. All are causes of passive pulmonary hypertension except
(a) Increase LVDP
(b) Mitral valve obstruction
(c) Pulmonary vein stenosis
(d) Anomolous pulmonary venous drairage nonobstractive

146. Use of thiazide diuretic in pregnant women may result in all the following except
(a) Hemolytic anemia
(b) Thrombocytopenia
(c) Hyponatremia
(d) Tachycardia

147. β-blockers are indicated in all following cardiac disorders except
(a) SA
(b) Post myocardial infarction
(c) HT
(d) HCM
(e) RCM

148. The LV involvement in cor pulmonale is manifested by
(a) LVH
(b) Low voltages in precordial lead
(c) Prolonged QRS duration
(d) Left atrial enlargement

149. All the following cardiomyopathies present with LVH on echo except
(a) Hypertensive cardiomyopathy
(b) Hypertrophic cardiomyopathy
(c) Restrictive cardiomyopathy
(d) Idiopathic dilated cardiomyopathy

150. Which cardiomyopathy presents with asymmetrical pattern of LVH?
(a) Hypertensive
(b) HCM
(c) RCM
(d) None of the above

151. Heart failure with normal sized heart is present in all the following except

(a) Acute myocardial infarction
(b) Cor pulmonale
(c) Constrictive pericarditis
(d) RCM

152. Which of the following is usually most reliable method of detecting cardiomyopathy?

(a) Clinical (b) ECG
(c) X-ray chest (d) All the above

153. Which is the last physical finding in heart failure to appear?

(a) Cardiomegaly (b) Increase JVP
(c) Large tender liver (d) Pedal edema

154. Therapeutic digoxin level is

(a) 0.8 – 1.6 mg/ml (b) 1.6 – 2 mg/ml
(c) 2.1 – 3 mg/ml (d) > 3 mg/ml

155. DCM is characterized by all except

(a) Intracardiac thrombus
(b) Mitral regurgitation
(c) Endocardial thickening
(d) Decrease LVEF

156. Myocardial mass is maximally increase in which cardiomyopathy

(a) DCM (b) RCM
(c) HCM (d) RV dysphasia

157. Endocardial plaque is a feature of

(a) RCM (b) HCM
(c) DCM (d) All the above

158. Maximum increase in end diastolic LV pressure occurs in

(a) DCM (b) HCM
(c) RCM (d) All the above

159. Edema with PND is most likely due to

(a) Right heart failure
(b) Left heart failure
(c) Renal failure
(d) Anemia and hypoproteinemia

160. Face is usually spared in which edema?

(a) Renal
(b) Anemia and hypoproteinemia
(c) Cardiac edema
(d) Hypothyroidism

161. Edema confined to upper limb, neck and face suggests

(a) Superior vena cava obstruction
(b) Myxoedema
(c) Renal failure
(d) Anemia and hypoproteinemia

162. Which S2 character is seldom present in dilated cardiomyopathy?

(a) Wide split (b) Single S2
(c) Reversed split (d) Normal split

163. Mitral regurgitation in dilated cardiomyopathy usually has following features except

(a) Mild to moderate
(b) Annular dilatation
(c) Present in 2/3 of cases
(d) Present in all cases

164. All the following are pointers of Ischemic dilated cardiomyopathy except

(a) Angina pain
(b) Q wave in ECG
(c) Diabetes mellitus
(d) Ejection fraction increases with exercise

165. All the following are reversible causes of dilated cardiomyopathy except

(a) Hypocalcaemia
(b) Iron storage disease
(c) Phaeochromocytoma
(d) Idiopathic dilated cardiomyopathy

166. All are hemodynamic features of restrictive cardiomyopathy except

(a) Increase RAP
(b) Increase LV and RV filling pressure
(c) RVP > LVP
(d) Moderate to severe pulmonary hypertension

167. LV apex is involved in which echo type of HCM?

(a) Type I (b) Type II
(c) Type III (d) Type IV

168. Cardiac performance chiefly depends on all the following except

(a) Ventricular contraction
(b) Ventricular relaxation
(c) Preload
(d) After load

169. All following nutritional deficiencies may causes dilated cardiomyopathy except

(a) Boron (b) Carnitine
(c) Selenium (d) Vitamin E

170. Ventricular arrhythmia commonly occurs in following cardiomyopathy except

(a) Arrhythmiogenic RV dysplasia
(b) Restrictive cardiomyopathy
(c) Dilated cardiomyopathy
(d) Hypertrophic cardiomyopathy

171. EUROPA Trial (2003) major points were except

(a) Perindopril vs placebo
(b) In CAD with preserved left ventricular function
(c) 20% risk reduction on cardiovascular mortality
(d) No effect on total mortality

172. In hope (2003) trial, the major point were all except

(a) Patients at high cardiovascular risk were included
(b) 220% risk reduction from cardiovascular cause
(c) Ramipril vs placebo
(d) No significant change in total mortality

173. Diastolic heart failure has all the following features except

(a) End-diastolic pressure-volume altered

(b) Impaired LV inotropic state
(c) Atrial booster function impaired
(d) Relaxation indices impaired

174. Which cause of pulmonary hypertension is associated with left atrial enlargement on ECG?
(a) Primary pulmonary hypertension
(b) Passive pulmonary hypertension caused by mitral stenosis
(c) Pulmonary veno occlusive disease
(d) Pulmonary embolism

175. Pedal edema in chronic cor pulmonale is due to all except
(a) Increase systemic venous pressure
(b) Acidosis
(c) Hypoxemia
(d) Hyper carbic

176. LV dysfunction in cor pulmonale is due to
(a) Associated CAD
(b) Associated HT
(c) Dilated hypertensive RV reduces LV compliance
(d) All the above

177. All the following trials related to LV dysfunction demonstrated decrease in over all mortality except
(a) Consensus
(b) Solvd
(c) SAVE
(d) Solvd–Prevention arm

178. All are 3rd generation β-blockers except
(a) Carvedilol (b) Labetalol
(c) Bucindalol (d) Bisoprolol

179. Which chromosome is not involved in HCM?
(a) Chromosome 1 (b) Chromosome 14
(c) Chromosome 19 (d) Chromosome 4

180. Commonest variety of HCM is
(a) ASH (b) Apical
(c) Mid ventricular (d) Symmetrical

181. Which is the dominant mechanism of diastolic heart failure in HCM?

(a) Decrease relaxation
(b) Chamber stiffness
(c) Both of the above
(d) None of these

182. Chamber stiffness in HCM is due to which of the following?

(a) Increase muscle mass
(b) Decrease volume
(c) Increase muscle stiffness
(d) All of the above

183. Decrease relaxation in HCM is due to which of the following?

(a) Increase contraction load
(b) Decrease relaxation load
(c) Decrease inactivation
(d) All of the above

184. All following may occur in HCM except

(a) Diastolic heart failure
(b) Atrial fibrillation
(c) Syncope
(d) Early pedal edema

185. Predominant hemodynamic abnormality in HCM is

(a) Systolic dysfunction
(b) Diastolic dysfunction
(c) LVOT obstruction
(d) Mitral regurgitation

186. Which drug may reduce sudden cardiac death in HCM?

(a) β-blocker (b) Ca-blocker
(c) Amiodarone (d) Disopyramide

187. Central cyanosis with clubbing occurs in all except

(a) Right–Left shunt (b) Pulmonary disease
(c) Heart failure (d) All the above

188. All the following statements are true regarding EEITE study except

(a) Comparison of losartan vs captoproil in heart failure (symptomatic)

(b) In elderly patients
(c) Losartan was superior than captopril (mortality and hospitalization rate)
(d) Side effects were more with losartan

189. Which of the dilated cardiomyopathy present as acute onset?

(a) Cobalt cardiomyopathy
(b) Alcohol cardiomyopathy
(c) Peripartum cardiomyopathy
(d) None of the above

190. Which of the following Dilated cardiomyopathy present initially with hypertension?

(a) Idiopathic (b) Peripartum
(c) Alcoholic (d) None of the above

191. Anthracycline cardiomyopathy has all the following features except

(a) Usually reversible on stoppage of drug
(b) Usually irreversible
(c) Non progressive
(d) All of the above

192. Which feature of heart failure is highest predictive accuracy?

(a) Paroxysmal nocturnal dyspnea
(b) S3
(c) Basal rales
(d) Tachycardia

193. Which feature of heart failure has least predictive accuracy?

(a) Orthopnea (b) Dyspnea
(c) Edema (d) Rales

194. Following are the criteria resynenronization therapy except

(a) Repeated hospitalization with no known precipitating factor and with full medical TF
(b) EF < 30% class III IV NYHA
(c) LBBB QRS demotion > 130 ins or > 150 ins
(d) Sims node dysfunction

195. Possible benefits of cardiac resyrichronization therapy are all following except

(a) Reduced rate of hospitalization
(b) Modest mortality reduction
(c) Inpranes exe tolerance
(d) Sudden cardiac death are reduced

196. All are correct statement regarding carvedilal except

(a) a1 & Beta-blockers
(b) Antioxidant
(c) Anti protiferative
(d) Increase endothelial levels

197. Which is the best procedemia for diagnosis of doxorebicium induced cardiomyopathy?

(a) Echo
(b) ECG
(c) Angiocardiography with radiolabeled antimyosin antibody
(d) Endomyocardial biopsy

198. All are ECG features of poor prognosis in idiopathic dilated CMP except

(a) Atrial fibrillation (b) LBBB
(c) VT (d) RBBB

199. All are poor biochemical features predictors in dileded CMP except

(a) Increase adranative
(b) Increase noradremaline
(c) Increase angiolesion
(d) None of the above

200. Which valvular heart disease does not cause dilated cardiomyopathy?

(a) Mitral regurgitation
(b) Aortic regurgitation
(c) Aortic stenosis
(d) Mitral stenosis

201. All following drugs cause dilated cardiomyopathy except

(a) Anthracyclins
(b) Cyclophosphamide
(c) Chloroquine (d) Metanidazole

202. All following are risk factors for Doxorubicin induced cardiomyopathy except

(a) Age > 70 years
(b) Faculae SVF
(c) High connotative dose
(d) DM

203. Acute or subacute cardiotoxicity of anthracyclin therapy present with

(a) Dysplasia
(b) Cardiomegaly
(c) S3
(d) ST/T changes in ECG

204. Anemia in heart failure is due to all except

(a) Braun more no superior
(b) Poor installs
(c) Renal dysfunction
(d) Haemolysis

205. Commonest echocardiography finding in acute myocarditis is

(a) Pericarditis effusion
(b) Cardiomegaly
(c) Global hypokinesia
(d) Impaired diastolic dysfunction

206. Fluid restriction in heart failure is usually indicated in all the following situation except

(a) Refractory fluid retention
(b) Significant hyponatrema
(c) Renal insufficiency
(d) EF < 35%

207. All the following β-blockers may be used in heart failure except

(a) Bisoprolal (b) Metaprolal
(c) Carvedilal (d) Atenolal

208. When β-blockers are indicated in HF in all following situation except

(a) Class II or III with symptoms
(b) A symptomatic patients with decrease EF
(c) Stable class IV without fluid retention
(d) All class IV patients

209. Incidence of sudden cardiac death in heart failure is

(a) 10% (b) 20%
(c) 30% (d) 50%

210. Which β-blockers has maximum reduction in mortality in heart failure?

(a) Metoprolal (b) Bisoprolal
(c) Carvedilal (d) Bucindolal

211. Which is most important risk factors for sudden cardiac death in HCM?

(a) LVH (b) F/H of SCD
(c) NSVT on hotter (d) Syncope

212. All following act as cardioprotective for boxorubiun cardiotoxicity except

(a) Prolonged continuous infusion of drug
(b) Iron chelator
(c) VHE (d) β-blockers

213. All following are electrically determined disorder which can present as HCM except?

(a) Friederich's ataxia
(b) Noonan syndrome
(c) Down syndrome
(d) Ganadal dyxgenesis

214. Reversible HCM may occur in young infarcts with the use of which drug?

(a) Antibiotics (b) Steroids
(c) Both (a) and (b) (d) None of the above

215. All are common cause of RCM except

(a) Amyloidosis
(b) Idiopathic
(c) Tropical endomyocardial fibrosis
(d) Sclerodema

216. Neonatal arrdiomyopathy in newborn from diabetic muller has all following feature except

(a) It is HCM
(b) Induced by material hormones
(c) Induced by material hematological and/or metabolic disturbance
(d) It is irreversible

217. Dynamic cardiomyoplasty in heart failure results in all the following except

(a) Symptomatic improvement in class III patients
(b) No significant effect in haemodynamic
(c) No significant effects on physical sign
(d) Mortality is reduced

218. Ventricular assert devices in heart failure resents in

(a) Sustain EF
(b) May reverse activation of RAAS
(c) May reverse remodeling
(d) Improves long term mortality

219. VRT in heart failure cause what changes in QRS?

(a) Duration increase farther
(b) Duration decrease from baseline
(c) Duration remains Same
(d) All the above

220. How the weight loss in heart failure is best managed?

(a) High caloric diet
(b) Appetite stimulant
(c) Growth hormone
(d) Physical training and regular exercise

221. All following are risk of ACE inhibitors in heart failure except

(a) 1st dose hypotensive in patients receiving diameters
(b) May impair renal function
(c) Hyperkelemia (d) All the above

222. Which NYHA class ryamine heart failure therapy by ACE inhibitor?

(a) Class I (b) Class II
(c) Class III & IV (d) All the above classes

223. All following beneficial effects ACE inhibitors in heart failure except

(a) Improve haemodynamic
(b) Anti thrombotic
(c) Anti proliferative (d) All the above

224. Commonest cause of pulmonary hypertension is

(a) Passive
(b) Reactive
(c) Hyperbemetic
(d) Ostrichive and abdicative

225. Most common cause of cor pulmonale is

(a) COPD
(b) Pulmonary embolism
(c) Pneumotharax
(d) Obstructive sleep apnea

226. Tako–Tsubo cardiomyopathy is characterized by all the following except

(a) Often occurs in females > 60 years
(b) ECG evidence of anterior myocardial infarction (ST elevation + Q waves)
(c) Normal Epicardial Coronary Arteries
(d) Cardiac Enzymes Markedly Elevated

227. All the following are ST elevated cardiomyopathy except

(a) Coronary artery disease
(b) Chemotherapy induced
(c) Tako–Tsubo cardiomyopathy
(d) Peripartum cardiomyopathy

228. Which dilated cardiomyopathy has best prognosis?

(a) Alcoholic (b) Peripartum
(c) Familial (d) Idiopathic

229. Tachycardia induced cardiomyopathy occurs with all following tachycardia except

(a) AF with fast VR
(b) Atrial flutter
(c) Ectopic atrial tachycardia
(d) Sinus tachycardia

230. Hypertrophic cardiomyopathic type changes occurs in all the following except

(a) Hyperparathyroidism
(b) Hyperthyroidism
(c) Hypothyroidism
(d) SLE

231. ECG is most reliable for diagnosis of pulmonary hypertension of which etiology

(a) Alveolar hypoventilation
(b) COPD
(c) Thrombo embolic
(d) Left–right shunt

232. In which type of pulmonary hypertension vasodilators are cautiously used?

(a) LVF
(b) COPD
(c) Chronic thrombo embolic
(d) Left–right shunt with PH

233. Most sensitive and specific marker for alcohol abuse in alcoholic cardiomyopathy is

(a) g Glutamyl transferase
(b) MCV
(c) Carbohydrate dependent transferrin
(d) All of the above

234. Which type of cardiomyopathy occurs in neonates of diabetic mother?

(a) DCM (b) RCM
(c) HOCM (d) Any of the above

235. Best drug for post infarct CHF prevention is

(a) Nitrates (b) β-blockers
(c) Ca-blockers (d) ACE Inhibitors

236. Cardiac synchronizing therapy (CST) is indicated in heart failure

(a) NYHA class II heart failure
(b) NYHA class III – IV heart failure
(c) NYHA class III – IV with narrow QRS complex
(d) NYHA class III – IV with LBBB

237. Ultrafiltration in heart failure is done when

(a) NYHA Class III heart failure
(b) NYHA Class IV heart failure
(c) NYHA Class IV heart failure with diuretic resistant edema
(d) Heart failure with severe renal function impairment

238. Diuretics of choice in severe renal insufficiency is

(a) Thiazides (b) K sparing diuretics
(c) Frusemide (d) Any of the above

239. Diagnosis of dilated cardiomyopathy due to CAD is favoured in all the following except

(a) Coronary calcification
(b) Large thallium defect
(c) Exercise induced fall in EF
(d) Exercise induced no fall in EF

240. Most common cause of heart failure is

(a) Dilated cardiomyopathy
(b) Pericardial disease
(c) Congenital heart disease
(d) Arrhythmias

241. All the following points favour diagnosis of dilated cardiomyopathy due to coronary artery disease except

(a) History of chest pain and prior infarctions
(b) Q waves on ECG
(c) Diabetes mellitus
(d) Atrial fibrillation

242. Most common cause of diastolic heart failure is

(a) Hypertrophic cardiomyopathy
(b) Myocardial ischemia
(c) Hypertension
(d) Amyloid heart disease

243. High output failure has all the following features except

(a) warm Skin
(b) Bounding pulse
(c) Cardiac index is lower than normal
(d) Arterial–mixed venous O_2 difference exceeds than low output failure

244. Most common site of myocardial disarray in HCM.

(a) Left ventricular myocardium
(b) Atrial myocardium
(c) Right ventricular myocardium

(d) IVS (Interventricular septum)

245. Pathologic hall mark of HCM is

(a) Myocardial disarray
(b) Myocyte hypertrophy
(c) Interstitial fibrosis
(d) Medial thickening of intramural coronary arteries

246. Which β-blockers has intrinsic sympathomimetic activity?

(a) Propranolol (b) Pindolol
(c) Metoprolol (d) All of the above

247. Which is cardio selective β-blockers?

(a) Metoprolol (b) Propranolol
(c) Pindolal (d) Timolal

248. Which Ca-blocker is used in cardiac transplant patients prophyllaencally for coronary attieroma development?

(a) Verapamil (b) Diltiazem
(c) Nifedipine (d) Any of the above

249. The greatest risk of ACE inhibitors is in which trimester of pregnancy?

(a) Ist trimester
(b) IInd, IIIrd trimester
(c) Post delivery

250. Which Ca-blockers is contra indicated in HOCM with resting obstruction?

(a) Varapamil (b) Diltazen
(c) Nifedipine (d) None of these

251. All following qenohormonal changes occurs in heart failure except

(a) Upregulation of beta adrenergic receptors
(b) Up regulation of atrial notriuretic peptide
(c) Incresed endothlin-I
(d) Increased tumer necrosis factor

252. Deadly lipid quartite causist of all the following except

(a) High TG (b) Normal LDL–C
(c) Decrease HDL–C (d) Increase LP

253. When pulses alternance disappears?

(a) Improvement of heart failure
(b) Worsening of heart failure
(c) Both the above
(d) None of the above

254. All following are mechanisms of pulsus alterans except

(a) Localized electromechanical dissociation
(b) Alteration in diastolic volume
(c) Alteration in relaxation
(d) Sinus tachycardia

255. All following are haemodynamic features of heart failure except

(a) Elevated filling pressures
(b) Reduced cardiac output
(c) Decreased pulmonary vascular resistance
(d) Increased systemic vascular resistance

256. Which β-blockers has an antioxidant property and used in heart failure?

(a) Nebivilol (b) Metoprolol
(c) Bisoprolol (d) Carvidiolol

257. β-blocker of choice in treatment of systolic left ventricular dysfunction

(a) Atenolol (b) Metoprolol
(c) Bisoprolol (d) Carvidiolol

258. All following β-blockers usually reduce mortality in heart failure except

(a) Carvidiolol (b) Metoprolol
(c) Bisoprolol (d) Propranolol

259. Which of the following β-blockers reduces mortality in heart failure?

(a) Nebivilol (b) Propranolol
(c) Atenolol (d) None of the above

260. DHF is characterized by all the following except

(a) More common in females
(b) More common in elderly
(c) More common in patients with diabetes mellitus
(d) More common in coronary artery disease

261. DHF patients have higher prevalence of all the following than SHF except

(a) Atrial fibrillation
(b) Hypertension
(c) Renal insufficiency
(d) Poor prognosis

262. DHF are less responsive to all the following except

(a) ACE inhibitors (b) Digoxin
(c) β-blockers (d) Ca-blockers

263. Carvidiolol affects remodelling process by all following mechanism except

(a) Cardiac antiadrenergic
(b) Antioxidant
(c) Antiischemic
(d) Bradykin-in / NO medirated

264. ACE Inhibitors affect remodelling process by all following mechanism except

(a) Bradykin-in / NO
(b) RAS activation modulation
(c) SNS modulation
(d) α1 blockade

265. Amrinone affects which cell component of blood

(a) RBC (b) WBC
(c) Platelets (d) All of the above

266. Which ARB does not causes diarrhoea?

(a) Losartan (b) Valsartan
(c) Irbisartan (d) Telmesartan

267. Which ARB causes fatigue?

(a) Losartan (b) Irbesartan
(c) Candesartan (d) Telmesartan

268. Which ARB has maximum AT1 receptor affinity?

(a) Valsartan (b) Losartan
(c) Irbesartan (d) Olmesartan

269. Which ARB has maximum trough peak ratio?

(a) Telmesartan (b) Losartan
(c) Irbesartan (d) Valsartan

270. All the following ARB's can causes cough except

(a) Losartan (b) Irbesartan
(c) Eprosartan (d) Telmesartan

271. Which ARB may causes viral infection?

(a) Losartan (b) Valsartan
(c) Telmesartan (d) Candesartan

272. Which of the following β-blockers is not lipid soluble?

(a) Atenolol (b) Metoprolol
(c) Nebivolol (d) Propranolol

273. Which β-blockers has highest ISA?

(a) Pindolol (b) Penbatalol
(c) Acebatulol (d) Celeprolol

274. Which β-blockers has highest B1 selectivity?

(a) Acebutalol (b) Atenolol
(c) Bisoprolol (d) Metoprolol

275. Which β-blockers has α-blockers Activity?

(a) Nebivolol (b) Carvidilol
(c) Metoprolol (d) Bisoprolol

276. Excessive tachycardia is found in which type of dilated cardiomyopathy?

(a) Idiopathic
(b) Periparturum
(c) Alcoholic CMP
(d) Anthracyclone induced CMP

277. Retadine absence of hypertrophy and dilation of LV is found in which dilated CMP?

(a) Idiopathic
(b) Peripatum
(c) Alcoholic CMP
(d) Anthracycline induced CMP

278. OS in mitral stenosis is best heard in which location?

(a) Apex
(b) Base
(c) Lower left sternal border
(d) Midway between left sternal border and apex

279. Which of the following is not found in severe mitral stenosis?

(a) Loud S1 (b) OS
(c) MDM (d) S3

280. All are clinical predictors of poor prognosis in heart failure except?

(a) NYHA IV (b) Signs of RHF
(c) Signs of LHF (d) S3 LV

281. All are electrocardiographic predictors of poor prognosis in heart failure except

(a) Atrial fibrillation (b) LBBB
(c) VT (d) PAT

282. All are hemodynamic predictors of poor prognosis in heart failure except

(a) PCWP > 20 mmHg
(b) Cardiac index < 2.5 L/min/m² BSA
(c) Low mean arterial pressure
(d) Sinus bradycardia

283. All are poor predictor on echocardiography in heart failure except

(a) Low EF
(b) Markedly increase LVEDD
(c) Diffuse wall motion abnormality
(d) Increased ventricular mass/volume ratio

284. Which Beta-blocker is avoided during lactation?

(a) Atenolol (b) Metoprolol
(c) Propranolol (d) All of the above

285. All the following drugs used in heart failure have arrhythmogenic potential except

(a) Digoxin (b) Diuretics
(c) Anti arrhythmic (d) β-blockers

286. Heart failure may causes anemia by following ways except

(a) Aspirin intake
(b) Malabsorption
(c) Cytokine induced BM suppression
(d) Diuretics therapy

287. Most common form of cardiomyopathy is

(a) Dilated
(b) Restrictive
(c) Hypertrophic nonobstructive
(d) Hypertrophic obstructive

288. Ischemic dilated cardiomyopathy most commonly occurs in

(a) Following anterior myocardial infarction
(b) Following posterior myocardial infarction
(c) Following inferior myocardial infarction
(d) Following superior myocardial infarction

289. Most powerful predictor of prognosis in heart failure is

(a) Clinical severity of heart failure
(b) Underlying heart disease
(c) Persistence of compensatory mechanisms
(d) EF

290. Most common form of dilated cardiomyopathy is

(a) Ischaemic (b) Idiopathic
(c) Nutritional (d) Metabolic

291. Hypertensive cardiomyopathy presents as all the following types except

(a) Dilated (b) Restrictive
(c) Unclassified (d) Hypertrophic

292. All the following are characteristic finding on microscopy in idiopathic dilated cardiomyopathy except

(a) Marked myocyte hypertrophy
(b) Myocytes with small nuclei
(c) Marked interstitial fibrosis
(d) Myocytes atrophy

293. Which of the following dilated cardiomyopathy has bad prognosis than others?

(a) Idiopathic (b) Ischemic
(c) Peripartum (d) Hypocalcemic

294. In IDC following HLA antigen are increased except

(a) HLA – A2 (b) HLA – DR4
(c) HLA – DQ4 (d) HLA – DRw4

295. Which β-blocker is preferred in pregnancy?

(a) Propranolol (b) Atenolol
(c) Metoprolol (d) Any of above

296. Pathognomonic sign of complete endocardial cushion defect is

(a) CHB
(b) Holosystolic murmur of mitral regurgitation
(c) Holosystolic murmur of VSD
(d) Goose neck deformity on selective L-V angiography

297. Persistent symptoms after surgery in constrictive pericarditis are due to all the following except

(a) Inadequate operation
(b) Recurrence of constriction
(c) Diastolic dysfunction
(d) Arrhythmias

298. All following are risk predictors in hypertrophic cardiomyopathy except

(a) Young person
(b) History of syncope
(c) Family history of sudden cardiac death
(d) Exercise induced hypertension

299. Which dilated cardiomyopathy has best prognosis?

(a) Idiopathic (b) Alcoholic
(c) Peripartum (d) Ischemic

300. In which dilated cardiomyopathy atrial fibrillation is rare?

(a) Ischemic (b) Hypertensive
(c) Peripartum (d) Alcoholic

301. Most cases of high altitude pulmonary edema occurs by rapid a ascent to which altitude

(a) 7000–8000 feet (b) 8000–9000 feet
(c) 9000–10000 feet (d) > 10,000 feet

302. Which is best tool to diagnose right ventricular dysplasia?

(a) Echo (b) ECG
(c) Clinical (d) MRI

303. Which β-blocker is recommended in open angle glaucoma?

(a) Propranolol (b) Bisoprolol
(c) Timolol (d) Atenolol

304. Which β-blocker used to prevent migraine?

(a) Atenolol (b) Metoprolol
(c) Carteolol (d) Propranolol

305. Which is best drug for overdose of Beta-blockers?

(a) Atropine (b) Dobutamine
(c) Isoprenaline (d) Glucagons

306. Low voltage on ECG with marked hypertrophy of myocardium is found in

(a) Dilated cardiomyopathy
(b) Hypertrophic cardiomyopathy
(c) Amyloid cardiomyopathy
(d) None of the above

307. Chloroquine commonly causes which type of cardiomyopathy.

(a) Dilated (b) Restrictive
(c) Hypertrophic (d) None of the above

308. Cardiac failure in anemia without underlying disease when hemoglobin is reduced to

(a) < 10 G% (b) < 8 G%
(c) < 7 G% (d) < 5 G%

309. All following causes of heart failure are potentially reversible except

(a) Ischemic
(b) Lymphocytic myocarditis
(c) Tachycardia induced CMD
(d) Idiopathic dilated CMP

310. Dopaminergic activity is found with which sympathomimetic amine?

(a) Norepinephrine (b) Epinephrine
(c) Dobutamine (d) Dopamine

311. All following drugs produce cardiomyopathy except

(a) Doxorubicin (b) Daunorubicin
(c) Epirubion (d) 5-Flourouraul

312. Which inotropic agent does not require dose adjustment in renal failure (GFR < 10) except?

(a) Amrinone (b) Dobutamine
(c) Milrinone (d) All of the above

313. All following drugs need no adjustment of dose in renal failure (GFR < 10) except

(a) Calcium blocker (b) Clonidine
(c) Captopril (d) Amiodarone

314. Which cardiac contractile protein has thick filament?

(a) Myosin (b) Actin
(c) Tropomyosin (d) Troponin

315. Which type of amyloid disease does not involve heart?

(a) Primary cryptogenic
(b) Non hodgkins lymphoma
(c) Multiple myloma
(d) Reactive secondary to chronic disease

316. All following drugs produce cardiomyopathy except

(a) Doxorubicin (b) Interleukin II
(c) Interferon 2α (d) Ca-blockers

317. Most common cause of pleural effusion in heart failure

(a) RVF (b) LVF
(c) Ventricular failure (d) All the above

318. Most frequent site of pleural effusion in heart failure is

(a) Right sided (b) Left sided
(c) Both sided (d) None of these

319. Which is stronger indication in predicting CV mortality?

(a) Pulse pressure
(b) Systolic blood pressure
(c) Diastolic blood pressure
(d) Mean arterial pressure

320. If ST and T wall changes are found in ECG in HF it indicates usually all the following except

(a) Ischaemia
(b) Arrhythmogenic RV cardiomyopathy
(c) Hypertrophic CMP
(d) Electrolyte disturbance

321. If LVH is found in heart failure in ECG it frequency indicates all except

(a) Hypertension
(b) Aortic stenosis
(c) HCM
(d) Advanced stage of DCMP

322. If ECG show in heart failure < B3 + RAD it indicates

(a) HCM (b) RCM
(c) AV disease (d) Advanced DCM

323. RBBB in heart failure indicates

(a) Mitral stenosis (b) Aortic stenosis
(c) VSD (d) Corpulmonale

324. Heart failure with low voltage complex indicator all the following except

(a) Pericardial disease (b) Hypothyroidisim
(c) Amyloidosis (d) Hypertension

325. Which diuretic takes shortest time to reach the peak effect when given orally in hours?

(a) Chlorthiazide (b) Metolazone
(c) Triamterine (d) Amiloride

326. Which diuretic has maximum duration of action?

(a) Spironolactone
(b) Acetazolamide
(c) Chlorothiazide
(d) Hydrochlorothiazide

327. Which diuretic acts on proximal tubule?

(a) Thiazide (b) Acetazolamide
(c) Ethacrynic acid (d) Triamterene

328. Which diuretic excretes HCO_3?

(a) Acetazolamide (b) Chlorothiazide
(c) Amiloride (d) Mercuride

329. Which diuretic does not cause loss of H+?

(a) Thiazides (b) Frusemide
(c) Amiloride (d) Acetazolamide

330. All are pharmacologic features of labetalol except

(a) Beta-blocker
(b) β-blocker
(c) Predominant route of elimination is kidney
(d) Noncardioselective

331. Which β-blocker does not need the dose adjustment in renal failure.

(a) Propranolol (b) Nadolol
(c) Atenolol (d) Esmolol

332. All following increase coronary/aretory circulation/cathalerial airctation except

(a) Nitrates (b) Nifedipine
(c) Verapamil (d) Diltiazem

333. Preload is maximally decreased by

(a) Nitrates (b) Nifedipine
(c) Verapamil (d) Diltiazem

334. All following are arterial dilators except

(a) Hydralazine (b) Minoxidil
(c) Amiodarone (d) Prazocin

335. Anticoagulation is indicated in heart failure in all the following except

(a) HF with EF < 35%
(b) HF with EF < 40%
(c) HF with AF
(d) HF with massile LV enlargement

336. Afterload is maximally decreased by

(a) Nitrates (b) Nifedipine
(c) Diltiazem (d) Verapamil

337. HR is maximally decreased by

(a) Nifedipine
(b) Verapamil
(c) Diltiazem
(d) β-blockers with ISA property

338. All are causes of high output failure except

(a) Anaemia (b) Hypothyroidism
(c) Beriberi (d) Liver cirrhosis

339. All following are mechanical alteration in myocardium in heart failure except

(a) Aligned inseries
(b) Decrease in velocity of shortening
(c) Decrease in force development
(d) Decrease in maximum rate of force development

340. Endocrinal toxicity of digoxin include all except

(a) Gynecomastica
(b) Enlargement of breast in females
(c) DM

341. Which receptors act by inhibiting adenyl cyclase?

(a) $\alpha 1$ (b) $\alpha 2$
(c) $\beta 1$ (d) $\beta 2$

342. Which chamber of heart has β-receptors?

(a) Left atrium (b) Right ventricle
(c) Left ventricle (d) All the above

343. Cardiac muscle has all following features except

(a) Mitochondria are present
(b) No oxygen debt
(c) No tetanus
(d) Intercalated disks absent

344. Go proteins in cardiovascular tissues are found in

(a) α-receptor
(b) β-receptors
(c) Muscarinic receptor
(d) a1 receptors

345. All are pathophysiologic mechanism of heart failure except

(a) Volume overload
(b) Presence overload
(c) Loss of muscle
(d) Ventricular extra systole

346. All are pathophysiologic mechanism of heart failure in CAD except

(a) Myocardial infarction
(b) Aneurysm
(c) Mitral regurgitation
(d) Sinus tachycardia

347. All following are true cause of heart failure except

(a) Cardiac tamponade
(b) Coronary artery disease
(c) Valvular heart disease
(d) Cardio myopathy

348. Which β-blocker has highest ISA activity?

(a) Propranolol (b) Oxprenolol
(c) Pindolol (d) Acebutolol

349. Which ion has highest cardiac ventricular concentration?

(a) Na^{+} (b) K^{+}
(c) Ca^{++} (d) Cl^{-}

350. Which ion has highest cardiac extracellular concentration?

(a) Na^{+} (b) K^{+}
(c) Ca^{++} (d) Cl^{--}

351. Which is early sign of heart failure in infant poor feeding with fatigue and?

(a) Dyspnea
(b) Enlarged tender liver
(c) Raised JVP
(d) Puffy eyelids

352. Which sign of heart failure is not found in with heart failure infants?

(a) Distended neck veins
(b) Enlarged liver
(c) Pedal edema (d) Tachycardia

353. All following present sudden cardiac death in heart failure except

(a) β-blocker
(b) Aldosterone antagonists
(c) ACE inhibitors (d) Aspirin

354. Diuretics are

(a) Antihypertensive
(b) Anti-ischemic
(c) Cardiovascular protection
(d) All of the above

355. Which type of HCM has been prognosis?

(a) Apical (b) ASM
(c) HCM (d) Mid ventricular

356. Most significant cardiovascular lesion in pseudoxanthoma elasticum is

(a) Increase in coronary artery disease
(b) MVP
(c) Endocardial fibroelastosis

357. ACE inhibitors have all the following features except

(a) Increase bradykinin
(b) Cause cough
(c) Angioedema
(d) Hyperkalemia in renal failure unlikely

358. What is the most often final diagnosis in unexplained cardiomyopathy?

(a) Idiopathic dilated CMP
(b) Myocarditis
(c) Peripartum cardiomyopathy
(d) Hypertensive cardiomyopathy

359. All following are important mechanism in Remodelling process by carvedilol except

(a) Cardiac adrenergic effect
(b) Antioxidant
(c) Anti-ischemia
(d) Bradykinin/nitric oxide

360. All following are important mechanism in remodeling process by ACE inhibitor except

(a) Bradykinin/nitric oxide
(b) Antioxidant
(c) SNS modulation
(d) HR reduction

361. Which is least common side effect with enalapril?

(a) Cough
(b) Angioedema
(c) Renal improvement
(d) Hypertension

362. At what level of RVSP, RV failure is inevitable in pulmonary hypertension?

(a) 30–50 mm Hg systolic
(b) 60–70 mm Hg systolic
(c) 70–80 mm Hg systolic
(d) When RVSP reaches to systemic systolic pressure

363. Atrial septo in severe RV overload in pulmonary hypertension results in following benefit except

(a) Improve exercise tolerance
(b) Improve RVF
(c) Lessen syncope
(d) Worsen hypoxemia

364. Most common site for infective endocarditis in hypertropic obstructive cardiomyopathy is

(b) IVS (b) AML
(c) PML (d) Papillary muscle

365. Which cardiomyoapthy demostrate low voltage in ECG despite hypertrophy on Echo?

(a) Post partum
(b) Hypertensive
(c) Amyloidosis
(d) Haemochromatosis

366. All following β-blockers have been used in treatment of heart failure except

(a) Metoprolol (b) Atenolol
(c) Bisoprolol (d) Carvidilol

367. Most common cardiomyopathy is

(a) Dilated (b) Hypertrophic
(c) Restrictive (d) ARV dysplasia

368. Common causes of dilated cardiomyopathy is

(a) Idiopathic (b) Myocarditis
(c) Hypertensive (d) Nutritional

369. Which ECG finding is rare in alcoholic cardio-myopathy?

(a) Peaked T wave
(b) ST Segment depression
(c) Ventricular arrhythmia
(d) Abnormal Q wave

370. Most specific finding of left heart failure is

(a) Interstitial edema on X-ray
(b) S3
(c) Cardiomegaly
(d) Basal rales

371. Most specific sign of RVF

(a) Jugular venous distension
(b) Liver enlargement
(c) Pleural effusion
(d) Edema

372. Which ACE inhibitors is balanced aerterio-venous dilator?

(a) Captopril (b) Quinapril
(c) Lisinopril (d) Enalapril

373. IV frusemide has which addition at haemodynamic effect which is useful in acute left ventricular failure

(a) Arterial dilator
(b) Reduces pulmonary wedge pressure
(c) Increase renal perfusion
(d) Increase peripheral perfusion

374. Which is balanced arterio venous dilator?

(a) Nitroglycerine
(b) Sodium nitroprusside
(c) Prazosin
(d) Lisinopril

375. All are confirmed sarcomere gene mutations in HCM except

(a) β-Myosin heavy chain
(b) Cardiac troponin T
(c) Cardiac troponin I
(d) Troponin C

376. All the following are ECG abnormalities in HCM except

(a) Pathologic Q
(b) Increase LV voltage
(c) Increase PR interval
(d) Left atrial enlargement

377. Method of choice in non obstructive HCM is

(a) β-blockers (b) Verapamil
(c) Disopyramide (d) Septal ablation

378. All are established risk factors for sudden cardiac death in HCM except

(a) Maximum wall thickness > 30 mm
(b) Abnormal BP response during exercise
(c) Resting outflow gradient > 50 mmHg
(d) Presence of significant mitral regurgitation

379. All following factors influence LV chamber stiffness except

(a) Myocardial relaxation
(b) RV infarction
(c) LV mass
(d) Atrial contraction

380. All are causes of LV diastolic dysfunction except

(a) Anaemia (b) Cirrhosis
(c) Thyrotoxicosis (d) Osteoporosis

381. All are causes of strain dependent LV dysfunction except

(a) Constriction pericarditis
(b) IHD
(c) HCM
(d) Atrial fibrillation

382. Which drug is not given in diastolic heart failure?

(a) Diuretics (b) β-blockers
(c) Verapamil (d) Digoxin

383. All following are the mechanism sinus of accelerated atherosclerosis is diabetes

(a) Endothelial dysfunction
(b) Dyslipidemia
(c) Impaired fibrinolysis
(d) All the above

384. All are non infiltrative CMP except

(a) Idiopathic
(b) Psendoxanthoma elasticum
(c) Sclerodema
(d) Gaucher's disease

385. All following antiarrhythmics increase defibrillation threshold in ICD patients except

(a) Class I (b) Verapamil
(c) Amiodarone (d) Class IA

386. Which antiarrhythmic agents has no effect on defibrillation threshold in ICD patients?

(a) Class IA (b) Class IB
(c) Class IC (d) Verapamil

387. All following arrhythmia have autosomal dominant inheritance except

(a) Atrial fibrillation (b) WPW
(c) Long QT (RW) (d) Long QT (JLW)

388. All are metabolic disease causing dilated CMP except

(a) Throtoxicosis
(b) Hypothyroidism
(c) Pheochromocytoma
(d) Addison's disease

389. RV enlargement is infrequent in which cardiomyopathy?

(a) Restrictive cardiomyopathy
(b) Dilated cardiomyopathy
(c) Endomyocardial fibrosis
(d) None of these

390. Low voltage ECG is often seen in all the following types of cardiomyopathy except

(a) HCM
(b) Idiopathic dilated CMP
(c) Amyloidosis
(d) Endomyocardial fibrosis

391. Biventricular pacing is usually indicated in medically refractory heart failure in all following situation except.

(a) LV ejection fraction < 35%
(b) NYHA class III – IV

(c) Normal QRS duration
(d) Wide QRS complex

392. Cardiac apex beat is displaced is which cardiomyopathy?

(a) HCM (b) RCM
(c) DCM (d) All of the above

393. Preload is increased in all the following conditions except

(a) Renal failure (b) Polycythemia
(c) Regurgitant lesions
(d) Left to right shunt

394. After load is increased in all the following except

(a) Aortic stenosis (b) Hypertension
(c) PS (d) Severe anaemia

395. Which of the following drug may be harmful in heart failure?

(a) Digoxin
(b) Non digitales inotropes
(c) ACE inhibitors (d) β-blockers

396. All following statements regarding use of ACE inhibitors in HF are correct except

(a) Reduce mortality
(b) Reduce ischaemic events
(c) Reduce arrhythmias
(d) Reduce hospitalizations

397. Which β-blocker has maximum duration of action?

(a) Oxprenolol (b) Bisoprolol
(c) Atenolol (d) Metoprolol

398. Which are is the water saluble β-blocker?

(a) Atenolol (b) Metoprolol
(c) Propranolol (d) Oxprenolol

399. Sudden worsening of cardiac dyspnoea is commonly due

(a) Increased in the basic lesion
(b) Anaemia
(c) Infective endocarditis
(d) Arrhythmia

400. Which of the following is incorrect?

(a) Highest venous O_2 saturation is 80%
(b) Lowest arterial O_2 saturation 90%
(c) Cyanosis cannot be detected if O_2 saturation is > 85%
(d) Arterial O_2 saturation ranges between 90 to 110%

401. All drugs are contraindicated HOCM except

(a) ACE inhibitors (b) Digoxin
(c) Diuretics (d) Disopyramide

402. Which ACE inhibitors has SH group?

(a) Captopril (b) Enalapril
(c) Lisinopril (d) Ramipril

403. PAP is < 50 mmHg in which of the following condition?

(a) Constrictive pericarditis
(b) Endomyocardial fibrosis
(c) Amyloid heart disease
(d) Primary restrictive cardiomyopathy

404. In amyloid heart disease all are absent except

(a) Pulsus paradoxus (b) Kussmaul's sign
(c) S3 (d) Murmur

405. In endomyocardial fibrosis all are present except

(a) Kussmaul's sign (b) 3rd HS
(c) Murmurs (d) Pulses paradoxus

406. Cardiac muscle has all the feature except

(a) Mitochondria are more than skeletal muscle
(b) Sarcoplasmic reticulum are less than skeletal muscle
(c) Oxygen debt is present
(d) Jetanin does not occur

407. All are mechanical alterations in heart failure except

(a) Decreased in velocity of shortening
(b) Decreased in force development
(c) Decreased in maximum rate of force development

(d) Increased in passive length – tension relations

408. All are biochemical alterations in heart failure except

(a) Decreased actomyosin ATP activity
(b) Decreased collagen
(c) Decreased myocardial NE
(d) Decreased function of sarcoplasmic reticulum

409. All the following diuretics given once a day

(a) Ameloride (b) Chlorthalidone
(c) Furosemide (d) Indapamide

410. All following diuretic are given once time a day except

(a) Furosemide (b) Mannitol
(c) Spironolactone (d) Metolazone

411. All following diuretics major excreting throbinding except

(a) Ameloride (b) Furosemide
(c) Mannitol (d) Spironolactone

412. Which diuretic may causes ototoxicity?

(a) Furosemide (b) Spironolactone
(c) Ameloride (d) Thiazides

413. Which β-blockers decreased mortality in heart failure maximally?

(a) Bisoprolol (b) Metoprolol
(c) Carvedilol (d) None of these

414. Most common symptom of inflammatory cardiomyopathy is

(a) Dyspnea on exertion
(b) History of viral infection
(c) Palpitation
(d) Angina

415. All following arrhythmia commonly occurs in heart failure except

(a) Atrial and ventricular extasystoles
(b) Atrial fibrillation
(c) Non sustained VT
(d) AV block

416. All following neuroendocrine metabolic abnormalities are associated with cardiac cachexia except

(a) Neuroendocrine activation
(b) Immune activation
(c) Development of metabolic syndrome
(d) Haemodynamic factors

417. All are common causes of restrictive cardiomyopathy except

(a) Amyloid
(b) Idiopathic
(c) Tropical endomyocardial fibrosis
(d) Scleroderma

418. Most sensitive and specific risk factors of sudden cardiac death in HCM

(a) Family history of sudden cardiac death
(b) LVH ≥ 30 mm
(c) Syncope
(d) NSVT drug holter

419. All are rare cause of restrictive cardiomyopathy except

(a) Scleroderma
(b) Storage diseases
(c) Radiation induced
(d) Haemochromatosis

420. Which is most sensitive finding on echo for cardiac amylodosis?

(a) Speckled appearance of IVS
(b) A–V regurgitation
(c) Enlarged atria
(d) EF < 25%

421. Which tissue biopsy is most sensitive for cardiac amylodosis?

(a) Rectal biopsy
(b) Skin biopsy
(c) Bone marrow biopsy
(d) Endomyocardial biopsy

422. Which is least sensitive test for cardiac amyloidosis?

(a) ECG
(b) Echo
(c) Tissue biopsy
(d) Radionuclide imaging

423. Radiological pattern of high altitude pulmonary edema has all following treatment except

(a) Supradiaphragmatic patch lung infiltrates
(b) Prominent pulmonary arteries
(c) Normal sized heart
(d) Diuretics causes resolution of infiltrates

424. Which sympatho mimetic agent acts only on β1 receptor?

(a) Dopamine (b) Dobutamine
(c) Propranolol (d) Levodopa

425. Most frequent arrhythmia with digitalis intoxication is

(a) PVC (b) PAT with block
(c) AV block (d) VT

426. Digoxin levels are increased by all following drugs except

(a) Quinidine (b) Verapamil
(c) Spironolactone (d) Neomycin

427. Which drug does not produce dilated cardiomyopathy?

(a) Anthracycline (b) Chloroquine
(c) Ephedrine (d) Ergotamine

428. Which contractive protein of heart located in thick filament?

(a) Myosin (b) Actin
(c) Tropomyosin (d) Troponin T

429. LBBB does not occurs usually in which type of cardiomyopathy

(a) Dilated (b) Restrictive
(c) Hypertrophic (d) All of the above

430. LV hypertrophy does not occurs in which cardiomyopathy

(a) Restrictive (b) Dilated
(c) Hypertrophic (d) All of the above

431. In which cardiomyopathy arrhythmias are less common?

(a) Restrictive
(b) Hypertrophic
(c) Dilated
(d) Arrhythmogenic right ventricular

432. Most common type of mechanical alternans

(a) 1 : 1 (b) 2 : 1
(c) 3 : 1 (d) 4 : 1

433. All are risk factors for heart failure except

(a) IHD (b) HT
(c) DM (d) Hyperlipidemia

434. Which type of cardiomyopathy is usually not the cause of sudden cardiac death?

(a) Idiopathic dilated CMP
(b) Peripartum CMP
(c) Hypertrophic CMP
(d) Right ventricular cardiomyopathy

435. Heart failure in elderly has all following features except

(a) High incidence
(b) Most commonly caused by CAD
(c) Diastolic dysfunction is prominent
(d) Drug of choice is high dose loop diuretics

436. Which diuretic does not cause myocarditis?

(a) Thiazide (b) Loop diuretics
(c) Acetazolamide (d) Spironolactone

437. All following nutritional deficiency are linked to dilated cardiomyopathy except

(a) Thiamine (b) Selenium
(c) Carnitine (d) Vit. D

438. All are reversible cause of heart failure except

(a) Ischemic
(b) Lymphocytic myocarditis
(c) Tachycardia induced cardiomyopathy
(d) Amyloid heart disease

439. Myocardial hypertrophy is due to all except

(a) Increased size
(b) Increased cell division
(c) Increased biosynthesis of protensis
(d) Increased surface area and cell volume

440. All are advantages of S–isomer metoprolol except

(a) Early reduction of blood pressure than racemic form
(b) Safe in COPD hypertension patients
(c) Safe in extensive metabolizers
(d) No advantage of OD Dose

441. Which is usual teratogenic effect of ACE inhibitor?

(a) PDA (b) PS
(c) Renal agenesis (d) HCM

442. Which β-blocker has maximal protein binding?

(a) Propranolol (b) Atenolol
(c) Metoprolol (d) Pindolol

443. Common causes of heart failure in elderly except

(a) Hypertension
(b) Coronary artery disease
(c) Amyloid heart
(d) Corpulmonale

444. Commonest causes of heart failure in elderly

(a) Coronary artery disease
(b) Calcific aortic stenosis
(c) Hypertension
(d) Idiopathic dilated cardiomyopathy

445. Nocturia occurs in all the following cardiac disorders except

(a) Cardiac edema (b) Hypertension
(c) During SVT (d) During CHBD

446. All the following endocrinal disorders lead to cardiac defect except

(a) Hypothyroidism
(b) Hypoparathyroidism
(c) Pheochromocytoma
(d) Addission's disease

447. All are true regarding mechanical prosthetic valve

(a) Opening click
(b) Closing click
(c) Absence of click indicate malfunction
(d) None of the these

448. Ischamic T wave has all the following features except

(a) Deep (b) Symmetrical
(c) Arrow head (d) Round head

449. Which of the following rarely produce atrial fibrillation?

(a) Coronary artery disease
(b) Cardiomyopathy
(c) Thyrotoxicosis
(d) Constrictive pericarditis

450. Which vasodilator are avoided in treatment of heart failure?

(a) Nitrate (b) ACE inhibitor
(c) ARBS (d) Ca-blockers

451. Mortality is reduced by all agents in heart failure except

(a) ACE inhibitor (b) Spironolactone
(c) Beta–blockers (d) ARBs

452. In heart failure sudden cardiac death is reduced by all except

(a) Spironolactone
(b) β-blocker
(c) AT receptor blocker
(d) ACE inhibitor

453. Which drug reduces sympts mortality sudden cardiac death in heart failure?

(a) β-blocker
(b) Diuretics
(c) Digoxin
(d) A2 receptor blockers

454. All following Beta-blocker are used to decrease intraoccular hypertension except

(a) Betaxalol (b) Carteolol
(c) Timolol (d) Metoprolol

455. Heart failure in diabetics is caused by all except

(a) Hypertension
(b) Coronary artery disease
(c) Thiazoindinediones
(d) Insulin

456. All are the cardiovascular complications of β-blockers except

(a) SSS
(b) High degree AV block
(c) Class II/III heart failure
(d) Raynaud's phenomena

457. Which Ca-blockers is associated more frequency of constipation?

(a) Verapamil (b) Diltiazem
(c) Nifedipine (d) Diltiazem XR

458. Dobutamine does not act on following receipts except

(a) α2 (b) DA1
(c) DA2 (d) B1

459. Isoprenaline does not act on all following receptors except

(a) α1 (b) α2
(c) DA2 (d) B2

460. Epinephrine does not act on all following receptors except

(a) β2 (b) DA1
(c) DA2 (d) B1

461. Norepinephrine does not act on following receptors except

(a) β2 (b) β1
(c) DA1 (d) DA2

462. Which is the commonest cardiomyopathy in India?

(a) Dilated cardiomyopathy
(b) HCM
(c) Enolomyocardial fibrosis
(d) Arrhythmogenic RV

463. Which is commonest complication of Untreated hypertension?

(a) LVH (b) Heart failure
(c) Angina (d) Stroke

464. All are atherosclerotic complications of hypertension except

(a) Cerebral thrombosis
(b) Coronary artery disease
(c) Clandicalin syndrome
(d) Renal failure

465. All are common features of diastolic heart failure except

(a) Frequently in elderly
(b) Usually with concentric LVH
(c) Pulmonary congestion
(d) S3

466. Ankle edema is most with

(a) Verapamil (b) Diltiazem
(c) Nifedipine (d) All of the above

467. Isoprenaline does not act on all following receptors except

(a) α1 (b) α2
(c) DA2 (d) B2

468. Epinephrine does not act on all following receptors except

(a) β2 (b) DA1
(c) DA2 (d) B1

469. Norepinephrine does not act on following receptors except

(a) β2 (b) β1
(c) DA1 (d) DA2

470. Which antiarrhythmic does not increase PR interval?

(a) Flecainide (b) Propaphenone
(c) Verapamil (d) Lidocaine

471. All following are electrophylogical parameters for poor prognosis in heart failure

(a) LBBB (b) Atrial fibrillation
(c) VT (d) 1° AV block

472. Which is most important funding ECG in diastolic heart failure?

(a) Low voltages (b) LVH
(c) Q wave (d) 'P' pulmonale

473. Which of the following antihypertensive reduces initially cardiac output?

(a) Ca-blocker (b) β-blocker
(c) ACE inhibitor (d) α-blocker

474. Drug of choice in hypertension with BPH

(a) α-blocker (b) β-blocker
(c) Ca-blockers (d) Thiazide

475. Drug of choice for hypertension with cerebrovascular disease.

(a) Thiazide (b) ACE inhibitors
(c) β-blockers (d) Ca-blockers

476. Flushing does not occur with which Ca-blocker

(a) Diltiazem (b) Verapamil
(c) Nifedipine (d) None of theses

477. All following ARBs have active metabolite except

(a) Candesartan (b) Losartan
(c) Olmesartan (d) Telmisartan

478. All following ARBS have no active metabolite except

(a) Irbesartan (b) Telmisartan
(c) Valsartan (d) Losartan

479. How frequent is hypertension in takayasu's Arteritis?

(a) 10% (b) 20%
(c) 30% (d) 50%

480. Which Ca-blocker does not cause constipation?

(a) Nifedipine (b) Diltiazem
(c) Verapamil (d) All of the above

481. β-blockers use in pregnancy results in neonate

(a) Sinus bradycardia (b) SSS
(c) AVB (d) BBB

481. Which cause of right heart failure persists with RVS3?

(a) Cardiac tamponade
(b) Mitral stenosis
(c) TS
(d) Corpulmonale

483. Which of the following change with aging does not occurs?

(a) Increased LV wall thickness
(b) Increased myocytes size
(c) Increased myocytes number
(d) Increased callagen

ANSWERS

1. (*c*)	2. (*d*)	3. (*a*)	4. (*d*)	5. (*d*)
6. (*d*)	7. (*d*)	8. (*b*)	9. (*d*)	10. (*c*)
11. (*d*)	12. (*a*)	13. (*d*)	14. (*b*)	15. (*d*)
16. (*b*)	17. (*d*)	18. (*d*)	19. (*d*)	20. (*a*)
21. (*c*)	22. (*a*)	23. (*a*)	24. (*a*)	25. (*c*)
26. (*b*)	27. (*a*)	28. (*a*)	29. (*d*)	30. (*b*)
31. (*d*)	32. (*d*)	33. (*d*)	34. (*d*)	35. (*d*)
36. (*c*)	37. (*c*)	38. (*c*)	39. (*b*)	40. (*c*)
41. (*d*)	42. (*a*)	43. (*c*)	44. (*c*)	45. (*b*)
46. (*d*)	47. (*d*)	48. (*d*)	49. (*d*)	50. (*a*)
51. (*d*)	52. (*d*)	53. (*c*)	54. (*d*)	55. (*a*)
56. (*d*)	57. (*d*)	58. (*d*)	59. (*c*)	60. (*d*)
61. (*b*)	62. (*c*)	63. (*d*)	64. (*a*)	65. (*d*)
66. (*d*)	67. (*a*)	68. (*c*)	69. (*d*)	70. (*c*)
71. (*a*)	72. (*c*)	73. (*d*)	74. (*a*)	75. (*d*)
76. (*d*)	77. (*a*)	78. (*a*)	79. (*d*)	80. (*d*)
81. (*c*)	82. (*d*)	83. (*d*)	84. (*d*)	85. (*a*)
86. (*d*)	87. (*a*)	88. (*c*)	89. (*d*)	90. (*b*)
91. (*c*)	92. (*a*)	93. (*d*)	94. (*d*)	95. (*c*)
96. (*d*)	97. (*b*)	98. (*c*)	99. (*b*)	100. (*c*)
101. (*d*)	102. (*d*)	103. (*d*)	104. (*c*)	105. (*a*)
106. (*d*)	107. (*a*)	108. (*c*)	109. (*c*)	110. (*d*)
111. (*b*)	112. (*c*)	113. (*c*)	114. (*d*)	115. (*c*)
116. (*d*)	117. (*a*)	118. (*d*)	119. (*d*)	120. (*a*)
121. (*d*)	122. (*d*)	123. (*d*)	124. (*a*)	125. (*d*)
126. (*b*)	127. (*a*)	128. (*a*)	129. (*a*)	130. (*a*)
131. (*d*)	132. (*a*)	133. (*a*)	134. (*b*)	135. (*d*)
136. (*a*)	137. (*a*)	138. (*d*)	139. (*a*)	140. (*d*)
141. (*d*)	142. (*d*)	143. (*d*)	144. (*a*)	145. (*d*)
146. (*d*)	147. (*c*)	148. (*d*)	149. (*d*)	150. (*b*)
151. (*d*)	152. (*c*)	153. (*d*)	154. (*a*)	155. (*c*)
156. (*a*)	157. (*b*)	158. (*a*)	159. (*b*)	160. (*c*)

161. (*a*)	162. (*b*)	163. (*d*)	164. (*d*)	165. (*d*)
166. (*c*)	167. (*d*)	168. (*b*)	169. (*d*)	170. (*b*)
171. (*d*)	172. (*d*)	173. (*c*)	174. (*b*)	175. (*b*)
176. (*d*)	177. (*d*)	178. (*d*)	179. (*d*)	180. (*a*)
181. (*a*)	182. (*d*)	183. (*d*)	184. (*d*)	185. (*b*)
186. (*c*)	187. (*c*)	188. (*d*)	189. (*a*)	190. (*a*)
191. (*a*)	192. (*b*)	193. (*a*)	194. (*d*)	195. (*d*)
196. (*d*)	197. (*d*)	198. (*d*)	199. (*d*)	200. (*d*)
201. (*d*)	202. (*d*)	203. (*d*)	204. (*d*)	205. (*a*)
206. (*d*)	207. (*d*)	208. (*d*)	209. (*d*)	210. (*c*)
211. (*b*)	212. (*d*)	213. (*c*)	214. (*d*)	215. (*d*)
216. (*d*)	217. (*d*)	218. (*d*)	219. (*b*)	220. (*d*)
221. (*d*)	222. (*d*)	223. (*d*)	224. (*a*)	225. (*a*)
226. (*d*)	227. (*d*)	228. (*b*)	229. (*d*)	230. (*d*)
231. (*a*)	232. (*d*)	233. (*c*)	234. (*c*)	235. (*d*)
236. (*d*)	237. (*c*)	238. (*c*)	239. (*d*)	240. (*a*)
241. (*d*)	242. (*b*)	243. (*c*)	244. (*d*)	245. (*a*)
246. (*a*)	247. (*a*)	248. (*b*)	249. (*b*)	250. (*c*)
251. (*a*)	252. (*b*)	253. (*c*)	254. (*d*)	255. (*c*)
256. (*d*)	257. (*d*)	258. (*d*)	259. (*a*)	260. (*d*)
261. (*d*)	262. (*d*)	263. (*d*)	264. (*d*)	265. (*c*)
266. (*b*)	267. (*b*)	268. (*a*)	269. (*a*)	270. (*d*)
271. (*b*)	272. (*a*)	273. (*a*)	274. (*c*)	275. (*b*)
276. (*d*)	277. (*d*)	278. (*d*)	279. (*d*)	280. (*c*)
281. (*d*)	282. (*d*)	283. (*d*)	284. (*a*)	285. (*d*)
286. (*d*)	287. (*a*)	288. (*a*)	289. (*d*)	290. (*a*)
291. (*d*)	292. (*b*)	293. (*b*)	294. (*d*)	295. (*c*)
296. (*d*)	297. (*d*)	298. (*d*)	299. (*c*)	300. (*c*)
301. (*d*)	302. (*d*)	303. (*c*)	304. (*d*)	305. (*d*)
306. (*c*)	307. (*b*)	308. (*d*)	309. (*d*)	310. (*d*)
311. (*d*)	312. (*b*)	313. (*c*)	314. (*a*)	315. (*a*)
316. (*c*)	317. (*c*)	318. (*c*)	319. (*a*)	320. (*d*)
321. (*d*)	322. (*d*)	323. (*d*)	324. (*d*)	325. (*b*)
326. (*a*)	327. (*b*)	328. (*a*)	329. (*c*)	330. (*c*)
331. (*d*)	332. (*c*)	333. (*a*)	334. (*d*)	335. (*b*)
336. (*b*)	337. (*b*)	338. (*b*)	339. (*a*)	340. (*c*)

341. (*b*) 342. (*b*) 343. (*d*) 344. (*c*) 345. (*d*)
346. (*d*) 347. (*a*) 348. (*c*) 349. (*b*) 350. (*a*)
351. (*a*) 352. (*c*) 353. (*d*) 354. (*a*) 355. (*a*)
356. (*a*) 357. (*d*) 358. (*b*) 359. (*d*) 360. (*d*)
361. (*b*) 362. (*d*) 363. (*d*) 364. (*b*) 365. (*c*)
366. (*b*) 367. (*a*) 368. (*a*) 369. (*d*) 370. (*a*)
371. (*a*) 372. (*d*) 373. (*b*) 374. (*b*) 375. (*d*)
376. (*c*) 377. (*b*) 378. (*d*) 379. (*b*) 380. (*d*)
381. (*d*) 382. (*d*) 383. (*d*) 384. (*d*) 385. (*d*)
386. (*a*) 387. (*d*) 388. (*d*) 389. (*b*) 390. (*a*)
391. (*c*) 392. (*c*) 393. (*b*) 394. (*d*) 395. (*b*)
396. (*c*) 397. (*b*) 398. (*a*) 399. (*d*) 400. (*d*)
401. (*d*) 402. (*a*) 403. (*a*) 404. (*b*) 405. (*d*)
406. (*c*) 407. (*d*) 408. (*b*) 409. (*c*) 410. (*d*)
411. (*d*) 412. (*a*) 413. (*c*) 414. (*a*) 415. (*d*)
416. (*d*) 417. (*d*) 418. (*d*) 419. (*d*) 420. (*a*)
421. (*d*) 422. (*d*) 423. (*d*) 424. (*c*) 425. (*a*)
426. (*d*) 427. (*d*) 428. (*a*) 429. (*b*) 330. (*b*)
431. (*a*) 432. (*a*) 433. (*d*) 434. (*b*) 435. (*d*)
436. (*b*) 437. (*d*) 438. (*d*) 439. (*b*) 440. (*d*)
441. (*c*) 442. (*a*) 443. (*d*) 444. (*a*) 445. (*d*)
446. (*b*) 447. (*d*) 448. (*d*) 449. (*d*) 450. (*d*)
451. (*d*) 452. (*c*) 453. (*a*) 454. (*d*) 455. (*d*)
456. (*c*) 457. (*a*) 458. (*d*) 459. (*d*) 460. (*d*)
461. (*b*) 462. (*a*) 463. (*a*) 464. (*d*) 465. (*d*)
466. (*c*) 467. (*d*) 468. (*d*) 469. (*b*) 470. (*d*)
471. (*d*) 472. (*b*) 473. (*b*) 474. (*a*) 475. (*d*)
476. (*a*) 477. (*d*) 478. (*d*) 479. (*d*) 480. (*a*)
481. (*a*) 482. (*d*) 483. (*c*)

SECTION–3

ARRHYTHMIAS AND SUDDEN CARDIAC DEATH

1. External cardiac massage is usually done in the

(a) Lower 1/3 of sternum
(b) Xiphisternum
(c) Middle of sternum
(d) Manubrium

2. Atrial fibrillation is seen in all of the following except

(a) Constrictive pericarditis
(b) Atrial septal defect
(c) Mitral stenosis
(d) Myocardial infarction
(e) Ventricular septal defect

3. All of the following are ECG manifestations in wolf parkinson white syndrome except

(a) Narrow QRS
(b) Initial slurred upstroke
(c) Short PR interval
(d) Normal QT interval

4. The commonest arrhythmia encountered in digitalis toxicity is

(a) Complete heart block
(b) Sick sinus syndrome
(c) Bigeminus rhythm
(d) Atrial fibrillation

5. The drug of choice in paroxysmal supraventricular tachycardia is

(a) Digoxin (b) Dilantin
(c) Propranolol (d) Adenosine

6. Which is the most common arrhythmia in myotonic dystrophy?

(a) Paroxysmal atrial fibrillation
(b) Paroxysmal complete heart block
(c) Paroxysmal atrial tachycardia
(d) Ventricular tachycardia

7. Atrial fibrillation is most commonly present in

(a) Severe chronic mitral regurgitation
(b) Mitral stenosis (Severe)
(c) Aortic stenosis (Severe)
(d) Aortic regurgitation(Chronic Severe)

8. Risk of sudden cardiac death is most common in which of the following surgically corrected lesions?

(a) Atrial septal defect
(b) Ventricular septal defect
(c) Patent ductus arteriosus
(d) Tetralogy of fallots

9. 1st degree AV-block particularly occurs in chronic aortic regurgitation

(a) Rheumatic
(b) Syphilitic
(c) Congenital
(d) Ankylosing spondylitis

10. Which drug is found to decrease mortality in heart failure?

(a) Thiazides
(b) Loop diuretics
(c) Aldosterone antagonist
(d) None of the above

11. All the following are contraindication to β-blockers except

(a) Left Bundle branch block
(b) High degree AV-block
(c) Sick sinus syndrome
(d) Severe bradycardia

12. Best β-blocker in treatment of re-entry arrhythmia is

(a) Propranalol (b) Atenolol
(c) Nebivolol (d) Sotalal

13. Verapamil is contraindicated in all of the following except

(a) Sick sinus syndrome
(b) Ventricular tachycardia
(c) Atrial fibrillation with WPW syndromes
(d) Exercise induced VT

14. Commenest cause of atrial fibrillation is

(a) Hypertension
(b) Restrictive cardiomyopathy
(c) Pericardial disease
(d) Heart failure

15. Adenosine is contraindicated in all except

(a) Advanced AV-block
(b) Acute myocardial infarction
(c) Asthma
(d) Heart failure

16. Median time for termination of AVNRT by adenosine is

(a) 60 sec
(b) 40 sec
(c) 80 sec
(d) 20 sec

17. Burgada syndrome is characterized by

(a) RBBB
(b) ST segment elevation in V1-V3
(c) Ventricular fibrillation
(d) All of the above

18. Commonest arrhythmia in digitalis toxicity is

(a) Multifocal PVC
(b) 1 degree AVB
(c) Ventricular tachycardia
(d) Complete heart block

19. All the β-blockers causes reduction in sudden cardiac death except

(a) Metoprolol (b) Atenolol
(c) Propranolol (d) Timolol

20. Most common arrhythmia by digitalis toxicity is

(a) Atrial fibrillation (b) AVB
(c) Bigeminal rhythm (d) VT

21. Most distinctive digitalis induced arrhythmia is

(a) VT (b) PVC
(c) PAT with block (d) Sinus bradycardia

22. Which of the following arrhythmia is commonest in athelete heart?

(a) Sinus bradycardia
(b) 1 degree AV block
(c) II degree AV block
(d) None of the above

23. Which of the ECG finding is most common in athlete's heart?

(a) ST segment elevation
(b) ST segment depression
(c) Biphasic T waves
(d) RBBB

24. Which arrhythmia is most common in HCM?

(a) Atrial fibrillation (b) RBBB
(c) LBBB (d) All of the above

25. Recurrences of atrial fibrillation depends on following except

(a) Duration > 1 year
(b) Age of patient > 60 years
(c) Large left atrial size > 55mm
(d) Lone atrial fibrillation

26. All are ECG evidences of pacemaker malfunction except

(a) Increase in height of pacing artifact
(b) Decrease in pacemaker generator rate
(c) Increase in pacemaker generator rate
(d) None of the above

27. Parasystole is diagnosed by all ECG features except

(a) Varying coupling intervals
(b) Constant short inter ectopic intervals

(c) Presence of fusion beats
(d) Presence of captured beats

28. Reversed bigeminy has all of the following features except

(a) Junctional escaped beat is paired with sinus impulse
(b) 'P' wave is sandwiched between two QRS complexes
(c) P wave is upright
(d) P wave is inverted

29. Amiodarone is definitely contraindicated in

(a) WPW syndrome with rapid atrial fibrillation
(b) Ventricular arrhythmias during pregnancy
(c) Arrhythmias with thyroid dysfunction
(d) None of the above

30. All of the following are urgent indication for cardioversion and defibrillation except

(a) VF (b) Hypertensive VT
(c) AF with rapid VR (d) Torsade depontes

31. Which arrhythmia requires least energy for cardioversion and defibrillation?

(a) VF (b) VT
(c) Atrial flutter (d) Atrial fibrillation

32. Which of the following is commonest SVT?

(a) AVNRT
(b) AVRT
(c) Atrial tachycardia
(d) Intra atrial re-entry tachycardia

33. Which tachycardia is frequently terminated by vagal maneuvers?

(a) AVNRT (b) AVRT
(c) VT (d) Sinus tachycardia

34. All of the following are indications for electrophysiological study except

(a) VT
(b) WPW with rapid atrial fibrillation
(c) 1degree AVB
(d) Sustained VT

35. Which of the SVT is not associated with AV block?

(a) Atrial flutter (b) SNRT
(c) AVNRT (d) AVRT

36. DDD pacing with short PR may be indicated in following except

(a) HOCM symptomatic
(b) HOCM with subaortic significant gradient
(c) Asymptomatic HCM
(d) All of the above

37. All are most frequentchanges in neurogenic heartsyndrome except

(a) Prolonged QT interval
(b) Wide T wave
(c) Atrial fibrillation
(d) VT

38. Prolonged resuscitation (for hours) should be done in all the following conditions except

(a) Hypothermia
(b) Barbiturate over dose
(c) Electrocution
(d) Drowning

39. Low energy cardioversion is effective in (10.50 w/s)

(a) Atrial flutter (b) Atrial fibrillation
(c) SVT (d) VT

40. Anticoagulation in atrial fibrillation the INR is recommended at

(a) 1-2 (b) 2-3
(c) 3-4 (d) Any of these

41. MFT has all the following features except

(a) Rate < 150/m
(b) Commonly occurs in chronic lung diseases
(c) under laying diseases
(d) No rate for cardiovascular

42. Treatment of choice in hemodynamically compromised atrial flutter is

(a) Carotid sinus massage
(b) Digoxin
(c) Verapamil
(d) Low energy cardioversion

43. NSVT in following sit native is all high for VT/VF except

(a) DCMP non ischemia
(b) Ischemia DCMP
(c) No inter lying heart diseases
(d) MVP

44. Patient with pence inabens are recommended which of the cellular phones except

(a) Ordaining cellular (b) Analog cellular
(c) Digital cellular (d) All of these

45. Which SVT is often associated with syncope?

(a) AVRT (b) AVNRT
(c) AAT (d) Atrial fibrillation

46. Most common underlying heart disease of sudden cardiac death is

(a) Idiopathic ischemic cardiomyopathy
(b) Hypertrophic cardiomyopathy
(c) Coronary artery disease
(d) Aortic stenosis

47. Which anti arrhythmic is avoided in pregnancy?

(a) Amiodarone (b) β-blocker
(c) Verapamil (d) All of them

48. Commonest arrhythmia in congenitally corrected transposition of great vessels is

(a) Varying duration of AV-block
(b) Atrial fibrillation
(c) WPW
(d) ANRT

49. Cardiac arrhythmia are more common in which part of brain lesion?

(a) Cerebral cortex
(b) Internal capsule lesion
(c) Brain stem lesion
(d) Basal ganglia

50. Diltiazem is contraindicated in all except
- (a) Systolic heart failure
- (b) 2 degree and 3 degree AV-block
- (c) 1 degree AV-block
- (d) Sick sinus syndrome

51. Arrhythmias are best assessed by
- (a) Holter
- (b) X-ray
- (c) ECG
- (d) Physical examination

52. Which during dose not coattail VR in atrial fibrillation?
- (a) Digoxin (b) Verapamil
- (c) Amiodarone (d) Nifedipine

53. All the following are indications for pacing except
- (a) Symptomatic persistent or intermittent CHB
- (b) Asymptomatic patients with VR < 40/min
- (c) Asymptomatic 1 degree AVB
- (d) Asymptomatic II degree AVB with prolonged HV interval

54. Commonest risk factor for sudden cardiac death is
- (a) Coronary artery disease
- (b) Coronary artery disease with left ventricle failure
- (c) Mitral valve disease
- (d) Pericardial disease

55. Brugada syndrome has all the following features except
- (a) ST elevation in V1-V3
- (b) RBBB
- (c) Sudden cardiac death
- (d) Underlying structural heart disease is present

56. Most effective antiarrhythmic agent for both supra ventricular and ventricular arrhythmias is

(a) β-blockers (b) Quinidine
(c) Xylocaine (d) Amiodarone

57. Which electrolyte abnormality is not associated with sudden cardiac death?
(a) Hypokalemia
(b) Hyperkalemia
(c) Hypocalcemia
(d) Hypomagnesaemia

58. All the following drugs may cause sudden cardiac death except
(a) Erythromycin (b) Clarithromycin
(c) Pentamidine (d) Theophylline

59. In arrhythmogenic right ventricular dysplasia the usual arrhythmic sites are all except
(a) RVOT (b) Apex
(c) RV inflow (d) Any part of RV

60. All following congenital heart disease are predominantly associated with sudden cardiac death except
(a) Congenital AS (b) TOF
(c) TGA (d) PDA

61. All the following are the mechanism of Cardiac arrest except
(a) Electromechanical dissociation
(b) Ventricular fibrillation
(c) Asystole
(d) Ventricular tachycardia

62. All following arrhythmias usually precipitate heart failure except
(a) Atrial fibrillation
(b) Ventricle tachycardia
(c) Multifocal atrial tachycardia
(d) 1° AV-block

63. Exertional syncope occurs in all the following except
(a) Aortic stenosis
(b) Hypertrophic cardiomyopathy
(c) Pulmonary hypertension
(d) Pulmonary stenosis

64. Symptomatic sinus tachycardia is treated with all of the following except

(a) Tranquilizers (b) Reserpine
(c) Propranolol (d) Digitalis

65. Which is the common tachyarrhythmia encountered in WPW syndromes?

(a) Paroxysmal SVT
(b) Atrial fibrillation
(c) Atrial flutter
(d) Ventricular tachycardia

66. Commonest block which precedes CHB is?

(a) LBBB
(b) 1° AVB
(c) Mobitz decrease AVB
(d) Bilateral bundle branch block

67. In which of the following supraventricular tachycardia verapamil is first choice drug?

(a) AVNRT (b) AVRT (wide QRS)
(c) MFAT (d) AT

68. Shock with out tachycardia occurs in all the following except

(a) Complete heart block
(b) Diabetes mellitus
(c) Intracranial surgery
(d) Myocarditis

69. Shock with atrial fibrillation can occurs in all the following except

(a) Acute myocardial infarction
(b) Mitral stenosis
(c) Acute pulmonary embolism
(d) Cardiac tamponade

70. Which anti anginal agent prevents sudden cardiac death in IHD?

(a) β-blockers (b) Diltiazem
(c) Amlodipine (d) Nitrates

71. Commonest digitalis induced arrhythmia is

(a) Non paroxysmal A-V junctional tachycardia
(b) VT

(c) CHB
(d) Since bradycardia

72. Torsades de pointes is commonly caused by all the following except

(a) Quinidine (b) Procainamide
(c) Flecanide (d) Amiodarone

73. Most common cause of sudden death in young is

(a) Aortic stenosis (b) HCM
(c) PS (d) Congenital CHB

74. Commonest supraventricular arrhythmia in acute myocardial infarction

(a) Aitrial fibrillation
(b) Atrial flutter
(c) Ectopic atrial tachycardia
(d) AVNRT

75. Which supraventricular arrhythmia is rare in acute myocardial infarction?

(a) AVNRT
(b) Atrial flutter
(c) Sinus tachycardia
(d) Ectopic atrial tachycardia

76. All following suggest WPW rcentrant SVT except

(a) wide QRS
(b) inverted 'P' in L1
(c) Electrical QRS alternans
(d) Syncope does not occurs

77. Vasopressin is effective in all except

(a) Ventricular fibrillation
(b) Asystole
(c) Electromechanical dissociation
(d) All of these

78. Hall mark ECG manifestation of quinidine effect

(a) Prolonged QT
(b) Widening or notching of 'P' wave
(c) ST & T wave changes
(d) Atrial flutter

79. All are toxic manifestation of quinidine except

(a) Prolongation of PR interval
(b) Atrial standstill
(c) Diffuse inter ventricular block
(d) Atrial flutter

80. Most common congenital heart disease associated with WPW syndrome

(a) Ebstein's anamoly
(b) Hypertrophic cardiomyopathy
(c) ASD
(d) All the above

81. Which is called as chung's phenomenon?

(a) Ventricular abberant conduction
(b) Atrial abberant conduction
(c) Wandering atrial pacemaker
(d) Junctional escape beat

82. Electrical alternans most commonly indicates

(a) QRS complex (b) 'P' wave
(c) ST segment (d) T wave

83. Common alternating ratio in electrical alternans is

(a) 2 : 1 (b) 3 : 1
(c) 4 : 1 (d) 4 : 2

84. Which is the commonest cause of electrical alternans?

(a) Pericardialeffusion
(b) Heart failure
(c) Hypocalcemia
(d) SLE

85. Commonest cause of atrialventricular dissociation is

(a) Intractable heart failure
(b) Digitalis intoxication
(c) Critically ill palients
(d) Pneumonia

86. Most common cause of chronic CHB is

(a) Degenerative process
(b) Coronary artery disease
(c) Digitalis intoxication
(d) Congenital

87. Most common cause of atrial stand stillis

(a) Digitalis intoxication
(b) Quinidine toxicity
(c) Hyperkalemia
(d) Hypercapnia

88. Most common cause of coarse atrial fibrillations

(a) Mitral stenosis
(b) Thyrotoxicosis
(c) Hypertensive heart disease
(d) Coronary artery disease

89. All the following tachyarrhythmia by acute myocardial infarction are benign and self limited except

(a) Idio ventricular tachycardia
(b) Para systolic ventricular tachycardia
(c) Junctional tachycardia
(d) Ventricular flutter

90. Following are the physical signs in CHB except

(a) Cannon 'a' wave
(b) Reytand murmur (mitral mid diastolic murmur)
(c) Cardiomegaly
(d) Mitral regurgitation murmur (systolic)

91. Cardio toxicity of quinidine include all except

(a) Sinus arrest (b) AV block
(c) VT (d) Atrial fibrillation

92. Lone atrial fibrillation has all the following features except

(a) Commonly occurs after age 40 years
(b) No underlying heart disease
(c) Heart failure may occurs
(d) Often associated with fast ventricular rate

93. Regular VR in atrial fibrillation occurs in all following except

(a) CHB
(b) VT
(c) Nodal tachycardia
(d) Digoxin with its toxicity

94. Cardiogenic embolism occurs is which of the following arrhythmia?

(a) Ventricular extrasytole
(b) Ventricular tachycardia
(c) Complete heart block
(d) Sick sinus syndrome

95. All the following anti arrhythmic increases digoxin levels except

(a) Quinidine (b) Propatenone
(c) Amiodarone (d) Fleicanide

96. Clinical clues for AV dissociation are all except

(a) Irregular cannon 'a' wave
(b) Variable intensity of S1
(c) Beat to beat changes in systolic blood pressure
(d) Variable splitting of S2

97. Multi focal atrial tachycardia is usually seen in all the following except

(a) COPD (b) IHD
(c) Myocarditis
(d) Valvular heart disease

98. Most common cause of sudden cardiac death in young

(a) HCM (b) Aortic stenosis
(c) Aortic regurgitation
(d) Mitral stenosis

99. Best drug for management of atrial fibrillation with heart failure

(a) Digoxin (b) Carvedilol
(c) Combination of digitalis + Carvedilol
(d) Atenolol

100. Which of the following arrhythmia originate in purkinje fibers?

(a) VT
(b) Idio ventricular tachycardia
(c) Torsade de points (d) RVOT tachycardia

101. In which ventricular arrhythmia the catholic ablution may be used?

(a) Sustained monomorphic ventricular tachycardia
(b) Palymorphic VT
(c) Ventricular fibrillation
(d) Polymorphic VT (non sustained)

102. Commonest arrhythmia in athletes is

(a) Sinus bradycardia
(b) 1 Degree AVB
(c) Mobitz type 1 block
(d) Sinus arrhythmia

103. All are electrical diseases related to atrial fibrillation except

(a) SSS
(b) Tachycardia induced
(c) Familial
(d) Brady cardia induced

104. Common valves diseases associated with Atrial fibrillation are all except

(a) Mitral stenosis
(b) Mitral regurgitation
(c) TR
(d) Aortic stenosis

105. All following SVT have long PR interval except

(a) Atrial tachycardia
(b) Permanent junctional tachycardia
(c) Atypical AVNRT
(d) Typical AVNRT

106. All are mechanisms of cardiac arrest except

(a) Asystolic (b) VF
(c) AF
(d) Electromechanical dissociation

107. Recovery from cardiac arrest following hours of resuscitation may occurs in all the following conditions except

(a) Hypothermia
(b) Barbiturate overdose
(c) Electrocution
(d) Following acute massive pulmonary embolism

108. 1 Degree AVB in infective endocarditis is caused by all except

(a) Extension of infection in conducting system
(b) Focal myocarditis
(c) Ring abscess
(d) Enhanced parasympathetic activity

109. Which anti lipidemic agent may cause torsades depontes?

(a) Gemfibrozil (b) Fenofibrate
(c) Statins (d) Probucal

110. All are risk factors for sudden cardiac death except

(a) Multiple infarctions
(b) LVEF < 35%
(c) LVH
(d) Atrial fibrillation

111. Presence of atrial fibrillation in aortic regurgitation suggest all the following except

(a) Infective endocarditis
(b) Mitral stenosis
(c) Heart failure
(d) Mitral regurgitation

112. Which is most pro arrhythmic antiarrhythmic drug?

(a) Quinidine (b) Amiodarone
(c) β-blockers (d) Mexiletin

113. Which anti arrhythmic has no pro arrhythmic effect?

(a) β-blockers (b) Mexiletin
(c) Propafenone (d) Amiodarome

114. Ischemic VT most commonly arises from

(a) Left ventricular and left ventricular side of IVS
(b) Right ventricular side of IVS
(c) RBBB
(d) LBBB

115. Most effective drug for letral ventricular arrhythmia is

(a) β-blocker (b) Amiodarone
(c) Procaenamide (d) Disopremide

116. Mono morphic repetitive VT has all following features except

(a) Usually benign
(b) More common in females
(c) Originate in right ventricular out flow tract
(d) Verapamil is contraindicated

117. Cardio version is only help full in which cardiac arrhythmia?

(a) AVNRT
(b) AVRT
(c) Ectopic atrial tachyarryhthmia
(d) Atrial fibrillation

118. Following anti arrhythmic are anti sympathetic except

(a) Propafenone (b) Bretylium
(c) Sotalol (d) Phenytion

119. High probability of induction of sustained VT on EP study are except

(a) Post myocardial infarction with unexplained syncope
(b) LVEF < 30%
(c) Left ventricularaneurysm
(d) Frequent VES

120. Most uncommon feature of vasode pressor syncope is

(a) Sudden fall in PVR thus blood pressure
(b) Return of consciousness if individual returns flat with legs elevated
(c) Injuries are uncommon
(d) Bradycardia < 50%

121. The most common cause of sino atrial block is

(a) Increasevagal tone in response to digoxin
(b) Acute infections
(c) Hyperkalemia
(d) Quinidine therapy

122. Most frequent mechanism of S-A attack in CHB is

(a) Asystole (b) VT
(c) VF
(d) Electromechanical dissociation

123. Epididymoorchitis can occur with which antiarrhythmic?

(a) Lidocanie (b) Quinidine
(c) Mexiletin (d) Amiodarone

124. Commonest tachycardia in WPW is

(a) AVRT (b) Atrial fibrillation
(c) Atrial flutter (d) VF

125. ECG finding diagnostic of VT in wide QRS tachycardia is

(a) Totally negative precordial concordance (V1–V6)
(b) A-V dissociation
(c) Positive concordance
(d) Fusion beat

126. Contraindication to lidocaine therapy are all except

(a) 1 degree AVB
(b) II / III degree AVB
(c) Idioventricular rhythm
(d) Sick sinus syndrome

127. Which neurological disease is contraindication to quinidine therapy?

(a) Polyneuritis
(b) G.B. syndrome
(c) Myasthenia gravis
(d) Muscular dystrophy

128. Which antiarrhythmic is contraindicated in porphyria?

(a) Quinidine (b) Procainamide
(c) Amiodarone (d) β-blockers

129. Which type of ventricular ectopic is associated with highest mortality?

(a) Salvs (b) Bigemini
(c) R on T (d) LV ectopics

130. All the following are late complications of pacemaker implantation except

(a) Pace maker failure
(b) Lead fracture
(c) Battery depletion
(d) Cardiac perforation

131. Which of the following does not damage the implanted pace maker?

(a) MRI
(b) Therapeutic radiation
(c) Digital cellular phones
(d) All of the above

132. All the following totally inhibit pace maker except

(a) MRI
(b) Cellular phones
(c) Electro cautery
(d) Radio frequency ablation

133. All the following increases pace maker rate except

(a) MRI (b) Cellular phones
(c) Electrocautery (d) Defibrillation

134. Most common AV conduction ratio in atrial-flutter is

(a) 1 : 1 (b) 2 : 1
(c) 3 : 1 (d) 5 : 1

135. Commonest cause of bi-directional tachycardia is

(a) Digitalis
(b) Acute myocardial infarction
(c) Cardiomyopathy
(d) Myocarditis

136. Idioventricular tachycardia is found in all except

(a) Acute myocardial infarction
(b) Digitalis toxicity
(c) During reperfusion
(d) DCMP

137. In which of the following arrhythmia carotid sinus massage has no effect?

(a) RBBB (b) LBBB
(c) II Degree AVB (d) CHB

138. What is optimal ventricular rate in atrial fibrillation by rate control drugs on rest?

(a) Resting VR 100/m
(b) Resting VR < 90/m
(c) Exercise VR < 100/m
(d) Exercise VR < 110/m

139. Atrial fibrillation after cardiac surgery has all the following features except

(a) Occurs in 30% cases
(b) For precaution β-blockers most effective
(c) Related to long cross clamp time
(d) Digoxin is most effective for termation of aortic failure

140. Which of the following anti arrhythmic has maximum negative inotropic effect?

(a) Quinidine (b) Disopyramide
(c) β-blocker (d) Procainamide

141. All the following arrhythmia can occur in young with out heart disease except

(a) VT
(b) SVT
(c) SB
(d) Sinus pauses < 2 sec

142. In atrial fibrillation all the following are correct except

(a) Atrial rate > 400/m
(b) Atrial rhythm regular
(c) AVB is variable
(d) VR is usually 100 – 140/m

143. Low risk atrial fibrillation following feature except

(a) No recent heart failure
(b) No previous embolism
(c) No hypertension
(d) < 60 years of age

144. What is the target INR value for oral anticoagulation in atrial fibrillation?

(a) < 2 (b) 2.5 – 2.9
(c) 3 (d) > 5

145. Auscultatory hall mark of CHB

(a) Variable intensity of S1
(b) Mid systolic murmur
(c) Normal splitting
(d) Normal intensity of S2

146. Which class of drugs are choice for conversion of acute paroxysm of atrial fibrillation?

(a) Class IA (b) Class IB
(c) Class IC (d) Class IV

147. All the following factors are involved for recurrence of atrial fibrillation except

(a) Duration > 1 – 3 years
(b) Age > 60 years
(c) Large LA size > 55 mm
(d) Underlying for acute myocardial infarction

148. Drug of choice for prevention of post cardiac surgery atrial fibrillation is

(a) β-blockers (b) Ca-blockers
(c) Disopyramide (d) Amiodarone

149. All the following of PVCS suggest cardiac abnormality except

(a) QRS duration of 0.18 seconds or more
(b) Variable coupling and interectopic interval
(c) Multifocal VES
(d) VES with LBB patters and vertical axis

150. Which of the following feature of atrial premature best is likely to initiate atrial fibrillation?

(a) Inter palated
(b) 'P' wave with abnormal common
(c) P–R interval is longer than P–R interval
(d) Coupling index is < 0.50

151. Atrial paroxysmal tachycardia with block occurs in all except

(a) Digitalis toxicity
(b) CAD
(c) Rheumatic heart disease
(d) Pericarditis

152. All are common causes of total electrical alternans in cardiac tamponade except

(a) Malignancy (b) Tuberculosis
(c) SLE (d) Purulent

153. 1° AV block occurs in all the following congenital heart disease except

(a) PDA (b) VSD
(c) ASD (d) Ebsteins anomaly

154. Which of following drug can induce torsedes de pointes?

(a) Quinidine (b) Lidocaine
(c) Propafenone (d) Mexiletine

155. Vagal maneuvers are not tried in which SVT?

(a) A symptomatic
(b) With mild heart failure
(c) With moderate heart failure
(d) With severe heart failure

156. Commonest arrhythmia after mustard procedure is

(a) Sick sinus disease (b) Atrial flulter
(c) VPS (d) VT

157. Which arrhythmia is frequently terminated by vagal manvoevours?

(a) Atrio ventricular node recentry tachycardia
(b) AVRT
(c) VT
(d) Atrial flutter

158. All the following arrhythmia need urgent cardioversion/ defibrillation except

(a) VF (b) Hypotension VT
(c) AF with fast VR (d) Asystolic

159. Which arrhythmia requires least energy shock as effective procedure?

(a) VT
(b) Atrial fibrillation
(c) Atrial flutter
(d) Ventricular fibrillater

160. QT interval is prolonged in which ventricular tachycardia?

(a) Bundle branch block re-etry tachycardia
(b) RVOT tachycardia
(c) Polymorphic VT
(d) Torsade – depointes

161. Verapamil is effective in which type of VT?

(a) RVOT VT (b) Polymorphic
(c) Torsade depointes (d) Scan related VT

162. Which of the following SVT is AV node dependence?

(a) Atrial tachycardia
(b) Atrial fibrillation
(c) Multifocal atrial tachycardia
(d) AVNRT

163. 3 or more types of 'P' wave morphology is found in which of the following?

(a) Atrial fibrillation
(b) Atrial flutter
(c) Multi focal atrial tachycardia
(d) All the above

164. DC shock is not required in all the following VTS except

(a) Sustained monomorphic with no symptoms / no hemodynamic compromise
(b) Non sustained VT
(c) Idioventricular tachycardia
(d) Sustained polymorphic VT

165. Which antiamythonic drug is removed likely by hemodialysis?

(a) Sotalol (b) Quinidine
(c) Lidocaine (d) Propafenone

166. Which antiarrhythmic has no proarrhythmia property?

(a) Sotalol (b) Quinidine
(c) Bretylium (d) Flecainide

167. Most potent Na-channel blocker is

(a) Quinidine (b) Procainamide
(c) Disopyramide (d) Flecainide

168. All following anti arrhythmics increase energy required for defibrillation except

(a) Lidocaine (b) Phenyloin
(c) Amiodarone (d) Procainamide

169. All following anti arrhythmics drugs have no effect on pacing-threshold except

(a) Amiodarone (b) Sotalol
(c) Tocainide (d) Propafenone

170. Most common mechanism of sustained VT is

(a) Enhanced automaticacity
(b) Re-entry
(c) Trigger activity early after depolarization
(d) Trigger activity–delayed after depolarization

171. Which is most common sustained cardiac arrhythmia?

(a) PVCS
(b) Atrial fibrillation
(c) 1 degree AV block
(d) AVNRT

172. Most common mechanism for paroxysmal atrial fibrillation is

(a) Local ectopic activity
(b) Single circuit re-entry
(c) Multiple circuit re-entry
(d) None of above

173. Atrial fibrillation in association with MV disease often has which mechanism

(a) Local ectopic activity
(b) Multiple circuit re-entry
(c) Single circuit re-entry
(d) All the above

174. Which arrhythmia requires least energy Shock as effective procedure?

(a) VT
(b) Atrial fibrillation
(c) Atrial flutter
(d) Ventricular fibrillation

175. Which adrenergic receptors indicate pro-arrhythmia response?

(a) β1 (b) B2
(c) α1 (d) All the above

176. All following arrhythmia have cannon 'a' waves except

(a) AVNRT (b) AVRT (WPW)
(c) Ventricular flutter (d) 1° AV block

177. Which arrhythmia has highest ventricular Rate (VR)

(a) Atrial flulter
(b) VT
(c) Reciprocating tachycardia due to COPW
(d) Ventricular failure

178. Normal ventricular rate (60–100/m) are usually found with all following except

(a) 1° AV block (b) RBBB
(c) LBBB (d) Aortic failure

179. Which arrhythmia has paradoxical splitting of S2?

(a) RBBB (b) LBBB
(c) 1° AV block (d) Atrial flutter

180. Hypertension in new born is caused by all except

(a) Renal artery stenosis
(b) Coarctation of aortic
(c) Broncho pulmonary dysplasia
(d) Wilm's tumor

181. Which CHB does not require permanent pacing in absence of symptoms?

(a) Congenital CHB
(b) AcquiredCHB
(c) Atrial flutter with CHB
(d) Neuromuscular disease with CHB

182. Carotid sinus massage may terminate which of the following arrhythmia?

(a) Sinus tachycardia (b) AVRT
(c) AVNRT (d) Atrial flutter

183. Mechanism for torsade pointes is

(a) Enhanced antormatierta
(b) Triggered activity
(c) Re-entry
(d) All the above

184. Commonest arrhythmia in digoxin intoxication extrasystole

(a) Ventricular (b) VT
(c) AVB 2 degree (d) Atrial flutter

185. Most common mechanism of ventricular arrhythmia is

(a) Increase antomaticity
(b) Triggered activity
(c) Re-entry
(d) All the above

186. Most common causes for re-entrant PVC is

(a) Ischemia (b) Druginduced
(c) Myocarditis (d) Physiological

187. All following are clinical presentations of SSS except

(a) Severe persistent sinus bradycardia
(b) sinus pauses > 3 sec
(c) BTS
(d) Aortic failure with VR between 100–140/m

188. Which valvular lesion does not causes sudden cardiac death?

(a) MVP (b) Aortic stenosis
(c) Mitral regurgitation
(d) All of the above

189. All following drugs can produce sudden cardiac death except

(a) Antiarrhythmics (b) Antidepressants
(c) Major tranquilisers
(d) β-blockers

190. All following congenital heart diseases produce sudden cardiac death except

(a) Fallots tetralogy
(b) Congenital long QT syndrome
(c) Congenital CHB
(d) ASD secondum

191. All following electrolyte disturbance produce sudden cardiac death except

(a) Hyperkalemia (b) Hypernatremia
(c) Hypomagnesaemia(d) Hypercalcemia

192. Supraventricular arrhythmia are commonly encountered in all the following congenital heart disease except

(a) ASD (b) VSD
(c) Ebstein's disease (d) MVP

193. In which SVT the organic heart disease is rare?

(a) AVRT
(b) Seversnode
(c) Atrial
(d) Automatic atrial techycardia

194. Functional BBB is common is

(a) AVRT (b) AVNRT
(c) SNRT (d) ART

195. All following antiarrhythmia are safe or relatively safe during pregnancy except

(a) Lidocain (b) Digoxin
(c) Quinidine (d) Phenytoin

196. Ischemia during gestation the treatment of choice is

(a) Nitrate (b) Ca-antagonists
(c) β-blockers (d) All of the above

197. Which cardiac arrhythmia is associated with S4?

(a) Supraventricular tachycardia
(b) Short PR interval
(c) Prolonged PR interval
(d) Sinus arrhythmia

198. Which diet may produce torsade de pointes?

(a) Single sodium diet
(b) High potassium diet
(c) low carbohydrate diet
(d) Liquid protein diet

199. Subnodal conduction is improved by

(a) Atropine
(b) Exercise
(c) Carotid sinus massage
(d) None of the above

200. AV nodal conduction is worsened by

(a) Atropine
(b) Exercise
(c) Carotid sinus massage
(d) None of the above

201. Mobitz II block never occurs due to block at

(a) AVN
(b) His bundle
(c) Right bundle branches
(d) None of the above

202. MAC frequently occur in all except

(a) Elderly male (b) Diabetic
(c) Hypertensive (d) Renal failure

203. Larger doses of digoxin is required in which atrial arrhythmia to block AVN?

(a) Atrial tachycardia
(b) Atrial flutter
(c) Atrial fibrillation
(d) All the above

204. Atrial flutter occuring without prior heart disease suggests

(a) Alcohol use
(b) Pregnancy
(c) Smoking
(d) Pulmonary embolism

205. All the following are medications for treatment of sinus bradycardia except

(a) Palpitation
(b) < 50 /m

(c) Hypertension
(d) Ventricular arrhythmia

206. The starting dose of atropine should be to avoid paradoxic bradycardia

(a) 0.2 mg (b) 0.3 mg
(c) 0.4 mg (d) 0.6 mg

207. Clinical cardioversion of atrial fibrillation with normal heart may be achieved by all except

(a) Flecainide (b) Propafenone
(c) Ibutilite (d) Sotalal

208. All the following are mechanism of abnormal impulse formation for genesis of cardiac arrhythmia except

(a) Abnormal automaticity
(b) Delayed after depolarization
(c) Early after depolarization
(d) Reflection

209. Which is most valuable part of cardiac cycle when if PVC falls may result in ventricular tachycardia / fibrillation

(a) Descending limb of QRS
(b) ST segment
(c) Beginning of T wave
(d) Apex of T wave

210. Which duration of sinus pause warrant careful clinical assesment of the patient

(a) 1.5 sec (b) 1.75 sec
(c) 2.5 sec (d) > 3.0 sec

211. Which anti arrhythmic drug has no effect on PR interval?

(a) Quinidine (b) Tocainide
(c) Flecainide (d) β-blockers

212. Maximum prolongation of PR interval occurs with

(a) IA (b) Ic
(c) II (d) III

213. QRS duration is prolonged by all the following except

(a) IA (b) Ic
(c) III (d) 1B

214. Atrial fibrillation is often found in which cause of pulmonary hypertension

(a) Eissenmenger syndrome
(b) Pulmonary veno occlusive disease
(c) Primary pulmonary hypertension
(d) Mitral stenosis

215. LBBB often found in which of the following causes of pulmonary hypertension?

(a) Mitral stenosis
(b) Dilated cardiomyopathy
(c) COPD
(d) Pulmonary veno occlussive disease

216. Most common sustained dysrrhthmic disorder is

(a) Atrial fibrillation (b) AVNRT
(c) Atrial flutter (d) 1° AV block

217. Patients with pacemakers should observe following precautions except

(a) MRI is contraindicated
(b) Analog cellular phone or digital cellular phone with power out < 300 at least 20 cm away from their pace maker
(c) Ultrasound is contraindicated
(d) None of the above

218. DDD pacing is indicated in which of the following?

(a) AV node disease
(b) Sinus node dysfunction
(c) Both of the above
(d) None of the above

219. AAI pacing is particularly indicated in

(a) AV block
(b) BTS with AVN disease
(c) Severe sinus bradycardia with AVN disease
(d) SSS with normal AVN

220. Biventricular pacing is indicated is

(a) HCM (b) DCM
(c) Both of the above (d) None of the above

221. Pace maker mediated tachycardia is treated by all the following except

(a) Spontaneous reversion
(b) Program DVI
(c) Program VVI
(d) Apply a magnet to block atrial tracking

222. In reciprocating tachycardia complicating WPW all the following agents are avoided except

(a) Digoxin (b) Verapamil
(c) Diltiazem (d) DC shock

223. Most frequent mechanism of digitalis induced arrhythmia is

(a) Enhanced automaticity
(b) Re-entry
(c) Delayed after depolarization
(d) Early after depolarization

224. Atrial premature depolarization may be treated with all except

(a) Sedation (b) β-blockers
(c) Digoxin (d) Qunidine

225. β-blockers are usually successful in treatment of symptomatic premature ventricular depolarization related to all the following except

(a) Occurs in stressful situation
(b) MVP
(c) Thyrotoxicosis
(d) Cardiomyopathy

226. All are reversible causes of bradycardia except

(a) Drug induced
(b) Electrolyte disturbance
(c) Sick sinus syndrome
(d) Hypothyroidism

227. All are features of atrial fibrillation in anterior myocardial infarction except

(a) Usually occurs after 24 hrs.
(b) Minimal preceding atrial ectopics
(c) After fast ventricular response
(d) Does not respond to anti arrhythmic

228. All are features of atrial fibrillation in inferior myocardial infarction except

(a) Often occurs early
(b) Frequent atrial ectopics preceding AF
(c) After fast ventricular rate
(d) Resistant to anti arrhythmia

229. Slow VT has all the following features except

(a) Occurs in acute myocardial infarction
(b) Usually resolves in 24–48 hrs.
(c) Treatment is always needed
(d) As a marker of reperfusion

230. RFA is least effective in which arrhythmias?

(a) Paroxysmal atrial fibrillation
(b) AVRT
(c) AVNRT
(d) Atrial flutter

231. RFA is most effective in all except

(a) AVRT
(b) AVNRT
(c) Uncerballced atrial fibrillation
(d) Sustained VT

232. Most common arrhythmia after coronary surgery is

(a) Atrial fibrillation (b) VE
(c) VT (d) AV-block

233. RBBB in coronary artery disease indicates

(a) Single vessel stenosis disease
(b) Multi vessel stenosis disease
(c) Good prognosis
(d) None

234. What is clinical importance of QRS duration in LBBB?

(a) No importance (b) Good prognosis
(c) Poor LVEF (d) All of the above

235. RAD with LBBB indicates

(a) LV enlargement (b) RV enlargement
(c) RA enlargement (d) None

236. Presence of coronary artery disease in LBBB is best known by

(a) Exercise stress testing or treadmill
(b) Exercise perfusion scintigraphy
(c) Pharmacologic stress echo
(d) None of these

237. LBBB usually occurs in the following conditions except

(a) LVH
(b) Myocardial infarction
(c) None of the above
(d) Both (a) and (b)

238. Clinical Signs of LBBB includes

(a) S1 increase
(b) S2 increase
(c) Reverse splitting of S2
(d) Presence of S3

239. Which murmur may be formed by LBBB

(a) ESM in AA
(b) EDM in AA
(c) PSM of mitral regurgitation
(d) PSM of TR

240. Poor prognosis in LBBB is related to

(a) Reverse splitting of S2
(b) Frontal plane QRS axis
(c) Absence of 8 weeks in left precordial leads
(d) Concordant ST–T wave changes

241. Cardiac syncope has all following feature except

(a) Time of convulsion after 30th sec
(b) Recovery rapid
(c) Post ictal amnesia present
(d) Pulse is present

242. rSR in V1 with LAD 'P' wave indicated which type of ASD

(a) SV defect (b) PFO
(c) OS ASD (d) OP ASD

243. rSR in V1 with LAD of QRS indicates which type of ASD

(a) OS ASD (b) OP ASD
(c) PFO (d) SV ASD

244. rSR in V1, LAD of 'P' and QRS indicates

(a) SV defect (b) OP defect
(c) OS defect (d) Single atrium

245. In which cardiac disorder sinus arrhythmia is absent?

(a) PDA (b) ASD
(c) PS (d) AS

246. Best drug to maintain normal sinus rhythm in patients with recurrent atrial fibrillation is

(a) β-blockers (b) Amiodarone
(c) Sotalol (d) Quinidine

247. Which is the distinctive combination ECG in gerboda's defect?

(a) Right and left atrial hypertrophy
(b) Left atrial hypertrophy with LVH
(c) RA hypertrophy with LVH
(d) RA hypertrophy with RVH

248. At present what is status of a rhythmic control or rate control in atrial fibrillation

(a) Rhythmic control is better
(b) Rate control is better
(c) Both are same
(d) None of the above

249. Recent onset atrial fibrillation < 48 hrs choice of treatment is

(a) Amiodarone (b) DC Shock
(c) Ibutilide (d) All of the above

250. Stroke rate in AF is reduced by oral anti-coagulation in which percentage of patients

(a) 30% (b) 40%
(c) 50% (d) 70%

251. In post operative atrial fibrillation when to give anticoagulation

(a) Immediately
(b) If atrial fibrillation persists for 12 hrs.
(c) If atrial fibrillation persists for 24 hrs.
(d) If atrial fibrillation persists more than 48 hrs.

252. All inchandes is up streamer therapy in atrial fibrillation except

(a) Targeting substrate development mechanism
(b) Reaming angiotensin systure nihilism present fibrosis this present AF
(c) ARBS also present promotion of AF by severe mechanism
(d) Prevention of AF by amiodarane

253. Which part of conducting system usually deprived of automaticity?

(a) SA node
(b) Atrial connecting tissue
(c) AV node
(d) His purkinje system

254. Prognosis in ventricular arrhythmia is linked to all the following except

(a) Sustained
(b) LV dysfunction degree of reduced EF
(c) Etiology of interlaying heart disease
(d) Age of patients

255. Best Anti arrhythmic in presence of EF < 30 %

(a) Amiodarone (b) Quinidine
(c) β-blockers (d) Mexiletine

256. Carotid sinus message is not rescanned in all the following except

(a) Carotid disease (b) Elderly
(c) Digitalis toxicity (d) Hyperthyroidism

257. Adenosin assist in diagnosis of all the following except

(a) Latest WPW type A
(b) Atrial flutter
(c) Wide QRS tachycardia to be ventricular or supraventricular
(d) Straggle line AF with atrial paralysis

258. Clinical defibrillator in VF is

(a) Quinidine (b) Lidoeaine
(c) Bretyeium tasylate (d) Amiodarone

259. Which hypolipidemic agent causes prolongation of QT interval?

(a) Statins (b) Fibrates
(c) Resins (d) Probucal

260. Which antibiotic prolongs QT interval?

(a) Penicillin (b) Streptomycin
(c) Sulphenamide (d) Erythromycin

261. Which of the following antihypertensive prolongs QT interval?

(a) Metoprolol (b) ACE inhibitor
(c) Atenolol (d) Sotalol

262. Effective drug for reducing VR in AF is

(a) β-blocker (b) Verapamil
(c) Diltiazem (d) Amioderone

263. Sinus bradycardia usually levels to which arrhythmia

(a) Atrial ectopies
(b) Ventricular ectopies
(c) Sinus tarchycardia
(d) Atrial fibrillation

264. Multifocal atrial tarchycardia is caused by all the following except

(a) Severe systemic hypoxia
(b) Hypercapnia
(c) Acidosis
(d) All the above

265. Av junctional rhythm may cause all the following except

(a) Loud S1
(b) Short PR interval
(c) Cannon A waves in jugular venous
(d) S2 Split is abname

266. Idioventricular tachycardia occurs in all the following except

(a) Digitalis intoxication
(b) Reperfusion after myocardial infection
(c) Acute myocardial infarction
(d) Cardiomyopathy

267. All following antiarrhythmia produce nenbopenia except

(a) Phenytoin (b) Propranolal
(c) Quinidine (d) Moricizine

268. Which antiarrhythmia may causes oplastic anemia?

(a) Quinidine (b) Cardiac tampon
(c) Amlodorane (d) Phenytion

269. Treatment of choice of hemodynamically unstable atrial flutter is

(a) High energy DC shock
(b) Low energy DC shock
(c) Verapamil (d) Class Ic agents

270. DC shock is not indicated is

(a) Atrial fibrillation
(b) VT
(c) Ventricular fibrillation
(d) Torsade De pointes

271. ECG changes in brugada syndrome are all except

(a) RBBB
(b) ST elevation V1–V3 (Particulary V2)
(c) Prolonged QT
(d) Polymorohic VT

272. Treatment of choice in bundle branch re-entrant ventricular tachycardia is

(a) Amiodarone (b) Procainamide
(c) Radio frequency ablation
(d) Sotalal

273. Which drug is used to unmask brugada syndrome ECG features?

(a) Procainamide (b) Mexiletine
(c) Phenytoin (d) Digitalis

274. Wandering atrial pacemaker has all the following features except

(a) Usually with lung disease
(b) In Elderly may be due to SSS
(c) HR > 100
(d) Significant respiratory arrhythmia

275. All are common arrhythmias in VSD in myocardial infarction except

(a) CHB (b) Sinus bradycardia
(c) Atrial fibrillation (d) BBB

276. Sinus bradycardia usually occurs in all the following except

(a) SSS
(b) Inferior myocardial infarction
(c) Post cardiac transplant
(d) Restrictive cardiomyopathy

277. Most common cause of PAT with block is

(a) IHD
(b) CMP
(c) Valvular heart disease
(d) Digoxin toxicity

278. Rare cause of non paroxysmal junctional tachycardia is

(a) Digoxin toxicity
(b) Congenital heart disease
(c) Inferior myocardial infarction
(d) Open heart surgery

279. Multifocal atrial tachycardia has all the following features except

(a) 3 or more different morphology of 'P' waves in single lead
(b) Variable PR interval
(c) Variable S1
(d) Variable S2 splitting

280. Most frequent digitalis effect on ECG is

(a) Reversed correct sign
(b) Increased U wave amplitude
(c) Shortened QT
(d) QT prolongation

281. Best drug for prevention of Ischemic VT

(a) ACE inhibitors (b) β-blockers
(c) Calcium blockers (d) All are similar

282. Which of the following drug is used for treatment of ischemic VT?

(a) Ca-blockers (b) β-blockers
(c) ACE inhibitors (d) All of the above

283. Increased LV potentials are found in all the following excepst

(a) LV enlargement (b) LBBB
(c) Elderly without heart disease
(d) Obese normal persons

284. Median time for termination of AVNRT by verapamil is

(a) 120 Sec. (b) 150 Sec.
(c) 80 Sec. (d) 100 Sec.

285. The most frequent digitalis induced sustained arrhythmia is

(a) Ventricular arrhythmia
(b) Atrio ventricular block
(c) Atrial tachycardia (d) None of the above

286. Atropine increases which of the following block?

(a) 1° AV block (b) Mobitz type I
(c) Mobitz type II (d) All of the above

287. In exercise induced AV block the usual site of block is

(a) Atrial conducting system
(b) AV node
(c) Intraventricular conducting system
(d) All of the above

288. AV block during sleep is more often of which type?

(a) 1° AV block (b) Mobitz type I
(c) Mobitz type II
(d) Advanced AV block

289. Most common site of 1 degree AV block is

(a) Atrium (b) AV node
(c) Ventricle (d) All of the above

290. Brady tachycardia syndrome in SSS manifest most commonly as

(a) Sinus bradycardia with paroxysmal atrial fibrillation
(b) Sinus bradycardia with atrial flurtter
(c) Sinus bradycardia with sinus tachycardia
(d) Sinus bradycardia with atrial tachycardia

291. Class IV antiarrhythmic agent prolongs which of the following?

(a) PR internal
(b) QRS duration
(c) QT internal
(d) None of the above

292. Class IA agents maximally prolong which of the following

(a) PR interval
(b) QRS duration
(c) QT interval
(d) None of the above

293. Alternation of QRS in narrow QRS tachycardia is most likely due to

(a) Atrial tachycardia (b) Sinus tachycardia
(c) AVNRT
(d) AVRT using accessing pathway for ventriculoatrial conduction

294. Sudden cardiac death most often occurs in

(a) Dilated CMP
(b) Ist year following myocardial infarction
(c) HCM
(d) Large QT syndrome

295. Sudden cardiac death in asymptomatic aortic stenosis may be caused by all except

(a) Ventricular tachyarrhythmia
(b) Ventricular asystolic
(c) CHB (d) EMD

296. Best drug for preventing PSVT in WPW syndrome is

(a) Amiodarone (b) Sotalol
(c) Verapamil (d) Digoxin

297. In CHB the wide pulse pressure is due to

(a) Large stroke volume
(b) Decreased peripheral resistance
(c) Both of the above
(d) None of these

298. DC shock induced myocardial damage is minimized by all except

(a) IV Calcium gluconate
(b) Low energy shock
(c) Biphase wave form
(d) Antioxidants

299. Which antiarrhythmic is avoided during lactation?

(a) Amiodarone (b) Verapamil
(c) Digoxin (d) Diltiazem

300. Which SVT responds best to catheter ablation?

(a) Atrial fibrillation (b) AVNRT
(c) AAT (d) Atrial flutter

301. Which arrhythmia treated by catheter has highest recurrence rate?

(a) Atrial fibrillation
(b) Atrial flutter
(c) AV reciprocating tachycardia
(d) AVNRT

302. Commonest indication for permanent pacemaker implantation is

(a) Sinus node dysfunction
(b) AV block
(c) Hypersensitive carotid sinus
(d) Tachy arrhythmias

303. All are non cardiac causes of atrial fibrillation except

(a) Hyperthyroidism
(b) Hyperparathyroidism
(c) Idiopathic
(d) Pulmonary disease

304. All the following are the myocardial substrate of arrhythmogenesis in heart failure except

(a) Ischemia (b) Hypertrophy
(c) Fibrosis (d) Myocyte loss

305. Serum K+ levels should be in which range to prevent sudden cardiac death in ischemic cardiomyopathy

(a) 3.5 – 4 meq/L (b) 4.5 – 5 meq/L
(c) 4.0 – 4.2 meq/L (d) 5 – 5.5 meq/L

306. All the following arrhythmias are more common in females than males except

(a) ANRT
(b) Torsades de pointers
(c) Post MI AF
(d) AV blocks

307. Most common chronic arrhythmia is

(a) Atrial flutter
(b) Functional tachycardia
(c) 1 degree AV block
(d) Atrial fibrillation

308. Which arrhythmia does not need anticoagulation?

(a) Atrial fibrillation
(b) Atrial flutter
(c) Multifocal atrial tachycardia
(d) Bradytachycardia syndrome

309. Sinus rhythm is restored in atrial flutter by which drug

(a) Amiodarone (b) Propafenone
(c) Diltiazem (d) Disopyramide

310. Which type of atrial flutter is most common?

(a) Isthmus dependent counter clock wise rotation
(b) Isthmus dependent clock wise rotation
(c) Non isthmus dependent
(d) All the above

311. Which cardiovascular response is most common in carotid sinus hyper-sensitivity?

(a) Cardio inhibitor response
(b) Vasodepressor response
(c) Mixed
(d) All the above

312. Most sensitive marker of cardiac effect tricydic antidepressants is

(a) QT prolongation
(b) QRS prolongation
(c) Right word deviation of terminal to MS of QRS (terminal R wave in aVR)
(d) Ventricular arrhythmias

313. Goal of slowing of heart rate at rest in atrial fibrillation is

(a) 60 – 80/m (b) 50 – 70/m
(c) 85 – 90/m (d) 80 – 100/m

314. Goal of slowing the heart rate on moderate exercise in atrial fibrillation is

(a) 90 – 115/m (b) 116 – 120/m
(c) 70 – 80/m (d) 120 – 130/m

315. Which drug does not control exercise induced increased VR in atrial fibrillation?

(a) Digoxin (b) Diltiazem
(c) Verapamil (d) Beta–blockers

316. Most common site of electrical alternans is

(a) 'P' wave (b) QT interval
(c) QRS complex (d) 'T' wave

317. Fusion beats are Found in all except

(a) Parasystole
(b) VT
(c) Advanced AV block
(d) 1 degree AV block

318. All are frequent causes of A-V dissociation except

(a) Acute myocardial infarction
(b) Digitalis toxicity
(c) Acute rheumatic fever
(d) Myocarditis

319. Which ECG change strongly support the LVH in LBBB?

(a) SV2 + RV5 > 45 mm
(b) QRS duration ≥ 0.14 sec
(c) Left atrial enlargement
(d) Left axis deviation

320. Most frequent ventricular rate in VT is

(a) 100/m (b) ≤ 80/m
(c) 130 – 170/m (d) > 200/m

321. Majority of SVT's are

(a) Reentrant (b) Ectopic
(c) Triggered Activity (d) All the above

322. Which tachycardia is little or not affected by exercise?

(a) Atrial flutter
(b) Atrial fibrillation
(c) Automatic atrial tachycardia
(d) All the above

323. Which drug does not cause CHB?

(a) Digoxin (b) Quinidine
(c) Procainamide (d) Mexiletine

324. Which valvular heart disease is associated with CHB?

(a) Mitral stenosis
(b) Aortic stenosis
(c) Tricuspid regurgitation
(d) Pulmonary regurgitation

325. Most common type of AV block is?

(a) 1 Degree AV block
(b) 2 Degree mobitz I
(c) 2 Degree mobitz II
(d) CHB

326. Shortening of PR interval occurs with all following except

(a) Exercise
(b) Sympathmimetic drugs
(c) Atropine
(d) Atrial pacing

327. Sick sinus syndrome usually manifest by all the following except

(a) Angina (b) Syncope
(c) Heart failure (d) Fatigue

328. Which cardiac vascular disorder is not usually associated with advanced AV block?

(a) Aortic stenosis
(b) Aortic regurgitation
(c) Mitral stenosis
(d) Hypertension

329. All following arrhythmia cause thrombo-embolism except

(a) Atrial fibrillation
(b) Atrial flutter

(c) Complete AV block
(d) Sick sinus syndrome

330. Spontaneous Diastolic Depolarization is the Result of the following except

(a) Interval current of Na^+
(b) Interval current of Ca^{++}
(c) Interval current of a + b
(d) Interval current of K^+

331. Normally sinus bradycardia occurs in all the following except

(a) Athletes (b) Elderly
(c) Pregnancy (d) None of the above

332. Which endocrine disorder causes sinus bradycardia?

(a) Hyperthyroidism
(b) Hypothyroidism
(c) Diabetes mellitus
(d) Hyperparathyriodism

333. All following antiarrhythmics have hepatic route of elimination except

(a) Amiodarone (b) Diltiazem
(c) Beta-Blocker (d) Bretylium

334. All are clinical signs of VT except

(a) Intermittent cannon a wave in neck veins
(b) Varying 1st heart sound
(c) Varying systolic blood pressure
(d) Pressure of murmur

335. Small pulse volume with bradycardia is found in

(a) SSS (b) Myxedema
(c) CHB (d) All the above

336. Best lead of choice for identifying frequency PVC'S

(a) L11 (b) L111
(c) V1 (d) aVL

337. All following are intriric causes of sinus node dysfunction except

(a) Degenerative (b) Ischemic
(c) Hypertension (d) Hypothyroidism

338. All following antiarrhythmics cause sinus node dysfunction except

(a) Class IA (b) Class IB
(c) Class IC (d) Class II

339. Most Common mechanism of monomorphic VT is

(a) Triggered (b) Focal
(c) Re-entry (d) All the above

340. All following electrolytes abnormalities may cause sudden cardiac death except

(a) Hypokalemia
(b) Hypomagnesaemia
(c) Hypermagnesemia
(d) Hypernatremia

341. All following valvular heart disease may cause sudden cardiac death except

(a) Aortic stenosis
(b) Aortic regurgitation
(c) Mitral valve prolapse
(d) Mitral stenosis

342. All following electrolytes abnormalities are associated with sudden cardiac death except

(a) Hypokalemia (b) Hypernatremia
(c) Hypomagnesaemia (d) Hypocalcaemia

343. All following agents can cause sudden cardiac death except?

(a) Cisapride (b) Cocaine
(c) Chloroquine (d) Statins

344. Which antiarrhythmia are concentrated in Breast Milk?

(a) Nadalol (b) Sotalol
(c) Atenolol (d) Tocainide

345. Which antiarrhythmic has maximum protein binding property?

(a) Amiodarone (b) Lidocaine
(c) Flecainide (d) Procainamide

346. All following cardiomyopathy cause sudden cardiac death except

(a) Right ventricular cardiomyopathy
(b) Idiopathic dilated cardiomyopathy
(c) Hypertrophy cardiomyopathy
(d) None of the above

347. In accelerated idioventricular rhythm the site of origin is

(a) AV node (b) Pulmonary veins
(c) Bundle branches (d) Purkinje fibres

348. Site of origin in torsades de-pointes is

(a) Atria (b) AV node
(c) Ventricles (d) Bundle branches

349. Amiodarone should be combine with which drug?

(a) Digoxin
(b) Thiazide diuretics
(c) Amiodipine
(d) All the above

350. Which anti arrhythmia is choice during pregnancy and ventricular tachycardia?

(a) Mexiletine (b) Amiodarone
(c) β-blockers (d) Lidocaine

351. DDDR Pacemaker is Indicated in

(a) AV block advanced
(b) SN dysfunction
(c) Hypersensitive carotid sinus
(d) Combined SN and AV node disease

352. Write function of pacemaker has following features except

(a) Voltage threshold high
(b) Current threshold variable
(c) Lead impedance high
(d) Electrocardiogram normal always

353. Insentation break in pacemaker system has all following features except

(a) Voltage threshold low
(b) Current threshold high
(c) Lead impedance low
(d) Electrogram normal (always)

354. All are complication of AICD use except

(a) Lead dislodgement
(b) Lead fracture
(c) Insulation defect
(d) Ventricular fibrillation

355. All are cardiac indication for AICD implantation

(a) Old myocardial infraction
(b) Recurrent myocardial infarction
(c) Frequent episodes of tachycardia
(d) Non sustained tachycardia

356. Leads dislodgment of pacemaker system featured by all except

(a) Voltage threshold high
(b) Current threshold low
(c) Lead impedance low
(d) Electrogram low

357. Exit block in pacemaker system is featured by all except

(a) Voltage threshold normal
(b) Current threshold high
(c) Lead impedance normal
(d) Electrogram normal

358. Electrophysiological effects of digoxin at toxic concentration is to increase effective refractory period all following except

(a) Atrium (b) AVN
(c) Purkinje fibres (d) Ventricles

359. Triboelection phenoment has all following features except

(a) High voltage deflection gestated by static electricity
(b) Usually wider than pacemaker stimulus
(c) Usually inregular than pacemaker stimulus
(d) Short over stoot

360. Paced QRS duration (≥ 190 m sec) in RV pacing is indicative of

(a) Predictor of heart failure
(b) Predictor of mortality
(c) Predictor of development of atrial fibrillation

(d) Predictor of development of VT

361. Prolangation of spike to QRS onset occurs in all following except

(a) Development of anterior myocardial infarction
(b) Severe myocardial disease
(c) Hyokalemia
(d) Variant angina

362. Paced QRS alternans occurs in all the following except

(a) Respiratary fluctuations
(b) Pericardial effusion
(c) Mechanical pulsus alternance
(d) All the above

363. All following antiarrhythmic block sympathetic nerves system activity except

(a) Bretylium (b) Amiodarone
(c) Mexiletime (d) Verapamil

364. All following antiarrhythmics prolong refractoriness of accessory pathways except

(a) Quinidine (b) Procainamide
(c) Disopyramide (d) Verapamil

365. Atrial refractoriness is prolonged by all the following except

(a) Quinidine (b) Procaniamid
(c) Disopyramide (d) Verapamil

366. Hisbundle refractoriness is prolonged all the following except

(a) Bretylium (b) Amiodarone
(c) Verapamil (d) Sotalol

367. Which antiarrhythmic drug decrease refractory period of ventricles?

(a) Quinidne (b) Procaniamid
(c) Disopyramide (d) Mexiletine

368. Which drug decrease refractiveness of AV node?

(a) Quinidine (b) Procainamide
(c) Disopyriamide
(d) Propranolol/Propafenone

369. Which drug has maximum protein brinding capacity?

(a) Diltiazem (b) Procainamide
(c) Propranolol (d) Doleazem

370. Most common arrhythmia by digitalis intoxication is

(a) Premature ventricular beats
(b) Premature atrial beats
(c) Atrial tachycardia with block
(d) Ventricular tachycardia

371. Which antiarrhythmic drug shortens action potential duration?

(a) Quinidine (b) Procainamide
(c) Disopyramide (d) Propranolol

372. All following antiarrhythmics shortens action potential duration except

(a) Lidocaine (b) Phenytoin
(c) Eucaenide (d) Amiodarone

373. All the following metabolic and electrolyte disorders are commonly associated with supraventricular tachycardia except

(a) Thyrotoxicosis
(b) Phaechromocytoma
(c) Hypokalemia
(d) Hyperkalemia

374. All the following neoplastic disorders are associated with SVT except

(a) Leukemia (b) Lymphoma
(c) Breast cancer (d) Liver tumors

375. Fast in ward current of action potential has all following characteristics except

(a) Main ion is Na^+
(b) Rate of activation and deactivation is Rapid
(c) Resting membrane potential is 60–70 mv
(d) Recovery prompt

376. Slow in ward current of action potential has all fallowing features except

(a) Main ion is Ca^{++}
(b) Rate of activation and deactivation is slow
(c) Resting membrane potential is –30 to –40 mv
(d) Recovery outlast forte repolarization

377. Calcium blockers are used in all the following except

(a) Hypertension (b) HCM
(c) DCM (d) Cardiac arrhythmia

378. AVN effective refractory period is most affected by

(a) Verapamil (b) Nifedipine
(c) Nimodipine (d) Felodipine

379. Ventricular effective refractory period is affected by

(a) Bepridil (b) Verapamil
(c) Diltiazem (d) All of there

380. Which Ca antagonist prolongs QRS interval?

(a) Verapamil (b) Nifedipine
(c) Diltiazem (d) Bepridil

381. Which Ca antagonist prolong QTc interval?

(a) Bepridil (b) Diltiazem
(c) Verapamil (d) Nimodipine

382. HV interval is prolonged by which calcium antagonists?

(a) Verapamil (b) Diltiazem
(c) Bepridil (d) Nimodipine

383. Effective refractory period of his purkinge is affected by

(a) Bepridil (b) Diltiazem
(c) Verapamil (d) All the above

384. In all following AV block the common type of block is

(a) Wide QRS III degree
(b) Wide QRS II degree or greater
(c) Type second degree
(d) I Degree AV block

385. All following are the metabolic causes of chronic infranodal block except

(a) Myxedema (b) Thyrotoxicosis
(c) Pagets disease (d) Diabetes

386. All are ECG signs indication of electrical arrhythmogenic disease except

(a) Long QT syndrome
(b) Short QT syndrome
(c) Brugada syndrome
(d) Decrease global T

387. Site of block in congenital complete heart block is

(a) Above his bundle
(b) His bundle
(c) Bundle branches
(d) Purkinje system

388. Which is the auscultating hall mark of complete heart block?

(a) Systolic murmur
(b) Slow rate
(c) Regular rhythm
(d) Variation in intensity of first heart sound

389. Which prokinetic agent prolongs QT interval?

(a) Cisapride (b) Mozapride
(c) Etopride (d) All the above

390. Which electrolyte disorder does not prolong QT internal?

(a) Hypokalemia (b) Hypocalcaemia
(c) Hypomagnesaemia (d) Hyponatremia

391. All following antibiotics prolong QT interval except

(a) Erythromycin
(b) Trimethoprin – Sulfamethoxazole
(c) Ampicillin
(d) Levofloxacin

392. All following antihistaminic prolong QT interval except

(a) Astemizole (b) Levocetrizine
(c) Terfinadine (d) None of these

393. All following antipsychotics prolong QT interval except

(a) Haloperidol (b) Chlorpromazine
(c) Thioridazine (d) Duloxitine

394. Which arrhythmia is uncommon in aortic regurgitation?

(a) Bundle branch block
(b) Ventricular arrhythmia
(c) AV blocks
(d) Atrial fibrillation

395. Major mechanism of paroxysmal atrial fibrillation is

(a) Focal source around pulmonary veins
(b) Multiple wavelets
(c) Nodal re-entry
(d) None of above

396. Commonest complication of catheter ablation in atrial fibrillation

(a) CVA
(b) Pulmonary vein stenosis
(c) Atrial macro re-entrant tachycardia
(d) None of these

397. Most common cause of sudden death in young athlete is

(a) Aortic stenosis
(b) HCM
(c) Long QT syndrome
(d) Primary pulmonary hypertension

398. In all following arrhythmia role of cardio versionis little or none except

(a) Ectopic atrial tachycardia
(b) Multifocal atrial tachycardia
(c) Torsade de pointes
(d) AVNRT

399. Arrhythmia in arrhythmogenic right ventricular dysplasia usually arise from all following sites except

(a) RVOT (b) RVIT
(c) Apex (d) LV

400. Arrhythmias are very common in

(a) Cortical brain lesion
(b) Internal capsule lesion
(c) Caudate lesion
(d) Brain stem lesion

401. Which is arrhythmogenic cardiogenic brain embolism?

(a) PAT (b) CHB
(c) SSS (d) 1 degree AV block

402. All are non gastrointestinal presentation of cardiac disease except

(a) Osteoporosis (b) Long stature
(c) Delayed puberty (d) Arthritis

403. Electrical alternans is a good prognosis sign in

(a) Slow sinus rhythms
(b) Rapid sinus rhythms
(c) Ectopic tachycardia
(d) Follow premature systolic

404. The most common alternating ratio in electrical alternans is

(a) 2 : 1 (b) 3 : 1
(c) 4 : 1 (d) 5 : 1

405. Which is the most common form of electrical alternans?

(a) QRS (b) P
(c) T wave (d) ST segment

406. Total electrical alternans is found in all the following except

(a) Malignant effusion (b) Tuberculosis
(c) SLE effusion (d) Viral effusion

407. The alternation is related to all the following except

(a) Cardiac position
(b) Alternation of cardiac output
(c) Alternating progression of refractory phase of heart
(d) Respiratory variation in HR

408. The hall mark of PAC is

(a) PR interval long
(b) PR[1] interval short
(c) Compensatory pause in less than full
(d) Compensatory pause often full

409. Commonest cause of ventricular tachycardia is

(a) IHD (b) CMP
(c) Valvular heart disease
(d) Myocarditis

410. Which is the commonest arrhythmia in holiday heart syndrome?

(a) Ventricular extrasystoles
(b) AVNRT
(c) AV block
(d) Atrial fibrillation

411. Most important clinical significance of prolonged QT interval is

(a) Ventricular fibrillation
(b) CHB
(c) Supraventricular tachycardia
(d) Electromechanical dissociation

412. All following VTS don't require electrical shock except

(a) Accelerated idioventricular rhythm
(b) Non sustained VT (with in 48 hr. MI)
(c) Sustained VT without haemodynamic compromise
(d) Sustained polymorphic VT

413. Which VT presents with prolonged QT interval?

(a) RVOT VT
(b) Arhythmogenic RV cardiomyopathy VT
(c) Scar related VT
(d) Torsade de points

414. Which SVT is AV node dependent?

(a) Sinus tachycardia (b) AVRT
(c) Atrial fibrillation (d) MAT

415. Drug of choice in idiopathic ventricular tachycardia from left ventricular septum

(a) IV β-blockers (b) IV Verapamil
(c) IV Amiodarone (d) IV Xylocaine

416. Which part of conducting system is not automatic?

(a) Sinus node
(b) AV node
(c) His purkinje system
(d) None of these

417. Which antiarrhythmic does not causes torsade depointes?

(a) Quinidine (b) Procainamide
(c) Lidocaine (d) Disopyramide

418. Which antiarrhythmic causes gingival hyperplasia?

(a) Lidocain (b) Phenytoin
(c) Amiodarane (d) Digoxin

419. In presence of atrial fibrillation the highest risk of thromboembolism is in which situation

(a) Previous TIA / Stroke
(b) DM
(c) Hypertension
(d) Heart failure

420. Most common cause of atrial stand strill

(a) Digitalis intoxication
(b) Quinidine toxicity
(c) Terminal stages of myocardial infarction
(d) Carbon dioxide toxicity

421. At which ventricular rate cardiac output usually drops

(a) 120/m (b) 140/m
(c) 160/m (d) > 180/m

422. Most common cause of atrial dissociation

(a) Intractable heart failure
(b) Hypertension
(c) Uraemia
(d) Rheumatic heart disease

423. Which congenital cardiac disease produce LBBB

(a) Aortic stenosis
(b) Aortic regurgitation
(c) VSD
(d) PDA

424. All are functions of magnet in patient of AICD system except

(a) Defibrillator activation
(b) No deactivation of defibrillator
(c) Routine battery checkup
(d) Creation of defibrillator backup mode to allow electrophysiological testing

425. PR interval is shortin all the following conditions except

(a) WPW syndrome
(b) Levine ganong syndrome
(c) Nodal rhythm
(d) CHB

426. All are K^+ Channel blockers except

(a) Amiodarone (b) Adenosine
(c) Bretyllium (d) Sotalol

427. Bradycardia/AVB maximally occurs with which drug

(a) β-blocker
(b) Diltiazem
(c) Verapamil
(d) Nitrates

428. Commonest arrhythmia for permanent pacing is

(a) SSS
(b) AVB
(c) Tachyarrhythmia
(d) Drug induced AV block

429. Atrial fibrillation most commonly occurs in

(a) Mitral stenosis
(b) Mitral regurgitation
(c) Mitral stenosis + Mitral regurgitation
(d) None of these

430. All following antiarrhythmic drugs need no adjustment of dose in renal failure except

(a) Quinidine
(b) Procainamide
(c) β-blocker
(d) Calcium channal blocker

431. Permanent pacing is indicated in congenital complete heart block in all the following situation except

(a) CHF
(b) Mide QRS escape rhythm
(c) H/o syncope
(d) Absence of ventricular arrhythmia

432. Commonest cardiac cause of sudden cardiac death is

(a) IHD (b) HCM
(c) Dilated CMP (d) RV dysplasia

433. All are narrow QRS tachycardia except

(a) Atrial fibrillation
(b) Atrial flutter
(c) Multifocal atrial tachycardia
(d) Paraxysmal atrial tachycardia

434. All following are safe agents in patients with EF < 30% except

(a) Amiodarone (b) Mexiletine
(c) β-blockers (d) Verapamil

435. Which of the following agents has least proarrhythmia incidence?

(a) Encainide (b) Flecainide
(c) Amiodarone (d) Quinidine

436. Most common arrhythmia requiring treatment is

(a) Sinus tachycardia (b) SSS
(c) CHB (d) Atrial fibrillation

437. Loud AZ in VSD occurs in all the following except

(a) TOF
(b) Coarctation of aorta
(c) Bicuspid aortic valve
(d) None of the above

438. Which is rare parasystole?

(a) Atrial
(b) Ventricular
(c) Junctional
(d) Combined atrial and ventricular parasytole

439. Electrical alternans is grave prognostic sign in

(a) SB
(b) ST
(c) Ectopic tachycardial
(d) Normal rates

440. Which is commonest parasytole?

(a) Atrial (b) Ventricular
(c) Junctional (d) Double parasytole

441. Commonest cause of atrial flutter is

(a) Rheumatic heart disease
(b) IHD
(c) Hypertension
(d) ASD

442. Which of the following arrhythmia is not caused by digitalis toxicity?

(a) PAT with block (b) Alternating VES
(c) Atrial fibrillation
(d) Multifocal atrial tachycardia

443. Common cause of parasystole is

(a) CHF (b) HCM
(c) RCM (d) Pericardial disease

444. All following are the most frequent causes of AV dissociation except

(a) Digitalis toxicity
(b) Inferior myocardial infarction
(c) Anterior myocardial infarction
(d) Acute rheumatic fiver

445. Prior temporary pacing required in which type of A–V block prior to elective surgery

(a) 1 Degree AVB (b) Mobitz type I
(c) Mobitz type II (d) RBBB with LAHB

446. Drug induced sycope occurs by all except

(a) β-blockers (b) Gangtion blockers
(c) Bromocriptine (d) Ca-blocker

447. Which antiarrhythmic agent has maximum negative inotropic effect?

(a) Mexiletin (b) Amiodarone
(c) Disopyramide (d) Quinidine

448. Which cause of atrial fibrillation can cause sudden cardiac death?

(a) Valvular heart disease
(b) Cardiomyopathy
(c) IHD
(d) WPW

449. Crochetage patten in ECG is found in

(a) OS ASD (b) TAPVD
(c) PAPVD (d) PDA

450. Most common cause of paraxymal supraventricular tachycardia

(a) Atrial fibrillation
(b) AVRT
(c) AVNRT
(d) Atrial tachycardia

451. Commonest tachyarrhythmia in WPW syndrome

(a) AVRT (b) Atrial fibrillation
(c) Atrial flutter (d) Ventricular flutter

452. LBBB occurs more commonly in

(a) LVH (b) MI
(c) DCMP (d) Pericardial disease

453. Most cases of intermittent LBBB are due to

(a) Aortic stenosis (b) LVH
(c) Ischaemic (d) Dilated CMP

454. Drug of choice for ventricular arrhythmia due to digitalis

(a) Phenytion (b) Lidocaine
(c) KClIV (d) Quinidine

455. Which arrhythmia is related to degree of LV dysfunction?

(a) AV block (b) Atrial tachycardia
(c) Ventricular arrhythmias
(d) Atrial fibrillation

456. Which arrhythmia may cause polyurea?

(a) SVT
(b) Atrial fibrillation
(c) Ventricular tachycardia
(d) CHB

457. Typical ischaemic chest pain occurs with which arrhythmia?

(a) Sinus bradycardia
(b) Atrial fibrillation
(c) VES
(d) Ventricular tachycardia

458. Which arrhythmia likily causes syncope?

(a) Ventriclur extrasystole
(b) Ventricular tachycardia
(c) 1 Degree AV block
(d) AVNRT

459. Which is least common arrhythmia in athletes?

(a) Mobitz Type I block
(b) Mobitz Type II block
(c) Sinus arrhythmia
(d) Sinus bradycardia

460. Most common congenital heart disease associated with WPW

(a) HCM
(b) ASD
(c) Ebstein's anomaly
(d) None of these

461. Which atrial tachyarrhythmia is not caused digitalis toxicity?

(a) AVNRT
(b) Atrial flutter
(c) Atrial fibrillation
(d) Atrial tachycardia with block

462. Post tachycardia syndrome has all features except

(a) Wide spread T inversion
(b) Last for 2 – 7 days
(c) Mechanism not known
(d) Indicates underlying heart disease

463. All are indication of cardioversion in atrial fibrillation except

(a) Haemodynamic collapse
(b) VR controlled by drugs
(c) Systemic embolization
(d) VR uncontrolled by drugs

464. Which AV ratio is most common in multifocal atrial tachycardia?

(a) 1 : 1 (b) 2 : 1
(c) 3 : 1 (d) 4 : 1

465. Most common manifestation of SSS is

(a) SM
(b) Pauses
(c) Atrial fibrillation slow VR with out drug
(d) Brady – Tachy < Syndrome

466. How frequent is AV nodal disease with SSS?

(a) 20 % (b) 30 %
(c) 40 % (d) 50 %

467. Most common mechanism of stokes – adam attacks in CHB is

(a) Asystole (b) VT
(c) VF (d) EMD

468. All following ECG patterns are strongly suggestive of acute corpulmonale except

(a) S1, Q3, T3 pattern with T inversion right precordial leads
(b) S1, T3 pattern
(c) S1, Q3, T3 pattern with RBBB
(d) Normal QRS axis

469. All following may happen to Q wave in L1, L2 avL in uncomplicated LBBB except

(a) Absent in L1 and avL
(b) If present in L-1 physiological
(c) If present in avL – pathological
(d) In L2 present

470. LVH in presence LBBB ECG reveals all the following except

(a) V2S + V5R = 45 mm or more
(b) LAE
(c) QRS duration 0.14 in sec or more
(d) QRS duration ≥ 0.12

471. Which is the least common cause of syncope

(a) Metabolic (b) CNS
(c) Cardiac (d) Vasovagal

472. Drug of choice for ventricular arrhythmia in heart failure

(a) Quinidine (b) Disopyramide
(c) Procainamide (d) Amiodarone

473. Drug of choice for PSVT in haemodynamically unstable patient is

(a) Diltiazem (b) Adenosine
(c) β–blockers (d) Digoxin

474. Most SVTS are caused by

(a) Re-entry
(b) Enhanced automaticity
(c) Triggered activity
(d) None of these

475. Fine atrial fibrillation often occurs in all the following except

(a) Coronary heart disease
(b) Thyrotoxicosis
(c) Hypertensive heart disease
(d) None of these

476. Most common cause of atrial standstill

(a) Digoxin toxicity (b) Quinidine toxicity
(c) Hyperkalemia (d) O_2 toxicity

477. Which arrhythmia causes long QT interval?

(a) Sinus bradycardia (b) Sinus tachycardia
(c) Ventricular tachycardia
(d) AVNR

478. Which VT with LBBB pattern has good prognosis without treatment?

(a) Post MI VT
(b) Cardiomyopathic VT
(c) Sarcoidosis
(d) RVOT VT with normal heart

479. Which antilipidemic agent causes long QT interval?

(a) Statins (b) Fibrates
(c) Probucal (d) Resins

480. All are class III antiarrhythmic agents except

(a) Amiodarone (b) Sotalol
(c) Esmolol (d) Bretylium

481. Extremly high risk of complication with which mode pacing?

(a) Transvenous (b) Trancutancous
(c) Transthoracic (d) Transesophageal

482. Long PR interval is found in all following tachycardia except

(a) Atrial tachycardia
(b) Sinus node re-entry
(c) Inappropriate tachycardia
(d) Typical AVNRT

483. Most common cardiac cause of sudden cardiac death is

(a) IHD (b) CMP
(c) WPW (d) RV dysplasia

484. All following are causes of SCD except in patients of non structural heart disease

(a) Long QT syndrome
(b) WPW syndrome
(c) Brugada syndrome
(d) Idiopathic

485. Typical atrial flutter has all following features except

(a) Conduction occurring reentry in RA
(b) Conduction occurring in conilar clock wise dilation
(c) F waves sawtooth appearance
(d) Response to antiarrhythmics is good

486. Which is the fastest pacing mode?

(a) Transcutaneous (b) Transvenous
(c) Transtharacis (d) Transthoracic

487. Most reliable pacing mode is?

(a) Trans venous (b) Transesophageac
(c) Transvenous (d) Transthoracic

488. Which is the commonest arrhythmia in hyperthyroidism?

(a) Sinus tachycardia (b) Atrial fibrillation
(c) Atrial ectopics
(d) Ventricular ectopices

489. Which pacing system defect causes high lead impedance?

(a) Wire fracture (b) Insulation block
(c) Lead displacement (d) Exit block

490. Which pacing system causes normal electrocardiogram?

(a) Exit block (b) Lead dislodgement
(c) Insulation break (d) Wire fractures

491. VA conduction most frequently occurs in

(a) Fascicular block (b) 2 degree AV block
(c) 3 degree AV block
(d) Sinus node dysfunction

492. All are causes of acute complete AV block except

(a) Myocardial infarction
(b) Hyperkalemia
(c) Hypercalcemia (d) Corrected TGA

493. All following drugs may causes sinus node dysfunction except

(a) Methyldopa (b) Clonidine
(c) Lithium (d) ACE inhibitors

494. Which of the pacing system defect cause low voltage threshold?

(a) Wire fracture (b) Insulation break
(c) Lead dislodgement (d) Exit block

495. Which of the following pacing system defect causes low lead impedance?

(a) Insulation break (b) Wire fracture
(c) Exit block (d) Lead dislodgement

496. All following are the properties of fast current in cardiac muscle except

(a) Na dependent
(b) Threshold for activation –60 to –70 mv
(c) Action potential magnitude 100 – 130 mv
(d) Safety factor for conduction low

497. All are properties of slow current in cardiac muscle except

(a) Mainly Ca^{++} dependent
(b) Threshold for activation 30 to –40 mv
(c) Conduction velocity 0.01 to 0.1 m/sec
(d) Response to stimulus all or none

498. Short PR interval is found in all the following except

(a) WPW syndrome
(b) Ganong levine syndrome
(c) Low atrial rhythm
(d) Left atrial rhythm

499. In ischemic arrhythmia all fallowing mechanism play part except

(a) Enhanced automaticity
(b) Triggered activity
(c) Re-entery
(d) Enhanced conduction

500. Which is commonest arrhythmia?

(a) PVC (b) Atrial fibrillation
(c) APC (d) VT

501. Which is the commonest arrhythmia?

(a) Atrial fibrillation
(b) I degree AV block
(c) II degree AV block
(d) III degree AV block

502. All of the following are associated arrhythmia with atrial fibrillation except

(a) Partial AV block (b) CHB
(c) VES (d) VT

503. All are physical signs of atrial fibrillation except

(a) Changing HS
(b) Pulse deficit
(c) Irregularly irregular pulse
(d) Neck venues loaves farms are normal

504. In atrial fibrillation beat PR interval is

(a) Normal (b) Short
(c) Long (d) Any of the above

505. Which is most common type of electrical alternans?

(a) P wave (b) PR internal
(c) QRS (d) T

506. All following are causes of atrial stand still

(a) Hypothermia (b) Copoisoning

(c) Hypoxia (d) Beta-blockers

507. All are risk factors for atrial fibrillation except

(a) DM (b) HT
(c) HF (d) Pericardial disease

508. Congenital complete heart nlock in new born occurs with

(a) Maternal rubella
(b) Maternal thalidomide use
(c) Maternal lithium toxicity
(d) Maternal lupus

509. Serious ventricular arrhythmia commonly occurs is

(a) Congenital aortic stenosis
(b) VSD
(c) Pulmonary stenosis
(d) Fallot's tetralogy

510. Most common fetal tachyarrhythmia is

(a) AV NRT (b) Atrial fibrillation
(c) AVRT (d) VT

511. Most common fetal bradyarrhythmia is

(a) CHB
(b) Non conducted atrial ectopic
(c) Sinus bradycardia
(d) 1st degree AV block

512. Most syncopes are

(a) Neurocardiogenic
(b) Metabolic
(c) Orthostatic
(d) Carotid sinus hypersenstivity

513. Potentially reversible causes of cardiac arrest due to VF

(a) Primzmetal's angina
(b) Proarrhythmia
(c) Electrolyte abnomalitus
(d) Dilated cardiomyopathy

514. Rapid recovery occurs with which type of syncope?

(a) Cardiac (b) Vasovagal
(c) Neurogenic (d) Independences

515. Most extensively sustained arrhythmia is

(a) Atrial fibrillation (b) AVNRT
(c) VT (d) CHB

516. All following are cause of EMD except

(a) Hypovolemia
(b) Tension pheumothorax
(c) Cardiac rupture (d) Cardiomyopathy

517. Most common cause of sudden arrhythmia cardiac death

(a) Myocardial infarction
(b) HOCM
(c) Aortic stenosis
(d) Brugada syndrome

518. Idiopathic LV tachycardia has all following features except

(a) Relative narrow QRS
(b) High incidence of false tendons
(c) Sensitive to verapamil
(d) Increased incidence of sudden cardiac death

519. Accelerated idioventricular rhythm has all the features except

(a) Usually rate ranges from 40–120/m
(b) May cause isorrhythmic AV dissociation
(c) Marker for successful reperfusion after thrombolysis
(d) May be termination by β-blocker

520. Repetitive monomorphic VT has all following features except

(a) Associated with no heart disease
(b) Provoked by exercise or emotion
(c) Mostly occurs in young men
(d) Has RBBB morphology

521. Repetitive monomorphic VT has all the features except

(a) Excellent prognosis
(b) Best drug for treatment is β-blocker
(c) Multiple VT morphology
(d) Catheter ablation is most effective stralegy to treat

522. Ventricular tachycardia in arrhythmogenic right ventricular dysplasia has all following feature

(a) LBBB pattern (b) SCD occurs
(c) First line treatment is amiodarone
(d) Multiple morphologies of VT are absent

523. How frequent is atrial fibrillation in mitral regurgitation?

(a) 10% (b) 20%
(c) 30% (d) 50%

524. ST segment changes during supraventricular tachycardia has all the features except

(a) Probably due to rapid heart rate
(b) Incomplete filing related
(c) Due to action potential duration differences between subendo-cardium and epicardium
(d) Related to myocardial Ischemia

525. Ectopic atrial tachycardia is caused by all except

(a) Acute myocardial infarction
(b) COPD
(c) Quinidine toxicity
(d) CHF

526. All are causes of asystole except

(a) During induction of anesthesia
(b) Heart block
(c) VT (d) SSS

527. IV calcium chloride is used in all the following except

(a) For treatment of hypotension following over dose of Ca-blocker
(b) Treatment of hypotension following hyperkalemia
(c) For treatment of asystole
(d) None of these

528. Prevalance of atrial fibrillation maximum in which age group

(a) 20 – 40 years (b) 40 – 50 years
(c) 50 – 60 years (d) > 60 years

529. In indian setting most common cause of atrial fibrillation is

(a) Chronic rheumatic heart disease
(b) Coronary artery disease
(c) Hypertension
(d) Dilated CMP

530. Commonest risk factor for stroke in atrial fibrillation

(a) Previous stroke / TSA
(b) Hypertension
(c) Heart failure
(d) DM

531. Highest risk for embolization in atrial fibrillation is in which combination

(a) CHF + HT + Advanced age + DM
(b) CHF + HT + Advanced age + DM + Previous stroke /TIA
(c) CHF + HT + DM + Advanced age + Previous stroke /TIA
(d) CHF + HT + DM + Prior stroke / TIA

532. Which drug is known to prevent substantial chance of atrial fibrillation in hypertension?

(a) β-blocker (b) ACE inhibitor
(c) ARBS (d) Diuretics

533. First line drug for paroxysmal atrial fibrillation in HT without LVH

(a) Flecanide (b) Amiodarone
(c) Procainamide (d) Disopyramide

534. First line drug for paroxysmal atrial fibrillation with heart failure

(a) Amiodarone (b) Procainamide
(c) Quinidine (d) Dofetilide

535. First line drug for paroxysmal atrial fibrillation with LVH

(a) Quinidine (b) Procainamide
(c) Amiodarone (d) Flecanamide

536. Drug of choice for vagally mediated paroxysmal atrial fibrillation

(a) Disopyramide (b) Amiodarone
(c) Procainamide (d) Dofetilide

537. First line drug for lone paroxysmal atrial fibrillation

(a) Flecainide (b) Amiodarone
(c) Procainamide (d) Quinidine

538. First line drug of paroxysmal atrial fibrillation with coronary artery disease is

(a) Dofetilide (b) Quinidine
(c) Procainamide (d) Disopyramide

539. Chemical cardioversion of atrial fibrillation may be achieved by all except

(a) Class IA (b) Class Ic
(c) Class III (d) Class IV

540. Drug of choice for paroxysmal atrial fibrillation with renal failure

(a) Quinidine (b) Procainamide
(c) Dofetilide (d) Amiodarone

541. Drug of choice for paroxysmal atrial fibrillation with liver disease is

(a) Procainamide (b) Quinidine
(c) Sotalol (d) Dofetilide

542. Drug of choice for paroxysmal atrial fibrillation with lung disease

(a) Sotalol (b) Amiodarone
(c) Quinidine (d) Fluvastatin

543. In all following situation DC cardioversion is contraindicated except

(a) Digitalis toxicity
(b) Multifocal atrial tachycardia
(c) Automatic atrial tachycardia
(d) SVT of WPW syndrome

544 Which antiarrhythmic agent can produce macrocytic annemia?

(a) Quinidine (b) Phenyloin
(c) Lidocaine (d) Bretyllium

545. Which antiarrhythmic is maximally dominated from the body?

(a) Lidocaine (b) Procoinamide
(c) Disopyramide (d) Phemytom

546. Which of the antiarrhythmic drug has active metabolite?

(a) Quinidine (b) Disopyramide
(c) Phenytoin (d) Lidocaine

547. Which antiarrhytmic drug causes thrombocytopenia?

(a) Procainamide (b) Disopyramide
(c) Xylocaine (d) Quinidine

548. β-blocker has all the following electrophysiological effects except

(a) Increase AVN conduction time
(b) Increase effective refractory period of AVN
(c) Decrease automaticity in HP system
(d) Decrease HP system conduction time

549. Which of the following is correct regarding lidocaine?

(a) Decrease automaticity of HP system
(b) No effect on atrial conduction time
(c) No effect AVN conduction time
(d) No effect on effective refractory period

550. Digoxin has all following electrophysiology effects except

(a) Atrial contraction time decrease
(b) Atrial effective refractory period decrease
(c) AV-Nodal conduction is increased
(d) His purkinje ventricular conduction time decrease

551. Ca-antagonisis has all following electrophysiologic effects except

(a) His purkinje automaticity increase
(b) AVN aonduction time increase
(c) AVN effective refractory period increase
(d) No change in atrial conduction time

552. All following arrhythmias may occur when clacification involves the conduction tissue in aortic stenosis except

(a) 1 degree AV block (b) Sinus bradycardia
(c) LBBB (d) CHB

553. When cardioversion / defibrillation is not indicated

(a) VT
(b) VF
(c) Torsade De pointes
(d) AF with rapid VR

554. In all following arrhythmias cardioversion / defibrillation is not indicated except

(a) Torsade De pointes
(b) Automatic rhythms
(c) Toxic arrhythmia
(d) None of these

555. Organic heart disease is rare in which SVT?

(a) AVNR
(b) Concealed accessory by pass tract
(c) Sinus node re-entry
(d) Automatic atrial tachycardia

556. P-wave affects QRS in which SVT?

(a) Sinus node re-entry
(b) Atrial re-entry
(c) Automatic atrial tachycardia
(d) Concealed accessory by pass tract

557. Functional bundle branch block is common in which SVT?

(a) Concealed accessory by pass tract
(b) Sinus node re-entry
(c) Automatic atrial tachycardia
(d) AVNRT

558. AV-block never occurs in which SVT?

(a) SN re-entry
(b) Atrial re-entry
(c) Automatic atrial tachycardia
(d) AVNRT

559. Cessation of which SVT is unpredictable

(a) SN Re-entry
(b) AVNRT
(c) Concealed accessory by pass tract
(d) Automatic atrial tachycardia

560. Critical AV conduction time is needed for which SVT?

(a) AVNRT
(b) Automatic atrial tachycardia
(c) SN re-entry
(d) Atrial re-entry

561. Carotid sinus massage duration should be which one of following?

(a) 2 sec (b) 4 sec
(c) 6 – 8 sec (d) > 8 < 15 sec

562. AV nodal or intraventricular conduction coexist in how may patients of SSS

(a) 10 % (b) 25 %
(c) 30 % (d) 50 %

563. Which arrhythmia is not found in athlete heart syndrome?

(a) Sinus bradycardia (b) 1 Degree AV block
(c) Mobitz III degree (d) Mobitz IIII degree

564. Most common mechanism in of SVTS is

(a) Re-entry
(b) Enhanced automaticity
(c) Triggered activity
(d) None of these

565. Which arrhythmia is most successfully ablated?

(a) AVNRT (b) AVRT
(c) AAT (d) Idiopathic VT

566. Which arrhythmia frequently recurrs after ablation?

(a) AVNRT (b) AVRT
(c) AAT (d) Idiopathic VT

567. All are cardiac causes pacemaker mediated tachycardia except

(a) Atrial fibrillation
(b) PSVT
(c) Atrial flutter
(d) Ventricular conduction time is < the post ventricular atrial refractory period

568. All are risk factors for development of digitalis toxicity except

(a) Hypokalemia
(b) Hypercalcemia
(c) Acute pulmonary disease
(d) Addisons disease

569. All following are the high risk factors for sudden cardiac death except

(a) Sudden cardiac death survivors
(b) VT with syncope
(c) VT with EF < 40%
(d) EF < 40%

570. In which disease atrial fibrillation is associated with slow VR (not drug induced)?

(a) Red
(b) Thyrotoxicosis
(c) SSS
(d) Cardiomyopathy

571. Which anti arrhythmic causes Gynecomastia?

(a) Verapamil
(b) Digoxin
(c) Disopyramide
(d) Mexiletine

572. Which of the block frequently progress to CHB?

(a) 1 degree AV block
(b) LBBB
(c) RBBB
(d) RBBB < LPH

573. Which block prognosis least to CHB?

(a) LAH
(b) LPH
(c) 1 Degree AV block
(d) LBBB

574. Which antiarrhythmic may cause syncope?

(a) Procainamide
(b) Quinidine
(c) Digoxin
(d) Mexiletine

575. Which antiarrhythmia causes corneal deposits?

(a) Digoxin
(b) Verapamil
(c) Amiodarone
(d) Quinidine

576. All following arrhythmias may lead to atrial fibrillation except

(a) AES
(b) Atrial flutter
(c) SSS
(d) AVNRT

577. Treatment of choice for symptomatic complete heart block is

(a) Thiazide symptomatic
(b) Isoprenaline
(c) Theophylline
(d) Pacemaker

578. Systemic embolism is most common in

(a) Mitral stenosis with atrial fibrillation
(b) Mitral regurgitation with atrial fibrillation
(c) Atrial fibrillation alone
(d) Aortic stenosis with atrial fibrillation

579. Which antiarrhythmic agent can cause pulmonary hypertension?

(a) Quinidine (b) Procainamide
(c) β-blocker (d) Amiodarone

580. Which antiarrhythmic agent can produce SLE?

(a) Quinidine (b) Procanamide
(c) Disopyramide (d) Amiodarone

581. rS complex in avR with r ≥ 1 mm is found in

(a) Inferior myocardial infarction
(b) RVH
(c) Posterior myocardial infarction
(d) None of the above

582. Most frequent type of paraystole is

(a) Ventricular
(b) Junctional
(c) Atrial
(d) Atrial + Ventricular

583. All following statement regarding parasytole are correct except

(a) More common is females
(b) Peak incidence over age 60 years
(c) Majority of cases have organic heart disease
(d) Quinidine was arbalest this arrhythmia

584. Verapamil is indicated in all following arrhythmia except

(a) For termination of AVNRT
(b) For control of VR in atrial fibrillation

(c) For termination idiopathic RV out flow tract ventricular tachycardia

(d) Atrial fibrillation of WPW syndrome

585. Large biphasic spike are seen in

(a) Unipolar pacing (b) Bipolar pacing

(c) Both (a) and (b) (d) None of the above

586. Most common mechanism of stokesadams affects in CHB is

(a) Ventricular asystole

(b) VT

(c) VF

(d) Combination

587. Majority of mobitz 1 degree AV block are Located in

(a) AVN

(b) Bundle branch

(c) Purkinge system

(d) All the above equally

588. Mobitz type II 2 degree AV block is located in

(a) AVN

(b) His purkinje system

(c) Intra atrial tracks

(d) None of these

589. Captured beat usually has all following features except

(a) Premature

(b) Idential to normal

(c) Indicates ventricular origin of tachycardia

(d) Indicates supra ventricular tachycardia

590. Bradycardia after paroxysmal tachycardia usually does not indicate

(a) AAT (b) AVNRT

(c) AVRT (d) VT

591. Irregularity of VR in CHB is usually due to

(a) Ventricular persistence beat

(b) Parasystolic

(c) Two foci for ventricular activation

(d) Sinus arrhythmia

592. Antiarrhythmic of choice in post infarct patients is

(a) IV Esmolol (b) IV Digoxin
(c) IV Verapamil (d) IV Diltiazem

593. Postural tachycardia syndrome occurs in all the following except

(a) Day (b) Amyloidosis
(c) Alcoholism (d) Ageing

594. Most common cause sudden cardiac death in young athlete is

(a) HCM
(b) AS
(c) Congenital coronary anomaly
(d) Arrhythmogenic RV

595. Which sinus bradycardia carries a poor prognosis?

(a) Drug induced
(b) Post resuscitation
(c) SSS
(d) Inferior myocardial infarction

596. Which tachyarrhythmia is not responsive to cardiovascular?

(a) Atrial flutter
(b) Atrial fibrillation
(c) VT
(d) Ventricular fibrillation

597. Most common complication of radio frequency ablation of accessory pathway

(a) Cardiac tamponade
(b) Coronary artery thrombosis
(c) Pericarditis
(d) Mild aortic regurgitation

598. In which type of VT sudden cardiac death is rare?

(a) Idiopathic
(b) Polymorphic
(c) Sustained monomorphic VT
(d) None of the above

599. Wandering atrial pacemaker has all the following features except

(a) Benign
(b) Usually with underlying lung disease
(c) Variable S1
(d) Thealed by Ca-blocker

600. Ventricular tachycardia has all following features except

(a) Myocardial ischemia with compromised EV function
(b) Stable haemodynamics does not excludect
(c) Common 'a' waves in neck vein
(d) Irregular tachycardia

601. Which is the treatment of choice for guration receprocatary tachycardia (permant)?

(a) β-blocker
(b) Digoxin
(c) Verapamice
(d) Radiofrequancy ablation

ANSWERS

1. (*a*)	2. (*e*)	3. (*a*)	4. (*c*)	5. (*d*)
6. (*b*)	7. (*a*)	8. (*d*)	9. (*d*)	10. (*c*)
11. (*a*)	12. (*d*)	13. (*d*)	14. (*a*)	15. (*d*)
16. (*d*)	17. (*d*)	18. (*a*)	19. (*b*)	20. (*c*)
21. (*c*)	22. (*a*)	23. (*a*)	24. (*c*)	25. (*d*)
26. (*d*)	27. (*d*)	28. (*d*)	29. (*a*)	30. (*d*)
31. (*c*)	32. (*a*)	33. (*b*)	34. (*c*)	35. (*d*)
36. (*c*)	37. (*d*)	38. (*d*)	39. (*a*)	40. (*b*)
41. (*d*)	42. (*d*)	43. (*c*)	44. (*a*)	45. (*a*)
46. (*c*)	47. (*a*)	48. (*a*)	49. (*c*)	50. (*c*)
51. (*a*)	52. (*d*)	53. (*c*)	54. (*b*)	55. (*d*)
56. (*d*)	57. (*b*)	58. (*d*)	59. (*d*)	60. (*d*)
61. (*d*)	62. (*d*)	63. (*d*)	64. (*d*)	65. (*a*)
66. (*d*)	67. (*c*)	68. (*d*)	69. (*d*)	70. (*a*)
71. (*a*)	72. (*d*)	73. (*b*)	74. (*a*)	75. (*a*)
76. (*d*)	77. (*c*)	78. (*a*)	79. (*d*)	80. (*a*)
81. (*b*)	82. (*a*)	83. (*a*)	84. (*a*)	85. (*a*)
86. (*a*)	87. (*a*)	88. (*a*)	89. (*d*)	90. (*d*)
91. (*d*)	92. (*d*)	93. (*d*)	94. (*d*)	95. (*d*)
96. (*d*)	97. (*d*)	98. (*a*)	99. (*c*)	100. (*b*)
101. (*a*)	102. (*a*)	103. (*d*)	104. (*d*)	105. (*d*)
106. (*c*)	107. (*d*)	108. (*d*)	109. (*d*)	110. (*d*)
111. (*a*)	112. (*a*)	113. (*a*)	114. (*a*)	115. (*a*)
116. (*d*)	117. (*c*)	118. (*d*)	119. (*d*)	120. (*d*)
121. (*a*)	122. (*a*)	123. (*d*)	124. (*a*)	125. (*a*)
126. (*a*)	127. (*c*)	128. (*c*)	129. (*c*)	130. (*d*)
131. (*b*)	132. (*d*)	133. (*d*)	134. (*b*)	135. (*a*)
136. (*d*)	137. (*d*)	138. (*b*)	139. (*d*)	140. (*b*)
141. (*a*)	142. (*b*)	143. (*d*)	144. (*c*)	145. (*a*)
146. (*c*)	147. (*d*)	148. (*a*)	149. (*d*)	150. (*d*)
151. (*d*)	152. (*d*)	153. (*b*)	154. (*a*)	155. (*d*)
156. (*a*)	157. (*a*)	158. (*d*)	159. (*c*)	160. (*d*)

161. (*a*)	162. (*d*)	163. (*c*)	164. (*d*)	165. (*a*)
166. (*c*)	167. (*d*)	168. (*d*)	169. (*d*)	170. (*b*)
171. (*b*)	172. (*a*)	173. (*b*)	174. (*c*)	175. (*d*)
176. (*d*)	177. (*d*)	178. (*d*)	179. (*b*)	180. (*d*)
181. (*a*)	182. (*c*)	183. (*b*)	184. (*a*)	185. (*c*)
186. (*a*)	187. (*d*)	188. (*c*)	189. (*d*)	190. (*d*)
191. (*b*)	192. (*b*)	193. (*a*)	194. (*a*)	195. (*d*)
196. (*c*)	197. (*c*)	198. (*d*)	199. (*c*)	200. (*c*)
201. (*a*)	202. (*d*)	203. (*b*)	204. (*d*)	205. (*a*)
206. (*d*)	207. (*a*)	208. (*d*)	209. (*d*)	210. (*d*)
211. (*b*)	212. (*b*)	213. (*d*)	214. (*d*)	215. (*b*)
216. (*a*)	217. (*c*)	218. (*d*)	219. (*d*)	220. (*b*)
221. (*a*)	222. (*d*)	223. (*c*)	224. (*c*)	225. (*d*)
226. (*c*)	227. (*d*)	228. (*c*)	229. (*c*)	230. (*d*)
231. (*d*)	232. (*a*)	233. (*d*)	234. (*c*)	235. (*b*)
236. (*b*)	237. (*c*)	238. (*c*)	239. (*d*)	240. (*a*)
241. (*d*)	242. (*a*)	243. (*b*)	244. (*d*)	245. (*b*)
246. (*b*)	247. (*c*)	248. (*b*)	249. (*b*)	250. (*d*)
251. (*d*)	252. (*d*)	253. (*c*)	254. (*d*)	255. (*a*)
256. (*d*)	257. (*d*)	258. (*c*)	259. (*d*)	260. (*d*)
261. (*d*)	262. (*d*)	263. (*b*)	264. (*a*)	265. (*d*)
266. (*d*)	267. (*d*)	268. (*d*)	269. (*b*)	270. (*d*)
271. (*c*)	272. (*d*)	273. (*a*)	274. (*c*)	275. (*b*)
276. (*d*)	277. (*d*)	278. (*b*)	279. (*d*)	280. (*a*)
281. (*b*)	282. (*b*)	283. (*d*)	284. (*c*)	285. (*c*)
286. (*c*)	287. (*c*)	288. (*b*)	289. (*d*)	290. (*a*)
291. (*a*)	292. (*c*)	293. (*d*)	294. (*a*)	295. (*d*)
296. (*a*)	297. (*a*)	298. (*a*)	299. (*a*)	300. (*b*)
301. (*a*)	302. (*a*)	303. (*b*)	304. (*d*)	305. (*b*)
306. (*d*)	307. (*d*)	308. (*c*)	309. (*b*)	310. (*a*)
311. (*a*)	312. (*c*)	313. (*a*)	314. (*a*)	315. (*a*)
316. (*b*)	317. (*d*)	318. (*d*)	319. (*c*)	320. (*a*)
321. (*a*)	322. (*c*)	323. (*d*)	324. (*b*)	325. (*a*)
326. (*d*)	327. (*a*)	328. (*b*)	329. (*c*)	330. (*d*)
331. (*c*)	332. (*b*)	333. (*d*)	334. (*d*)	335. (*b*)

336. (*c*)	337. (*d*)	338. (*b*)	339. (*c*)	340. (*d*)
341. (*d*)	342. (*b*)	343. (*d*)	344. (*d*)	345. (*a*)
346. (*d*)	347. (*d*)	348. (*c*)	349. (*b*)	350. (*d*)
351. (*d*)	352. (*d*)	353. (*d*)	354. (*d*)	355. (*a*)
356. (*b*)	357. (*a*)	358. (*c*)	359. (*d*)	360. (*a*)
361. (*c*)	362. (*d*)	363. (*c*)	364. (*d*)	365. (*d*)
366. (*c*)	367. (*d*)	368. (*c*)	369. (*c*)	370. (*a*)
371. (*d*)	372. (*d*)	373. (*d*)	374. (*d*)	375. (*c*)
376. (*c*)	377. (*a*)	378. (*a*)	379. (*a*)	380. (*d*)
381. (*a*)	382. (*c*)	383. (*a*)	384. (*d*)	385. (*d*)
386. (*d*)	387. (*a*)	388. (*d*)	389. (*a*)	390. (*d*)
391. (*d*)	392. (*b*)	393. (*d*)	394. (*d*)	395. (*a*)
396. (*a*)	397. (*b*)	398. (*d*)	399. (*d*)	400. (*d*)
401. (*c*)	402. (*b*)	403. (*a*)	404. (*a*)	405. (*a*)
406. (*d*)	407. (*d*)	408. (*c*)	409. (*a*)	410. (*d*)
411. (*a*)	412. (*c*)	413. (*d*)	414. (*b*)	415. (*b*)
416. (*b*)	417. (*c*)	418. (*b*)	419. (*d*)	420. (*d*)
421. (*d*)	422. (*a*)	423. (*a*)	424. (*b*)	425. (*d*)
426. (*b*)	427. (*a*)	428. (*a*)	429. (*c*)	330. (*b*)
431. (*d*)	432. (*a*)	433. (*d*)	434. (*d*)	435. (*c*)
436. (*d*)	437. (*d*)	438. (*d*)	439. (*a*)	440. (*b*)
441. (*a*)	442. (*d*)	443. (*a*)	444. (*c*)	445. (*c*)
446. (*d*)	447. (*c*)	448. (*d*)	449. (*a*)	450. (*c*)
451. (*a*)	452. (*a*)	453. (*c*)	454. (*b*)	455. (*c*)
456. (*a*)	457. (*d*)	458. (*b*)	459. (*b*)	460. (*c*)
461. (*a*)	462. (*d*)	463. (*d*)	464. (*a*)	465. (*d*)
466. (*d*)	467. (*a*)	468. (*d*)	469. (*d*)	470. (*d*)
471. (*a*)	472. (*d*)	473. (*c*)	474. (*a*)	475. (*b*)
476. (*a*)	477. (*a*)	478. (*d*)	479. (*c*)	480. (*c*)
481. (*c*)	482. (*d*)	483. (*a*)	484. (*d*)	485. (*d*)
486. (*a*)	487. (*a*)	488. (*a*)	489. (*a*)	490. (*a*)
491. (*d*)	492. (*d*)	493. (*d*)	494. (*a*)	495. (*b*)
496. (*d*)	497. (*d*)	498. (*d*)	499. (*d*)	500. (*a*)
501. (*a*)	502. (*a*)	503. (*d*)	504. (*b*)	505. (*d*)
506. (*d*)	507. (*d*)	508. (*d*)	509. (*a*)	510. (*a*)

511. (*a*)	512. (*d*)	513. (*d*)	514. (*a*)	515. (*a*)
516. (*d*)	517. (*a*)	518. (*d*)	519. (*d*)	520. (*d*)
521. (*c*)	522. (*c*)	523. (*d*)	524. (*d*)	525. (*c*)
526. (*c*)	527. (*c*)	528. (*d*)	529. (*a*)	530. (*a*)
531. (*b*)	532. (*a*)	533. (*a*)	534. (*a*)	535. (*c*)
536. (*a*)	537. (*a*)	538. (*a*)	539. (*d*)	540. (*d*)
541. (*c*)	542. (*b*)	543. (*d*)	544. (*b*)	545. (*a*)
546. (*d*)	547. (*d*)	548. (*d*)	549. (*a*)	550. (*d*)
551. (*a*)	552. (*d*)	553. (*c*)	554. (*a*)	555. (*b*)
556. (*d*)	557. (*a*)	558. (*d*)	559. (*d*)	560. (*a*)
561. (*c*)	562. (*d*)	563. (*d*)	564. (*a*)	565. (*a*)
566. (*b*)	567. (*d*)	568. (*d*)	569. (*d*)	570. (*c*)
571. (*b*)	572. (*a*)	573. (*a*)	574. (*b*)	575. (*c*)
576. (*d*)	577. (*d*)	578. (*b*)	579. (*d*)	580. (*b*)
581. (*a*)	582. (*a*)	583. (*a*)	584. (*d*)	585. (*a*)
586. (*a*)	587. (*a*)	588. (*b*)	589. (*d*)	590. (*d*)
591. (*a*)	592. (*a*)	593. (*d*)	594. (*a*)	595. (*b*)
596. (*a*)	597. (*a*)	598. (*a*)	599. (*d*)	600. (*d*)
601. (*d*)				

SECTION–4

ATHEROSCLEROTIC HEART DISEASE, DISEASE OF AORTA AND HYPERTENSION

1. The complications of myocardial infarction are all except

(a) Pulmonary embolism
(b) Systemic embolism
(c) Dissection of aorta
(d) Ventricular fibrillation

2. Drug useful in acute myocardial infarction are all except

(a) Nifedepine (b) Aspirin
(c) ACE inhibitors (d) Metoprolol

3. Linked angina in patients of coronary artery disease is used for

(a) Emotion induced angina
(b) Gastrointestinal factors induced angina
(c) Stress induced angina
(d) None of the above

4. Nocturnal angina may be produced by all except

(a) Redistribution of intravascular blood volume
(b) Hypercapnia
(c) Augmented sympathetic discharge
(d) None of the above

5. The term angina means

(a) Chest pain (b) Burning in chest
(c) Strangling (d) None of the above

6. First treatment for angina was

(a) Amyl nitrite
(b) NTG (Nitroglycerine)
(c) β-blockers (d) Alcohol

7. **In stable angina electrocardiogram is abnormal during anginal pain in**
   (a) 20% (b) 40%
   (c) 50% (d) 100%

8. **Progeria is associated with**
   (a) Coronary atherosclerosis
   (b) Congenital heart disease
   (c) Valvular heart disease
   (d) Pericardial disease

9. **Risk of coronary artery disease is maximum with**
   (a) Cigarette smoking
   (b) Cigar smoking smoke not inhaled
   (c) Pipe smoking smoke not inhaled
   (d) Tobacco chewing

10. **Coronary artery plaque vulnerability to rupture depends on**
   (a) Plaque composition
   (b) Plaque size
   (c) Severity of stenosis
   (d) All of the above

11. **With which antihypertensive agent the sex life is better?**
   (a) Methyldopa (b) β-blockers
   (c) ACE Inhibitors (d) Diuretics

12. **Nitrates are contraindicated in all the following except**
   (a) Large acute anterior infarct
   (b) Acute myocardial infarction with hypotension
   (c) Right ventricular infarction
   (d) None of the above

13. **Which is the commonest presentation of Ischemic heart disease?**
   (a) Stable angina
   (b) Unstable angina
   (c) Acute myocardial infarction
   (d) Sudden cardiac death

14. **Commonest drug prescribed in stable angina is**

(a) Aspirin (b) β-blockers
(c) Statins (d) ACE inhibitors

15. All following statements regarding atorvastatin are correct except

(a) 4th generation statins
(b) Half-life is 14 hours
(c) Lipophillic
(d) Hydrophillic

16. Which of the following does not precipitates angina?

(a) Walking against cold wind
(b) Walking after major meals
(c) Coitus (d) Hot environment

17. Relief of angina by sublingual nitroglycerine occurs within

(a) 30 sec (b) After 1 min
(c) 1.5 min (d) 10.15 min

18. Anginal pain occurs in all of the following locations except

(a) Lower chest
(b) Between epigastrium and pharynx
(c) Lower cervical spinal
(d) Upper jaw

19. The quality of anginal pain are all except

(a) Gradual increase and gradual fall in intensity
(b) Burning
(c) Stabbing (d) Constricting

20. In variant angina all following statements are correct except

(a) Usually occur at night during rest
(b) Relieved by sublingual nitroglycerine
(c) Associated with severe coronary artery disease
(d) Associated with ST elevation

21. Which of the following cell accumulation determines the extent of ischemial myocardial damage?

(a) Lymphocytes (b) Neutrophils
(c) RBC (d) Monocyctes

22. Myocardial dysfunction is best assessed by

(a) History
(b) Physical examination
(c) Chest X-ray
(d) ECG

23. Myocardial ischemia is best assessed by

(a) Physical examination
(b) Resting ECG
(c) Exercise ECG
(d) Holter monitoring

24. Functional capacity of heart disease is best assessed by

(a) History
(b) Resting ECG
(c) Exercise ECG
(d) Physical examination

25. All are risk factors for abrupt closure following PTCA except

(a) Male gender
(b) Long lesion
(c) Lesion at branch point
(d) Lesion associated with thrombus

26. All are risk factors for restenosis following PTCA

(a) Male gender
(b) Diabetes mellitus
(c) Hypertension
(d) Unstable angina

27. All are mechanical complications of myocardial infarction except

(a) Mitral regurgitation
(b) Ventricular septal defect
(c) Rupture of free wall
(d) Pericarditis

28. All of the following factors occur in phaeochromocytoma except

(a) Severe headache
(b) Postural hypotension
(c) Profuse sweating
(d) None of the above

29. All of the following features regarding phaeochromocytoma are correct except

(a) 10% are unilateral
(b) 10% are malignant
(c) 10% are extra adrenal
(d) 10% familial

30. Which statement regarding statins in aortic stenosis is incorrect?

(a) Decreases progression of aortic stenosis
(b) The effect correlates with cholesterol
(c) Decreases gradient across aortic valve
(d) Decreases mortality

31. Conclusion of CASS trial include all the following except

(a) CABG did not prolong life in unstable angina
(b) CABG did not prevent myocardial infarction in mid angina
(c) Long term survival was improved in patients with baseline EF < 50%
(d) None of the above

32. SHEP trial cocludes except

(a) Stepped care approach in treatment of ISH reduced the incidence of stroke
(b) In older persons the LV mass was reduced with chlorithalidone based regimen
(c) Low dose chlorthalidone therapy had no effect on cardiovascular risk factor
(d) Reduced the major cardiovascular events

33. All are clinical complications of atherosclerosis except

(a) Ischemic heart disease
(b) Ischemic stroke
(c) Aortic abdominal aneurysm
(d) Hemorrhagic stroke

34. All are biomedical risk factors for atherosclerosis except

(a) Dyslipidemia (b) Hypertension
(c) Diabetes (d) Smoking

35. Which antihypertensive drug improves lipid profile?

(a) β-blockers
(b) α-blockers
(c) Calcium channel-blockers
(d) ARBs

36. Diuretics are drug choice in elderly hypertensive because of

(a) Good control of blood pressure
(b) Prevents osteoporosis
(c) Prevents dementia
(d) All of the above

37. Variant angina has all features except

(a) ST elevation during pain
(b) Occur usually at rest
(c) ST elevation persists after pain is over
(d) β-blocker are not given

38. Which drug is avoided in spasmodic angina?

(a) Vesapamil (b) Nitrate
(c) β-blocker (d) Asprin

39. Which β-blocker is not usually recommended in hypertension?

(a) Metoprolol (b) Propranolol
(c) Atenolol (d) Sotalol

40. All drugs are associated with hypersensitive myocarditis except

(a) Methyldopa (b) Streptomycin
(c) Tetracycline (d) Chloromycetin

41. All drugs causes toxic myocarditis except

(a) Emetine (b) Lithium
(c) Theophylline (d) Procanamide

42. All the statements regarding MR in myocardial infarction are correct except

(a) Affects the posteromedial papillary muscle
(b) Affects the anterolateral papillary muscle
(c) Occurs commonly in acute myocardial infarction
(d) Associated with loud systolic murmur

43. Earliest ECG change in mitral stenosis is

(a) Right axis deviation
(b) Left atrial enlargement
(c) R/S > 1 in V1
(d) Right atrial enlargement

44. Constrictive pericarditis has all features except

(a) Pulsus paradoxus (b) Kussmaul's sign
(c) S3 (d) Murmurs

45. Culture negative infective endocarditis occurs in

(a) 20% (b) 25%
(c) < 5% (d) 5.10%

46. Which of the following is a feature of active endocarditis?

(a) Increase ESR
(b) Leukocytosis
(c) Proteinuria
(d) Increased polyclonal immunoglobulin

47. All are major common risk factors for venous thromboembolism (VTE) except

(a) Previous VTE
(b) Lower limb orthopedic surgery
(c) Paralysis
(d) Varicose veins

48. All of the following increases risk of restenosis following angioplasty except

(a) Diabetes (b) Hypertension
(c) Hyperlipidemia (d) Young age

49. ACE inhibitors should not be given for hypertension during pregnancy because of

(a) Renal impairment in mother
(b) Renal failure in fetus
(c) Improper control of blood pressure
(d) All of the above

50. Which of the following condition has highest maternal mortality during pregnancy?

(a) VSD- left to right shunt
(b) Pulmonary stenosis
(c) Pulmonary hypertension
(d) ASD- left to right shunt

51. Aortic stenosis patients are fit for pregnancy with all the following factors except
(a) Moderate aortic stenosis
(b) Negative exercise test
(c) Left ventricle dysfunction
(d) Normal ECG

52. Higher INR (3-5-4) is recommended for which prosthetic valve?
(a) Bileaflet (b) Tilting discs
(c) Caged ball (d) All of the above

53. Long-term anticoagulation is done in all patients with bioprosthetic valve except
(a) With atrial fibrillation
(b) With atrial thrombus on echocardiography
(c) Previous history of embolism
(d) None of the above

54. Optimum duration of antibiotic therapy in majority of patients with Infective endocarditis is
(a) 2 week (b) 10 days
(c) 4 weeks (d) 6 weeks

55. Strong indication for surgical intervention in infective endocarditis includes all except
(a) Resistant heart failure
(b) Endocarditis caused by filamentous fungi
(c) Occlusion of valve by large vegetation
(d) Late onset prosthetic valve endocarditis

56. All are immunologically mediated lesion of Infective endocarditis except
(a) Glomerulonephritis
(b) Osler's node
(c) Roth spots
(d) Janeways lesion

57. Least common finding in lax pericardial effusion is
(a) Rub (b) Pulsas paradoxus
(c) Palpable apex (d) Soft heart sounds

58. Least common finding in constrictive pericarditis is

(a) Hepatomegaly (b) Raised JV pressure
(c) Pericardial knock (d) Ascites

59. All are found in constrictive pericarditis except

(a) Pericardium thickness > 5 mm
(b) Pericardial calcification
(c) Normal wall thickness
(d) Increased wall thickness

60. Average age of survival in severe aortic stenosis is

(a) < 2 years (b) 5 years
(c) 2 years (d) 3 years

61. Secondary hyperlipidemia is found in following except

(a) Hypothyroidism
(b) Billiary cirrhasis
(c) Hyperthyroidism
(d) Nephrotic syndromes

62. Hypertriglyceridemia is found in all except

(a) Alcoholism (b) Diabetes mellitus
(c) Pancreatitis (d) Cushing syndrome

63. Tissue ACE inhibitors are cardio protective because of all of the following except

(a) Antiproliferative effect
(b) Antiatherogenic effect
(c) Mantain endothelial function
(d) Thrombolytics effect

64. Nitrates in acute myocardial infarction cause all except

(a) Reduce pain
(b) Improve associated heart failure
(c) Reduce infarct size
(d) Improve survival

65. Sublingual nifedipine in hypertensive crisis causes all except

(a) Rapidily reduces blood pressure
(b) Causes subendocardial ischemia
(c) Causes left ventricular failure
(d) May cause myocardial infarction

66. All are established mechanism of cardio protection by ACE inhibitor except

(a) Prevention of remodelling
(b) Modification of heart rate variability
(c) Regression of LVH
(d) Prevention of reperfusion arrhythmia

67. All of the following arrhythmia in acute coronary syndrome are due to excessive sympathetic stimulation except

(a) Sinus tachycardia (b) Atrial fibrillation
(c) Paroxysmal SVT (d) AV blocks

68. All are manifestation of hypertensive heart disease except

(a) LVH on ECG
(b) Clinical LVH
(c) LVF
(d) A-V conduction defects

69. All of the following factors are associated with adverse prognosis after first myocardial infarction except

(a) Age > 70 years
(b) LVEF < 40 %
(c) Large anterior infarction
(d) Pericarditis

70. Thiazides act on the which part of nephron

(a) Loop of henle
(b) Cortical diluting segment
(c) Distal tubule
(d) All of the above

71. Calcium antagonist are dilators of

(a) Arterial (b) Venous
(c) Arterial + Venous (d) None of these

72. Prazosin is dilator of

(a) Arterial (b) Arterial + Venous
(c) Venous (d) None of these

73. Severe chest pain with murmur of aortic regurgitation the most likely diagnosis is

(a) Acute myocardial infarction
(b) Dissection of aorta

(c) Acute pulmonary embolism
(d) None of the above

74. All are additional benefits of Na restriction in hypertension except

(a) Regression of LVH
(b) Decrease in osteoporosis
(c) Decreased stroke mortality
(d) Decreased coronary artery disease mortality

75. Left ventricular hypertrophy in hypertension is related to

(a) Diastolic blood pressure
(b) Systolic blood pressure
(c) Both of them (d) None of these

76. Left ventricular hypertrophy more frequently occurs in hypertension in all following conditions except

(a) With obesity
(b) High dietary sodium
(c) Diabetes mellitus
(d) Coronary artery disease

77. All are atherosclerotic complications of hypertension except

(a) Cerebral thrombosis
(b) Coronary artery disease
(c) Claudication syndrome
(d) Aortic dissection

78. Acute myocardial infarction is suspected with which ECG finding in patients with pacemaker

(a) Marked ST elevation V1-V3
(b) Increase in latency period between pacing spike and onset of QRS
(c) Notched 'S' wave in V3-V5
(d) Both (a) and (b)

79. In posterolateral infarct most likely artery involved is

(a) Circumflex branch of LCA
(b) Distal circumflex branch of LCA
(c) Posterior marginal branch of Left circumflex
(d) Any of the above

80. In high lateral infarct which artery is likely to be involved

(a) Obtuse marginal branch of left circumflex
(b) High obtuse marginal branch of left circumflex
(c) Distal RCA
(d) Posterior descending branch of RCA

81. Inferior myocardial infarction is caused by occlusion all except

(a) Right coronary artery
(b) Post descending branch of RCA
(c) Left circumflex artery
(d) Distal circumflex branch of LCA

82. Treatment of hypertension is done in stroke patients in all following except

(a) BP > 200/100
(b) Haemorrhagic progression of ischemic stroke
(c) With left ventricular failure
(d) Hypertension < 180/100

83. Virchows triad include all except

(a) Venous stasis
(b) hypercoagulability
(c) Damage to vessel wall
(d) Thrombocytopenia

84. Which surgery is least risk factor for deep vein thrombosis?

(a) Spinal cord (b) Knee arthropathies
(c) Leg amputation (d) Neurosurgery

85. Drug of choice for prevention of DVT in patients undergoing orthopedic surgery

(a) LMWH
(b) Standard heparin (low dose)
(c) Oral anticoagulants
(d) Dextran

86. Best choice for preventing DVT during cardiovascular surgery is

(a) Low dose heparin
(b) Aspirin

(c) Oral anticoagulants
(d) Intermittent pneumatic compression

87. Which is least common site of DVT?

(a) Posterior tibial vein
(b) Common femoral vein
(c) Iliac vein
(d) Anterior tibial vein

88. Most established noninvasive test for deep veins thrombosis detection is

(a) Impedance plethyesmography
(b) Fibrinogen uptake test
(c) MRI (d) Thermography

89. Which is gold standard test for DVT diagnosis?

(a) Venography
(b) Impedance plethyesmography
(c) Doppler ultrasound
(d) B-mode ultrasound

90. All are most frequent manifestation of pulmonary embolism except

(a) Dyspea (b) Tachypnea
(c) Pleuritic chest pain
(d) Myocardial ischamic pain

91. Most widely used noninvasive method for diagnosis of pulmonary embolism is

(a) Perfusion lung scan
(b) X-ray chest
(c) ECG
(d) Arterial blood gas analysis

92. Most sensitive & specific test for diagnosis of pulmonary embolism is

(a) Pulmonary angiography
(b) Perfusion/ventilation scan
(c) ECG
(d) X-ray chest

93. Major cardiac risk for cocaine use is

(a) Myocardial ischemia
(b) Arrhythmia
(c) Dilated cardiomyopathy
(d) Myocarditis

94. All of the following are generally correct in women with acute coronary syndrome except

(a) Occurs in younger women
(b) Have multiple risk factors
(c) High risk of adverse outcome
(d) Occurs in older women

95. All the following aortic diseases are associated with myocardial ischamic except

(a) Aortic stenosis
(b) Aortic regurgitation
(c) Aortic dissection extending to coronaries
(d) Co-arctation of aorta

96. All are predictors of cardiogenic shock in Myocardial Infarction except

(a) Hyperglycemia (b) CK-MB > 160/L
(c) LVEF < 55% (d) Hypertension

97. All the following risk factors if eliminated lowers cardiovascular risk except

(a) Smoking (b) LDL-C
(c) LVH (d) Lp(a)

98. Thiazides causes following lipid abnormalities except

(a) Increases triglycerides
(b) Increases Total cholesterol
(c) Increases HDL-cholesterol
(d) Increases LDL-cholesterol

99. Thrombolytics are indicated in all except

(a) ST elevation anterior myocardial infarction
(b) ST elevation inferior myocardial infarction
(c) ST elevation superior nyocardial infarction
(d) ST elevation posterior myocardial infarction

100. Thrombolysis s done in all the following except

(a) ST elevation anterior myocardial infarction
(b) ST elevation lateral myocardial infarction
(c) ST depression anterior myocardial infarction
(d) ST elevation posterior myocardial infarction

101. All following are more common dihydiopyridine calcium channel blockers than non

dihydiopyridine calcium channel blockers except

(a) Hypotension (b) Constipation
(c) Ankle edema (d) Flush

102. Sudden development of electromechanical dissociation in acute myocardial infarction is a sign of

(a) Papillary muscle rupture
(b) Ventricular septal rupture
(c) Free wall rupture
(d) None of the above

103. Which neurological condition is associated with nocturnal hypertension?

(a) GB syndrome
(b) Benorecptor failure
(c) Alzheimer's diseases
(d) Parkinson's diseases

104. All the following heavy metal poisoning may cause hypertension except

(a) Lead (b) Gold
(c) Mercury (d) Thallium

105. Post operative hypertension occurs with all the following surgical intervention except

(a) After myocardial revascularisation Surgery
(b) Aortic valve replacement
(c) resection of aortic co-arction
(d) Balloon mitral valvotomy

106. Significant hypertension develop during following acute conditions except

(a) Acute pancreatitis
(b) Acute intermittent porphyria
(c) Acute respiratory distress
(d) Diabetic ketoacidosis

107. All the following neurological disorders are associated with hypertension except

(a) Quadriplegia following cervical injury
(b) Brain tumor
(c) Severe head injury
(d) Meningitis

108. Only systolic hypertension is found in which of the following condition

(a) Hypothyroidism
(b) Hyperthyroidism
(c) Acromegaly
(d) Hyperparathyroidism

109. All the following agents induce hypertension except

(a) Cyclophosphamide (b) Cyclosporine
(c) Disulfiram (d) Erythropoeitin

110. Nonsteroidal anti inflammatory drugs blunt the antihypertensive effect of all the following except

(a) ACE inhibitors
(b) β-blockers
(c) Calcium channel blockers
(d) Methyldopa

111. Which feature of chest pain is associated with most likelihood for myocardial infarction?

(a) Chest pain only
(b) Chest pain with radiation to right shoulder
(c) Chest pain with radiation to left shoulder
(d) Chest pain with radiation to both shoulders

112. Which feature of chest pain is associated with most lekily possibility of myocardial infarction?

(a) Pleuritic (b) Stabbing
(c) Positional (d) Squeezing

113. Features of inappropriate hypertension are all except

(a) Blood pressure > 180/110
(b) Left ventricular hypertrophy on ECG
(c) Abdominal bruit
(d) Adequate response to therapy

114. Commonest finding in reno vascular hypertension is

(a) Abdominal bruit
(b) Urinary casts
(c) Age of onset after 50 years
(d) Grade 3 or 4 fundoscopic changes

115. Most common location of pheochromocytomas is

(a) Unilateral adrenal (b) Bilateral adrenal
(c) Intra thoracic (d) In the risk

116. Most common clinical presentation of phaeochromocytoma is

(a) Paroxysmal hypertension
(b) Sustained hypertension
(c) Tremor
(d) Flushing

117. All the following peptides stenciled brown phoiochromocyronia are vasoconstriction except

(a) Endothelium (b) neropephidey
(c) Rennin (d) Adrenomednlta

118. All may be associated findings with phaeochromocytoma except

(a) Dyspnea on exertion
(b) Hypocalcaemia
(c) Polycythemia
(d) Anemia

119. All are more likely features of phaeochromocytoma in children except

(a) Familial
(b) Multiple tumors
(c) Extra abdominal
(d) Familial paroxysmal HTN

120. Mitral regurgitation after exercise in coronaty artery disease usually indicates

(a) SVD (b) LMCD
(c) DVD (d) TVD

121. All following statements are correct regarding coronary calcium except

(a) Presence of atherosclerotic plasma
(b) Presence of calcium indicates apophasis in polymer
(c) Presence of calcium indicates lipid content of plaque
(d) Indicates vulnerable plaque for reframe

122. Most specific and sensitive test for evaluation of coronary artery disease is

(a) Stress ECG (b) Stress echo
(c) Stress thallium (d) Ambulatory ECG

123. Detection of complication of coronary artery disease is best done by

(a) Stress ECG
(b) Stress echo
(c) Stress thallium
(d) Clinical examination

124. All the following lipid abnormality in obesity are commonly found except

(a) Increased triglycerides
(b) Increased HDL
(c) Increased apoB
(d) Increased small dense LDL

125. Commonest location of infarct from anamolous origin of left coronary artery from pulmonary artery is

(a) Inferior wall myocardial infarction
(b) Infero posterior wall myocardial infarction
(c) Antero septal myocardial infarction
(d) Antero lateral myocardial infarction

126. Microalbuminuria (M (d)) is best treated by

(a) ACE inhibitor
(b) Angiotensive receptor blockers
(c) Combination of ACE inhibitor & verapamil
(d) Verapamil

127. Best test for diagnosis of peripheral vascular disease is

(a) Colour wave doppler
(b) Ankle brachial index
(c) Transcutaneous perival pressure of oxygen
(d) Angiography

128. High total cholesterol is associated with all the following except

(a) Coronary artery disease
(b) Peripheral arterial disease
(c) Thrombotic strokes
(d) Rheumatic valve disease

129. Which of the following are the acronyms for percutaneous transmyocardial revascularization?

(a) PTMR (b) PMR
(c) DMR (d) PMLR
(e) TMR (f) None of these
(g) All of these

130. PTMR is indicated in patients if

(a) Angina is treatable by PTCA/CABG
(b) Angina is controllable on medical treatment
(c) Angina not treated by CABG/PTCA
(d) All of the above

131. Proposed mechanism of PTMR in treating angina

(a) Clears the plaque
(b) Improves supply through grafts
(c) Createsneoangiogenesis
(d) Decreases myocardial oxygen demand

132. Following PTMR the average hospital staysis

(a) 10-12 days (b) 15-20 days
(c) 1-2 days (d) 7 days

133. PTMR is done via

(a) Percutaneous femoral route
(b) Median sternotomy
(c) Lateral thorocotomy
(d) Heart port approach

134. The depth of channels created in PTMR are

(a) 2-3 mm (b) 4-5 mm
(c) 6-8 mm (d) 10-15 mm

135. The average duration for which the channels remain patent is

(a) Few minutes (b) Few days to 1 week
(c) 1 week to 1 month (d) $>$ 1 month

136. The average duration of a standard PTMR procedure is

(a) 2-5 minutes (b) 30-45 minutes
(c) 2-5 hours (d) > 5 hours

137. PTMR is done under

(a) LA (b) GA
(c) Spinal anesthesia (d) No anesthesia

138. The important randomized PTMR studies under investigations are

(a) Atlantic study
(b) Pacific and crimson study
(c) CASS trial
(d) PAMI trial

139. Angiographic thrombus is most common in

(a) Stable angina (b) Unstable angina
(c) Non Q myocardial infarction
(d) Q myocardial infarction

140. No clot is found is

(a) Stable angina
(b) Unstable angina
(c) Non Q myocardial infarction
(d) Myocardial infarction

141. Red clot is found is

(a) Stable angina
(b) Unstable angina
(c) Non Q myocardial infarction
(d) Q myocardial infarction

142. In elderly hypertension all are true except

(a) Direct arterial measurement frequently differs markedly from the cuff measurement
(b) Pseudo hypertension should be excluded by Osler's maneuver
(c) Radio femoral delay is frequent
(d) AV nipping is a non-specific

143. In elderly hypertensive which is the most important risk factor

(a) Systolic pressure
(b) Diastolic pressure

(c) Mean arterial pressure
(d) Both Systolic and diastolic pressure

144. In elderly subjects secondary hypertension frequently occurs due to

(a) Coarctation of aorta
(b) Secondary hyper aldosteronism
(c) Secondary renal artery stenosis
(d) Primary hyperaldosteronism

145. Elderly hypertensive are good responders to all of the following except

(a) Diuretics (b) β-blockers
(c) α-blockers
(d) Calcium channel blockers

146. Drug therapy in elderly hypertensives produces all of the following side effects except

(a) Depression (b) Anxiety
(c) Constipation
(d) Intermittent claudication

147. In USA, percentage of hypertensive who are aware that they have high blood Pressure is

(a) Less than 5% (b) 25–35%
(c) 65–75% (d) > 75%

148. In USA, the percentage of hypertensive whose blood pressure is effectively controlled in

(a) Less than 10% (b) 25–30%
(c) 35.60% (d) > 60%

149. In India figures for effectively controlled blood pressure at a national level are

(a) Not known (b) Less than 5%
(c) 10–20% (d) 20–30%

150. Which of the following environmental factors may increase blood pressure even if present temporarily?

(a) Noise
(b) Exposure to severe cold
(c) Pain
(d) Position of arm on which blood pressure is being measured
(e) All of the above

151. JNC VI (1997) has recommended the following as compelling indications for the use of low dose diuretics in hypertensive

(a) No compelling indication
(b) Isolated systolic hypertension (older patients)
(c) Hypertension associated with heart failure
(d) Hypertension associated with impotence as a side effect with β-blockers
(e) Both (b) and (c)

152. Which definition correctly depicts resistant hypertension?

(a) When blood pressure cannot be reduced to below 140/90 mm Hg inspite of full compliance of triple drug regime which also includes a diuretic at maximal doses
(b) When blood pressure remains ≥ 150/95 mm Hg inspite of maximal doses of at least two drugs
(c) When blood pressure remains ≥ 165/100 mm of Hg inspite of maximum tolerated antihypertensive therapy

153. The following are class 2 risk factors except

(a) Diabetes mellitus
(b) Thrombogenic factors
(c) Physical inactivity
(d) Postmenopausal status

154. Linear relationship of serum levels with CAD risk is found with

(a) HDL-C (b) VLDL-C
(c) LDL-C (d) Chylomycrons

155. Oleic acid is a

(a) PUFA (b) MUFA
(c) Saturated fat (d) None of the above

156. For each 1 mg/dl increase in HDL-C level the risk for CAD decreases by

(a) 1 to 2% (b) 2 to 3%
(c) 3 to 4% (d) 4 to 5%

157. Hypertriglyceridaemia is a proven coronary artery disease risk factor in

(a) Children (b) Men
(c) Women (d) All of the above

158. Syndrome-X has all the following components except

(a) Hyper insulinemia (b) Hyperlipidemia
(c) Hypertension (d) Hyperuricemia

159. All the following reduce homocysteine levels except

(a) Vitamin C (b) Vitamin B6
(c) Vitamin B12 (d) Folic Acid

160. All the following mediate direct endothelial damage except

(a) Glycosylated LDL (b) Oxidised LDL
(c) Homocysteine (d) Lipoprotein [a]

161. The following drugs increases HDL-C levels except

(a) Gemfibrozil (b) Bile acid resins
(c) Probucol (d) Statins

162. Anti thrombotic effect is a feature of

(a) Saturated fats (b) MUFAs
(c) Omega-6 PUFAs (d) Omega-3 PUFAs

163. Left ventricular hypertrophy regression is best obtained with

(a) Diuretics
(b) β-blockers
(c) ACE inhibitors
(d) Calcium channel blockers

164. Increased thrombus formation occurs in the deficiency of the following factors except

(a) Lipoprotein [a]
(b) Protein C
(c) Anti-thrombin III
(d) Protein S

165. The maximum risk to develop pulmonary embolism subsequent to setting of deep vein thrombosis is within

(a) First 12 hrs (b) First 24 hrs.
(c) First 48 hrs. (d) First 72 hrs.

166. Which one of the following is the most reliable diagnostic modality for deep vein thrombosis

(a) Venous plethysmography
(b) Real time B-mode compression ultrasonography
(c) Radioisotope fibrin uptake
(d) Doppler ultrasound

167. Which one of the following is the most reliable diagnostic method for pulmonary embolism?

(a) Chest X-ray
(b) Electrocardiography
(c) V/Q scan
(d) Surfactant test

168. Which is the commonest site of deep vein thrombosis?

(a) Lower limb below knee
(b) Lower limb above knee
(c) Ilio-femoral vein
(d) Upper limb

169. Which one of the following is an infrequent event in pathogenesis of pulmonary embolism?

(a) Atelectasis
(b) Pulmonary edema
(c) Pulmonary infarction
(d) Right ventricular failure
(e) Surfactant depletion

170. Which one of the following is not a sign or symptom of pulmonary embolism?

(a) Hemoptysis
(b) Wheeze
(c) Chest pain
(d) Diaphoresis

171. Resolution of emboli gets completed in

(a) 2-4 weeks
(b) 4-6 weeks
(c) 4-8 weeks
(d) After 8 weeks

172. In case of pregnancy the diagnosis of deep vein thrombosis is best made by

(a) Ultrasound
(b) Doppler ultrasound
(c) Real time B-mode compression ultrasonography
(d) Magnetic resonance imaging

173. Thrombectomy is best indicated in

(a) Acute cerebral thrombi
(b) Acute cervical thrombi
(c) Acute iliofemoral venous thrombi
(d) Acute upper limb thrombi

174. In which case low molecular weight heparin is not a suitable drug for the management of pulmonary embolism?

(a) Primary prophylaxis
(b) Acute treatment
(c) Long-term management
(d) All of the above

175. What does minimally invasive coronary artery surgery means?

(a) Avoidance of cardiopulmonary bypass and access through smaller incision
(b) CABG or cardiopulmonary bypass through mid sternotomy
(c) Not different from conventional surgery except that it requires video thoracoscope
(d) All of the above

176. What are the reasons for re-emergence and rapid acceptance of mimilally invasive coronary artery surgery?

(a) Increasing cost of conventional surgery, post operative discomfort of media sternotomy and damading effect of cardiopulmonary bypass
(b) Long operative time required for conventional surgery
(c) post-operative results are sub-optimal with conventional surgery
(d) All of the above

177. Upper mid-sternstomy approach is used for

(a) MIDCAB procedure
(b) Aortic and mitral valve surgery
(c) Conventional CABG
(d) All of the above

178. Right minithoracotomy approach is used for

(a) Revascularisation of circumflex system
(b) Conventional CABG
(c) For mitral valve surgery and ASD closure
(d) All of the above

179. Pharmacological agents most commonly used for stabilization of heart during minimally invasive CABG are

(a) Epinephrine and dobutamine
(b) Esmolol verapamil and adenosine
(c) Cordarone and Xylocard
(d) None of these

180. All are common emerging risk factor for atherosclerosis except

(a) Lipoprotein(a) (b) Fibrinogen
(c) Triglycerides (d) Insulin levels

181. Myocardial calcification most commonly occurs in

(a) Calcified thrombus
(b) Myocardial hydatid disease
(c) Healed myocardial infarction with out aneurysm
(d) Healed myocardial infarction with aneurysm

182. The effect of cholesterol reduction on IHD mortality occurs after

(a) 1 month (b) 1 years
(c) 2 years (d) 3 years

183. Liver function abnormality by statin which statement is incorrect?

(a) Occur in 0.5% of cases
(b) Dose dependent
(c) Depend on duration of treatment
(d) Should be stopped if transaminase levels exceed three times the upper limit of normal

184. RISC Trial Concluded

(a) Low dose aspirin reduces mortality in unstable angina/ none Q wave myocardial infarction

(b) Heparin reduces mortality in NQMI
(c) Both aspirins / Heparin reduces mortality
(d) Heparin reduces mortality in unstable angina

185. Ventricular aneurysm in myocardial infarction has following features except

(a) Develop mostly after large transmural acute myocardial infarction
(b) Associated with heart failure
(c) Myocardium around aneurysm is arrhythmogenic
(d) Associated with pericarditis

186. Which of the following mechanism is most important of HDL anti atherogenic effect?

(a) Reverse cholesterol transport
(b) Inhibition of LDL oxidation
(c) Inhibition of adhesion molecules
(d) All of the above

187. All features regarding primary aldosteronism are correct except

(a) Hyperkalemia
(b) Hypokalemia
(c) Commonly caused by adenoma
(d) 24 hours urinary aldosterone excretion is increased after salt loading

188. Most useful diuretic in hypertension of primary hyperaldosteronism is

(a) Furosemide (b) Thiazide
(c) Spiranslachore (d) All of the above

189. Pedal edema associated with calcium channel blockers is best managed by

(a) Adding ACE inhibitor
(b) Using S isomer of amlodipine
(c) Adding diuretic
(d) Replacing CCB by other agent

190. Acute arterial occlusion is featured by all the following except

(a) Pain (b) Redness
(c) Parasthesia (d) Pulselessness

191. The risk of myopathies is increased if Atorvastatin is used with all the following except

(a) Erythromycin (b) Verapamil
(c) Diltiazem (d) β-blockers

192. All are absolute contraindication to thrombolysis except

(a) Active internal bleeding
(b) Aortic dissection
(c) Pregnancy
(d) Diastolic pressure > 100 but < 120 mm/Hg

193. Septal rupture in acute myocardial infarction is characterized by all except

(a) Recurrence of chest pain
(b) Hemodynamic detoriation
(c) Short systolic murmur at left sternal border
(d) High prevalence in 2nd infarction

194. All the following statements are correct regarding goal controsl of BP except

(a) All uncomplicated BP < 140/90
(b) Type 2 DM with BP < 130/80
(c) HT with CAD BP < 140/88
(d) HT with type 2 DM & proteinuria (> 1 gm/ 24 hrs) < 125/75

195. Drugs aggravating angina or myocardial infarction are all except

(a) Nifedipine (b) Dipyridamole
(c) Hydralazine (d) Verapamil

196. All are causes of painless infarction except

(a) Diabetes mellitus (b) Dementia
(c) During anesthesia (d) Aspirin therapy

197. All drugs causes hypertension except

(a) Oral contraceptives
(b) Erythropoeitin
(c) Cyclosporine
(d) Quinidine

198. Which anti hypertensive does not cause AV block?

(a) Clonidine (b) Methyldopa
(c) Verapamil (d) α-blocker

199. Which of the renal artery lesion causing hypertension is least progressive?
(a) Atherosclerotic
(b) Fibromuscular dysplasia intimal type
(c) Fibromuscular dysphasia medial type
(d) Fibromuscular dysplasia periarterial type

200. Branch disease of normal artery is rare in which type of renal artery lesion?
(a) Atherosclerotic
(b) Fibromuscular dysplasia intimal
(c) Fibromuscular dysplasia medial
(d) Fibromuscular dysplasia periarterial

201. All are clinical characteristics of hypertensive crisis except
(a) Heart failure
(b) Renal failure
(c) Neurological disturbances
(d) Dystolic blood pressure usually < 120 mm Hg

202. Which is the leading cause of death in diabetes mellitus?
(a) Ischemic heart disease
(b) Renal dysfunction
(c) Diabetic cardiomyopathy
(d) Autonomic neuropathy

203. All following anti-hypertensives on sudden withdrawl cause rebound-phenomenon except
(a) Clonidine (b) Methyldopa
(c) β-blockers (d) ACE inhibitors

204. Which anti anginal agent is first line treatment in IHD?
(a) β-blockers (b) Amlodipine
(c) Nifedipine (d) Nitrates

205. Which anti anginal agent prevents ventricular fibrillation in IHD?
(a) β-blockers (b) Nifedipine
(c) Verapamil (d) Nitrates

206. Which anti anginal drug best prevents coronary spasm?

(a) β-blockers (b) Verapamil
(c) Nitrates (d) All of the above

207. Prevention of death in coronary artery spasm is possible by which drug?

(a) β-blockers (b) Ca-blocker
(c) Nitrate (d) None of the above

208. Coronary artery filling is best done by

(a) β-blockers (b) Nitrate
(c) Amlodipine (d) Nifedipine

209. All the following features are related to deep vein thrombosis except

(a) Contraceptive pill
(b) Diabetes mellitus
(c) Post partum period
(d) Hypertension

210. Diagnostic X-ray finding of dissecting aneurysm of aorta is

(a) Wide supra cardiac shadow
(b) Double aortic knob
(c) Spangling of aortic Arc CN
(d) Increase size of aorta

211. Commonest cause of secondary hypertension is

(a) Renal
(b) Pheochromocytoma
(c) Coarctation of aorta
(d) Primary aldosteronesm

212. All are most common underlying renal disease associated with hypertension except

(a) Chronic glomerulonephritis
(b) Diabetc nephropathy
(c) Polycystic kidney
(d) Hypernephroma

213. Complications of PCI includes all except

(a) Coronary artery dissection
(b) Coronary artery spasms
(c) Coronary artery thrombosis
(d) Coronary artery perforation

214. Drug of choice for hypertensive encephalopathy

(a) IV beta blockers (b) IV Nitroprusside
(c) IV Nitroglycerine (d) All of the above

215. AT1 receptors are located in all following places except

(a) Vessels (b) Brain
(c) Kidney (d) Liver

216. AT2 receptors are located at all following except

(a) Heart (b) Adrenal gland
(c) Myometrium (d) Nerves

217. AT4 receptors are located in all following except

(a) Heart (b) Brain
(c) Lungs (d) Nerves

218. Which ECG finding is persistent in pulmonary embolism?

(a) 'P' pulmonale (b) S1 Q3 pattern
(c) Q wave in inferior leads
(d) None of the above

219. Reducing systolic blood pressure reduces the risk of all except

(a) Ischemic events (b) Stroke
(c) Heart failure (d) All of the above

220. All the following are usually found in atrial infarction except

(a) No ventricular infarction
(b) Deviation of PR segment
(c) Sudden appearance of atrial arrhythmia
(d) Bizarre configuration of P wave

221. Normal value of serum cholesterol (total) in new born is

(a) 75 mg% (b) 100 mg%
(c) 150 mg% (d) 180 mg%

222. Incidence of coronary artery disease in urban India is

(a) 12% (b) 20%
(c) 25% (d) > 25%

223. Incidence of coronary artery disease in rural India is

(a) < 1% (b) 4%
(c) 10% (d) > 10%

224. All are coronary artery disease markers except

(a) Lipoproteins
(b) Blood sugar
(c) Intimamedia thickness
(d) Homocysteine levels

225. All following are correct regarding HDL-C except

(a) < 40 mg/dl definite risk factor
(b) 40 mg –50 mg/dl is normal
(c) 40 – 60 mg/dl is normal
(d) > 60 is a negative risk factor

226. Effective reduction of lipids in coronary artery disease mortality best achieved in

(a) 6 month (b) 1 yeas
(c) 2 years (d) After 3 years

227. Type 2 DM with hyperlipidemia which lipid lowering drug is avoided

(a) Statins (b) Niacin
(c) Fibrates (d) None of the above

228. Ideal blood pressure control for uncomplicated hypertension is

(a) < 140/90 (b) < 160/90
(c) < 150/90 (d) < 120/80

229. Ideal BP control of hypertension with DM with proteinuria >1gm/day is

(a) < 140/90 (b) < 130/80
(c) < 125/75 (d) < 150/80

230. Myocardial infarction in elderly has all the following features except

(a) More common
(b) Increased incidence of shock
(c) Increased incidence of heart failure
(d) ACE inhibitors do not reduce mortality as in young

231. ACE inhibitors are useful in all the following except

(a) Early acute myocardial infarction
(b) Chronic use in myocardial infarction with LV dysfunction
(c) Unstable angina
(d) Future cardiovascular events in post MI patients

232. Anti hypertensive of choice in subarachnoid haemorrhage is

(a) Nitroprusside (b) beta-blocker
(c) Nifedipine (d) Nitroglycerine

233. All are life threatening arrhythmias of digitalis toxicity except

(a) Complete heart block
(b) Ventricular tachycardia
(c) Asystole
(d) Multi focal ventricular premature complexes

234. Atheroma usually does not develop in following vessels except

(a) Vein
(b) Pulmonary artery with normal PAP
(c) Subclavian artery
(d) Iliac arteries

235. Which is major risk factor for development of metabolic syndrome?

(a) Obesity (Central)
(b) Hormonal imbalance
(c) Lack of exercise
(d) Ageing

236. All are indications of IABP in acute myocardial infarction except

(a) Selected cases of cardiogenic shock
(b) Post infarct angina (selected case)
(c) RVI with refractory hypertension
(d) Ventricular arrhythmia

237. LDL – Cholesterol is reduced most by which method?

(a) Reduction of saturated fat in diet
(b) Reduction of cholesterol in diet
(c) Weight loss
(d) Increase fiber in the diet

238. Systolic blood pressure is reduced most by which life style modification

(a) Desirable weight
(b) Sodium restriction
(c) Regular exercise
(d) Limitary alcohol consumption

239. IV Nitroglycerine is indicated in all the following myocardial infarction except

(a) Chest pain unresponsive to morphine and β-blocker
(b) Continued ischemia
(c) Myocardial infarction with left ventricular failure
(d) Inferior wall myocardial infarction with right ventricle infarction

240. ACE inhibitors are usually beneficial in all the following in acute myocardial infarction except

(a) Decreases mortality
(b) Decreases recurrent myocardial infarction
(c) Decreases heart failure
(d) Reduce incidence of arrhythmia

241. Highest mortality in acute myocardial infarction related to which of the following

(a) Cardiogenic shock (b) Severe heart failure
(c) EF < 30% (d) All the above

242. Which is best Beta blocker in myocardial infarction?

(a) Atenolol (b) Bisoprolol
(c) Metoprolol (d) Pindolol

243. LMCA occlusion may be suspected from which of the ECG finding

(a) ST elevation in aVR with ST depression in anterior leads
(b) Extensive anterior myocardial infarction
(c) Infero-Posterior myocardial infarction
(d) Anterolateral myocardial infarction

244. Best time for streptokinase therapy after symptoms of myocardial infarction as regards to survival is

(a) Within 1 hours
(b) Within 2-4 hours
(c) Within 4-6 hours
(d) > 6 hours to 12 hours

245. ST elevation in aVR is found in all except

(a) LMCA occlusion
(b) Circumflex occlusion
(c) Right ventricle overload
(d) Right ventricle infarction

246. Which of the following markers of myocardial infarction take maximum time to returns to normal?

(a) Trop I (b) Trop T
(c) Myoglobin (d) CPKMB

247. Troponins are increased in all the following except

(a) Heart failure (b) Hypertension
(c) Hyperthyroidism (d) Renal failure

248. All following are usual cardiac complications of hypertension except

(a) LVH
(b) Heart failure
(c) Coronary artery disease
(d) Valvular heart disease

249. All are physiological risk factors for venous thrombosis except

(a) Advanced age (b) Pregnancy
(c) Post partum (d) Post menopausal

250. Which statin is non lipoplytic?

(a) Atorvastatin (b) Rosuvustatin
(c) Simvastatin (d) Pravastatin

251. Nitrate is first choice in stable angina in following situations except?

(a) With left ventricular dysfunction
(b) Infrequent angina
(c) Stable angina with hypertension
(d) None of these

252. β-blocker is first choice is stable angina in all the following conditions except

(a) Post myocardial infarction SA
(b) Angina with HT
(c) Angina with migraine
(d) Angina with peripheral vascular disease

253. Ca-blocker (Non DPH) is first choice in stable angina in all the following except

(a) Beta-blockers contraindicated
(b) Where coronary spasm is suspected
(c) Associated diabetes mellitus
(d) Post myocardial infarction stable angina

254. Which of the following antiarrhythmics has anti anginal activity?

(a) Quinidine (b) Procainamide
(c) Lidocaine (d) Amiodarone

255. Atrial fibrillation in acute myocardial Infarction, all statements are correct except

(a) Increased embolization
(b) Increased infarct size
(c) DC shock is contraindicated
(d) Increased hospital mortality rate

256. β-blockers in post myocardial infarction patients are most effective for

(a) Decreases total mortality
(b) Decreases sudden cardiac death
(c) Decreases reinfarction rate
(d) Decrease in ventricular arrhythmia

257. Abdominal aortic aneurysm is likely to rupture if its size is

(a) 1 cm (b) 2 cm
(c) 4 cm (d) > 5 cm

258. Dissection of aorta most commonly involves

(a) Ascending aorta (b) Arch of aorta
(c) Thoracic aorta (d) Abdominal aorta

259. Coronary angiography is indicated in aortic stenosis in all except

(a) Age > 35 years
(b) Two or more risk factor for coronary artery disease
(c) Typical angina (d) No heart failure.

260. Deep venous thrombosis is characterized by all except

(a) Swelling (b) Redness
(c) Warm (d) Non tender

261. Which statin is known to increase fibrinogen level?

(a) Revastatins (b) Atorvastatins
(c) Simvastatins (d) Pravastatins

262. All following abdominal diseases cause hyperlipidemia except

(a) Biliary cirrhosis
(b) Pancreatitis
(c) Obstructive jaundice
(d) Malabsorption syndrome

263. All the following may cause angina with normal coronary arteries except

(a) Coronary artery spasm
(b) MVP
(c) Diabetic microangiopathy
(d) Pulmonary stenosis

264. Most common cause of syncope in angina is

(a) Sublingual nitrate
(b) Ischemia induced LVF
(c) Ischemia induced ventricular arrhythmia
(d) Ischemia induced arrhythmia complete heart block

265. All following may cause silent ischemia except

(a) Diabetics (b) Elderly
(c) Small mass of ischamic myocardium
(d) Ischemia with increases LVEDP

266. High prevalence of heart disease in elderly male is of

(a) Coronary artery disease
(b) Hypertension
(c) Valvular
(d) Congenital

267. Best antihypertensive agent in patients of hypertension with migraine is

(a) Selective β-blocker
(b) Non selective β-blocker
(c) ACE inhibitor
(d) α-blocker

268. Anti hypertensive of choice in patients with hypertension & osteoporosis

(a) β-blocker (b) Thiazide diuretics
(c) Aldactone (d) Loop diuretics

269. Most specific marker of acute myocardial infarction in 2 hours chest pain

(a) Total MB-CK activity
(b) Total MB-CK mass
(c) Troponin 'T'
(d) Myoglobin

270. Most specific & sensitive marker of acute myocardial infarction at 22 hours after chest pain

(a) Total MB-CK mass
(b) Trop –T
(c) Trop – I
(d) Myoglobin

271. Smoking causes atherosclerosis most in

(a) Peripheral arteries (b) Cerebral arteries
(c) Coronary arteries (d) Retinal artery

272. Blood pressure cause atherosclerosis most in

(a) Coronary arteries (b) Retinal arteries
(c) Peripheral arteries (d) Cerebral arteries

273. Cholesterol is involved in atherosclerosis mainly in which arteries systolic

(a) Peripheral (b) Cerebral
(c) Retmal (d) Coronaries

274. DM affects most which arterial systemic

(a) Peripheral (b) Retinal
(c) Coronary (d) Cerebral

275. Dietary cholesterol cause following changes in lipid profile except

(a) Increase TC (b) No effect on TG
(c) Increases LDL-C (d) Decreases HDL-C

276. Which saturated fatty acid has no effect on lipid profile?

(a) Pomitic acid
(b) Stearic acid
(c) Medium chain fatty acid
(d) Myristic acid

277. Which saturated fatty acid cause maximum risk of LDL-C?

(a) Lauric acid
(b) Myristic acid
(c) Medium chain fatty acid
(d) Palmitic acid

278. Which mono saturated fatty acid has no effect or lipid profile?

(a) Oleic acid
(b) Tran fatty-acid
(c) Both the (a) and (b)

279. Which disease least common with peripheral vascular disease?

(a) Coronary artery disease
(b) Hypertensive
(c) Hyperlipidemia
(d) Cerebro vascular disease

280. Best drug to prevent myocardial infarction in VA is?

(a) Nitrate (b) β-blockers
(c) Ca-blockers (d) Heparin

281. Mortality reduction in VA is best achieved by

(a) β-blockers (b) Nitrates
(c) Aspirin (d) Heparin

282. All following reduce in ventricular O_2 demand except

(a) Nitrate (b) b-blockers
(c) Ca-blockers (d) Aspirin

283. Single best way for predrecting severity of aortic stenosis is

(a) Pulsus parves et tardus
(b) Late perking murmur
(c) S4
(d) Paradoxical splitting

284. Reduced HDL-C by all except

(a) Smoking (b) Increase TG
(c) β-blockers (d) Increase TC

285. Yearly mortality rate in left main artery disease is

(a) 5% (b) 6%
(c) 7% (d) > 8%

286. Lipoprotein is a best reduced by

(a) Statin
(b) Niacin
(c) Resons
(d) Diet low in saturated fat

287. Statins therapy has all the following feature except

(a) work best with high level of LDL
(b) Aortic stenosis the LDL decrease their effect also shunts
(c) There is no rebound after stoppage
(d) Long duration lang lesion therapy favorable effect

288. Which statins has least hypothec effect?

(a) Lova statins (b) Smiver statins
(c) Carnba statins (d) Atorvastatin

289. Which in the commonest variety of acute arteritis?

(a) Type I (b) Type II
(c) Type III (d) TypeIV

290. Anecorysmia occur in aortoarterites

(a) Ascending aorta (b) Descending aorta

(c) Both (a) and (b) (d) None of these

291. All following occur in retinal vascular in aortoarteritis except

(a) Retinal vein distension
(b) Micro aneurysm formation
(c) Arterio venous anastomosis
(d) Retinal vein thrombosis

292. Which is commonest manifestation of aorta arteritis?

(a) Decrease or absent pulse
(b) Bruit
(c) Hypertension
(d) Heat failure

293. Heart failure aorta arteritis is due to all except

(a) Hypertension
(b) Valvular incompetence
(c) Cardiomyopathy
(d) Atrial fibrillation

294. Pulmonary artery involvement in aorta Arteritis featured by all except

(a) Lesion occur large and medium size
(b) Lesion at stenosis
(c) Right upper lope artery is frequently involved
(d) PH is common

295. Which statement is correct regarding angina equivalents?

(a) Dyspnoea (b) Fatigue
(c) Both A & B (d) None of the above

296. Coronary arteries most commonly involved in

(a) Poly arteritis nodosa
(b) Ankylosing spondylitis
(c) Rheumatic arttritis
(d) SLE

297. Most frequent cause for acute myocardial infarction in pregnancy is

(a) Hyper coagubility
(b) Enhance athero thrombosis
(c) Drug induced
(d) Coronary dissection

298. All following antihypertensive removed by haemodialysis except

(a) Methyl dopa (b) Nitropruside
(c) Minoxidil (d) Clonidine

299. All following antiarrthymia are remond by haemodralysis except

(a) Quinidine (b) Disopyramide
(c) Procanomide (d) Amiodarone

300. Worsing of angina may occur with which Ca-channel blockers

(a) Verapamile (b) Diltuzem
(c) Nitedifine (d) Bepridril

301. Which calcium channel blocker has least antihypertensive effect?

(a) Amlodipine (b) Diltiazem
(c) Verapamil (d) Nifedipine

302. Which calcium channel blocker has best anti anginal effect?

(a) Amlodipine (b) Nifedipine
(c) Verapamil (d) Diltiazem

303. Free wall rupture most commonly occurs in

(a) Lat wall infarction
(b) Septal infarction
(c) Inferior infarction
(d) Infero post wall infarct

304. Papillary muscle rupture most commonly occur

(a) Ant septal myocardial infarction
(b) Infero-Post myocardial infarction
(c) Lat wall myocardial infarction
(d) RVI

305. Left ventricular aneurysm most common develops in

(a) Anterior myocardial infarction
(b) Inferior myocardial infarction
(c) Post myocardial infarction
(d) Infero-post myocardial infarction

306. Ventricular septal rupture commonly occurs in

(a) Anterior myocardial infarction
(b) Inferior myocardial infarction
(c) Post myocardial infarction
(d) Infero-post myocardial infarction

307. Beneficial effect of clopidogrel may be multi-facet by all following statins except

(a) Lambastin (b) Atorvastatin
(c) Rosuvastatin (d) Lenavastatin

308. In comparison to Q wave myocardial infarction the non Q wave myocardial infarction has all the following features except

(a) Reinfarction is more
(b) Arrhythmias are less
(c) Post infarct angina is more
(d) Heart failure is more

309. IV Nitroglycerine usually more then in

(a) Hyporalemia
(b) RVI
(c) Cardiac temponade
(d) Uncomplicated inf-myocardial infection

310. All are least myocardial depressant except

(a) Quinidime (b) Mexilitine
(c) Amiodorone (d) Propafenone

311. Which is not lipid specific ACE inhibitor?

(a) Lisinopril (b) Perindopril
(c) Ramipril (d) Trandolapril

312. Most important risk for increased incidence of CAD in India is

(a) Hypertension (b) Insulin resistance
(c) DM (d) Dyslipidemia

313. Q wave MI has all the following feature more common than non QMI except

(a) Refraction is more
(b) Heart failure is more
(c) Arrhythmia are more
(d) Post infarction angina is Less

314. SVR is decreased most by

(a) Nifedipine (b) Diltiazem
(c) Verapamil (d) Amlodipine

315. Sinus node depression does occur with which CB?

(a) Nifedipine (b) Diltiazam
(c) Verapamil (d) Amlodipine

316. Difference of BP between two arms > 15 mmHg is found in all except

(a) Aortic aneurysm
(b) Aortic arch syndrome
(c) Coorctation of aorta
(d) Aortic stenosis

317. Headache may occur in hypertension at which diastolic blood pressure level

(a) 90 – 100 mm Hg
(b) 100 – 110 mm Hg
(c) 110 – 140 mm Hg
(d) > 140 mm Hg

318. All are major determinants of myocardial O_2 consumption except

(a) Myocardial mass
(b) Wall stress
(c) Contractility
(d) External work load

319. Which of the following is not the cause of hypertension?

(a) Hyperthyroidism
(b) Hypothyroidism
(c) Hyperparathyroidism
(d) Hypoparathyroidism

320. Which gene is unlikely to be related to hypertension?

(a) Renin (b) ACE
(c) Endothelin (d) ANP

321. Obstructive sleep apnea causes systemic hypertension by all the following mechanism except

(a) Increases sympathetic activity
(b) Increases erythropoetin
(c) Increases endothelin
(d) Volume expansion

322. All statins are lipophilin except

(a) Pravastatin (b) Atoravastatin
(c) Sirovastatin (d) Lovastatin

323. All the following drugs reduce cardiovascular events in CHD except

(a) Anti platelet agents
(b) Lipid lowering drugs
(c) Angiotensin converting enzyme inhibitors
(d) β-blockers

324. Annual mortality in high risk IHD patients is?

(a) 1% (b) 2%
(c) 3% (d) > 3%

325. The most sensitive index of ischemia (myocardial) is

(a) ECG changes
(b) Enzyme changes
(c) Cardiac protein changes
(d) Regional wall motion abnormalities

326. What is the incidence of silent myocardial infarction?

(a) < 5% (b) 5 – 10%
(c) 10 – 20% (d) > 25% to 35%

327. How often the reno vascular hypertension occurs in aortic dissection?

(a) 1% (b) 5%
(c) 10% (d) 20%

328. Which laboratory finding does not occurs in reno vascular hypertension?

(a) Increase plasma renin
(b) High serum K
(c) Low serum Na
(d) Proteinuria

329. All the following anti hypertensive does not require dose modification with renal insufficiency except

(a) Ca-blocker (b) Clonidine
(c) α-blocker (d) Nadolol

330. Which type of hypertension is known to preced microalbummunia?
(a) Day time systolic blood pressure
(b) Nocturnal systolic blood pressure
(c) Combined systolic & diastolic hypertension
(d) Diastolic hypertension

331. Which is the commonest fibro muscular dysplasia for reno vascular hypertension?
(a) Intimal (b) Medial
(c) Peripheral (d) All of them

332. All the following drugs require dose modification with renal insufficiency except
(a) Atenolol
(b) Nadalol
(c) ACE inhibitors
(d) Angiotension receptor blocker

333. Which divretic requires dose modification in renal insufficiency?
(a) Thiazide
(b) Loop diaretics
(c) Xanthines
(d) K^+ sparing diaretics

334. All the following statement are truce regarding MI during pregnancy except
(a) Commonly occurs during labour and deliving
(b) May be due to atherothrombosis
(c) May be due to thrombosis
(d) Thrombolydis is done

335. HELLP syndrome has all the following except
(a) Haemolysis
(b) Elevated liver enzyme
(c) Low platelet count
(d) Proteinuria

336. For acute severe hypertension in pre-ecclampsia which drug is more safe and effective
(a) Hydralazine IV
(b) Sod. nitroprusside IV
(c) Clonidine (d) Nifedipine

337. In comabass following conclusion ware draven except

(a) Scruples was comparable to streptokinase in ACMI in terms of total mortality

(b) Scruples caused sunitor traemorthyia strokes

(c) Scruples caused less thromboembolic strokes

(d) Scruples caused less allergic reaction

338. PAMI trial showed all the following except primary angioplasty causes lower occurrence of

(a) Non fatal recurrect infarction

(b) Primary angioplasty reduces mortality

(c) Increases rate of intracranual bleeding

(d) Decrease rate of intracranial bleeding

339. TIMI trail I demonstrate all the following except

(a) rtPA causes more rapid reperfusion than streptokinase

(b) Bleeding complication.are more with streptokinase

(c) Mortality was similar in both groups

(d) LV function was similar in both groups

340. ISIS2 trail demonstrated all the following except

(a) Aspirin reduces mortality in acute myocardial infarction

(b) Streptokinase reduces mortality in acute myocardial infarction

(c) Combination has no synergistic effect on mortality

(d) Combination did not increases the rate of status

341. ISIS III concluded the following except

(a) Heparin cause small improvement in acute myocardial infarction

(b) Reduces reinforcing

(c) No advantage of aspirin over streptokinase

(d) Strokes were decrease with PA

342. LATE trail demonstrated all the following except

(a) Thrombolysis was archeived by altepease
(b) Administered in 6–24 hours of chest pain
(c) No effect on mortality
(d) Mortality was reduced

343. CATS trail showed all the following except

(a) Decrease progression of heart failure (Caplopil)
(b) Decrease ischemia related events
(c) Increase exercise performance
(d) On with drauol of coptopril increases incidence of ischemic events

344. DAVIT II trail showed all the following except

(a) Verapamil after acute myocardial infarction reduce mortality
(b) Verapamil after ACMI reduce renifarction in patients of heart failure
(c) Verapamil after ACMI reduce mortality in patients of without heart failure
(d) Verapamil after ACMI reduce renifarction in patients without heart failure

345. TIMI-9 trail concluded all the following except-cardiac rupture following thrombolysis

(a) For acute myocardial infarction occur more commonly in young
(b) For acute myocardial infarction occur more commonly in old
(c) For acute myocardial infarction occur more commonly in women
(d) Anticoagulation does not influence its development

346. TRACE trail showed all the following except long-term with trandolupril in LV dysfunction

(a) After acute myocardial infarction reduce total mortality
(b) Reduce cardiovascular mortality
(c) No effect on sudden death
(d) Prevent progression of heart failure

347. Most common site for peripheral arterial aneurysm is

(a) Femoral (b) Radial
(c) Ulnar (d) Brachial

348. Splenic artery aneurysms has all the following features except

(a) Reaction is not done in female in clued bearing age more common in women
(b) Curvilinear shadow of calcification on X-ray
(c) Rupture may occur in last trimester of pregnency
(d) All of the above

349. Most common cause of peripheral arterial aneurysms is

(a) Athero sclerosis
(b) Penetrative trauma
(c) Blunt trauma
(d) Post stenotic dilatation

350. Which of the following does not cause raynauds phenomena?

(a) Scleroderma
(b) Rheumatoid arthritis
(c) Ankylosine spondylitis
(d) SLE

351. Raynaud's disease has all the following feature except

(a) More in femeles
(b) Occurs at age < 40 years
(c) Usually bilateral involvement
(d) Systemic symptoms are present

352. Avert trail concluded all the following except

(a) Aggressive lipid lowering with atriovastatin reduces ischemic events
(b) Reduced revasculausation procedure
(c) In coronary artery disease with hyperlidemia
(d) Dose of atria atorvastatin used was 60 mg/day

353. In prevent study following was concluded except

(a) Amlodipine in CAD patients reduced the carotid wall thickness carotid wall thickness
(b) No effect on quantitative angiography
(c) No effect on hospitalization for heart failure
(d) Reduced the need for revisualization

354. In patients of hypertension and essentials tremors which drug is the choice

(a) Atenodol (b) Metoprolol
(c) Propranalol (d) Nevibalol

355. Drug of choice in treatment of hypertension with osteoporosis

(a) β-blockers (b) Thiazide diuretics
(c) Loop diuretics (d) ACE inhibitors

356. All the following stimuli causes angina except

(a) Serotonin (b) H^+
(c) Kinins (d) Adenosine

357. Increased cardiovascular risk in hypertension is associated with all the following except

(a) Coronary artery disease
(b) DM
(c) Retinopathy
(d) Neuropathy

358. P Fox inhibitors in angina cause all the following except

(a) Increase myocardial ischemia
(b) No significant effect on HR
(c) No significant effect on blood pressure
(d) Decrease coronary flow

359. Which anti angial drug is avoided in patients with peripheral vascular disease?

(a) Nitrates
(b) β-blocker non selective
(c) Metabolic modulators
(d) Calcium blockers

360. Which antianginal drug is to be avoided in DM?

(a) Nitrates

(b) Non selective β-blockers
(c) Calcium blockers
(d) Metabolic modulators

361. Low dose oral anti coagulation is recommended in CAD in all the following situation except
(a) Ventricular aneurysm
(b) Inferior wall myocardial infection
(c) Atrial fibrillation
(d) Decreased LVEF

362. Focal strokes following CABG is most commonly caused by
(a) Intracracial vascular disease
(b) Embolic from atrium ventricle
(c) Post operative atrial fibrillation
(d) Atheroembolism from aorta

363. Angina with ventricular arrhythmia which is the drug of choice for angina?
(a) Nitrates
(b) β-blockers
(c) Metabolic modulator
(d) Dihydropyridine Ca-blocker

364. Angina with sinus tachycardia the choice of antianginal is
(a) β-blockers
(b) Dihydropyridine Ca-blockers
(c) Nitrates
(d) Metabolic

365. Angina with thyrotoxicosis the drug of choice is
(a) β-blockers
(b) Ca-blockers
(c) Nitrates
(d) Metabolic modulator

366. Angina with depression which antianginal to avoid?
(a) Nitrate
(b) β-blockers
(c) Long acting Ca-blockers
(d) Metabolic modulartor

367. Which is the best way to differentiate adenoma from hyperplasia of adrenals?

(a) Basal plasma 18-hydroxycortisone
(b) Adrenal CT
(c) Adrenal MRI
(d) Adrenal venous aldosterone cortisol ratio

368. Best treatment option for adrenal hyperplasia is

(a) Spironolectone (b) Amiloride
(c) Surgery (d) all of them

369. All are features of adosterone producing edema except

(a) Hypokalemia frequent
(b) Plasma renin using low
(c) Plasma aldosteron levels very high
(d) Surgical removal rarely help

370. Bilateral adrenal hyperplasia is characterised by all except

(a) Hypokalemia less common
(b) Plasma rennin levels low
(c) Surgical removal usually causes gives relief
(d) Occurs in old age

371. All are common manifestation of phochromocytoma except

(a) Paroxysmal hypertension
(b) Persistent hypertension
(c) Sweating
(d) Palpitation

372. All are less common manifestation of phochromocytoma except

(a) Tremor (b) Flushing
(c) Dysnea (d) Pallor

373. Which is most rapidly acting drug in hypertensive emergencies?

(a) Captopril (b) Clonidine
(c) Frusemide (d) Propranolol

374. Which drug has longest duration of action in hypertensive emergencies when given orally?

(a) Captopril (b) Clonidrine
(c) Labetalol (d) Propranolol

375. Which antihypertensive is contraindicated in patients with postural hypotension?

(a) α-blockers (b) β-blockers
(c) Ca-blockers (d) ACE inhibitors

376. While treating hypertension in elderly all the following statements are correct except

(a) β-blocker are choice
(b) Use long acting drug
(c) Start with small dose
(d) Check the postural and post Prondial hypotension before staling the drug

377. Recurent strock prevention which drug is given

(a) ACE inhibitors (b) Ca-blockers
(c) AR Bs (d) β-blockers

378. Vasodilatation occurs with all the following drugs except

(a) Ca-blockers (b) β-blockers
(c) ACE inhibitor (d) α-blockers

379. Hypertension with high coronary risk all the following are indicated except

(a) Aldostecone antagonist
(b) β-blockers
(c) ACE-inhibitors (d) Ca-blockers

380. In diabetic hypertension all are Tried except

(a) ACE Inhibitors
(b) AR Bs
(c) Calcium-blockers
(d) Aldosterone antagonist

381. Which ARB has uricosuric effect?

(a) Losartan (b) Telmesatan
(c) Erbesartan (d) Olmisartan

382. In post myocardial infarction all the following are indicated except

(a) β-blockers (b) Ca-blockers
(c) Aldostenosis antagonism
(d) ACE inhibitors

383. Which antihypertensive improve lipid profile?

(a) β-blockers (b) ACE inhibitors
(c) α-blockers (d) Diuretics

384. What is equilibrium level for LDL-C at which progression and regression of the plaque is ouanerage siam low?

(a) 75 mg% (b) 80 mg%
(c) 90 mg% (d) 100 mg%

385. Nitrates are given in acute myocardial infarction in all the following except

(a) Recurrent or ongoing ischemia
(b) Hypertension
(c) LVF
(d) Right ventricular infarction

386. All the following dietary changes improve lipid profile except

(a) Purple or red grape juice
(b) Tea with milk
(c) Nuts
(d) Almonds

387. Which statin is associated with hypertension?

(a) Senvastatin (b) Atorvastatin
(c) Rosuvastatin (d) Fluvastatin

388. Which drug is given in hypertension caused by phaechromoeytoma?

(a) Sotalol (b) Methyldopa
(c) Propranalol (d) ACE inhitors

389. Ca-blockers in hypertension causes reduction in all the following except

(a) Cardiovascular deaths
(b) Total mortality
(c) Heart failure
(d) Stroke

390. Commonest complication of untreated hypertension

(a) LVH
(b) Proteinuria
(c) Going to accelerated phase
(d) Heart failure

391. Survival is most reduced by which complication of hypertension?

(a) Accelerated phase (b) Stroke
(c) Proteinuria
(d) Left ventricular hypertrophy

392. Combined systolic + Diastolic hypertension has all the following features except

(a) Age of onset 30–50 years
(b) Multi factorial etiology
(c) Progress is rapid contimans
(d) Often cause CAD & renal insufficiency

393. All the following are feature of isolated systolic hypertension except

(a) Age of onset > 55 years
(b) Due to arterial stiffness
(c) Progress is slow variable
(d) Leads to heart failure/stroke

394. All are atherosclerotic complication of hypertension except

(a) Heart failure (b) Claudication
(c) Coronary artery disease
(d) Cerebral thrombosis

395. All are hypertensive complications of HT except

(a) Aortic dissection (b) Heart failure
(c) Encephalopathy
(d) Myocardial infarction

396. Tangiers disease has all the following feature except

(a) Dyslipidemia
(b) High incidence of coronary artery disease
(c) Increase HDL
(d) Orange large lobulated tonsils

397. All the following are found on X-ray chest in aortic rupture except

(a) Widening of superior mediastinum
(b) Depression of left bronchus
(c) Displacement of trachea on right side
(d) Aortic knuckle prominent

398. What is abnormal blood pressure while awake on ambulatory blood pressure measurement?

(a) 130/80 (b) 135/85
(c) 140/80 (d) > 140/90

399. What is abnormal blood pressure at sleep on ambulatory blood pressure measurement?

(a) > 125/75 (b) 130/80
(c) > 140/90 (d) > 126/86

400. Insulenemia causes hypertension by all the following mechanism except

(a) Sympathetic stimulation
(b) Increase production of angiotension II
(c) Endothelial dysfunction
(d) Increase viscosity of blood

401. Which location of coronary occlusion after I month of successful reperfusion has highest mortality?

(a) Proximal LAD (before 1st septed perforator)
(b) Mild LAD
(c) RCA
(d) Left circunflex

402. Hypertensive retinopathy rarely occurs in which etiological type of hypertension?

(a) Renovascular hypertension
(b) Renal parenchymal disease
(c) Coarctation of aorta
(d) Essential hypertension

403. Peripheral arterial thrombosis has all following features except

(a) Gradual onset of symptoms
(b) Claudication (Prior) common
(c) Physical finding of vascular disease common
(d) Temperature level demarcation well defined

404. Peripheral arterial embolism has all the following features except

(a) Sudden onset
(b) Prior claudication absent
(c) Temperature level demarcation sharp
(d) Arterragraphy reveals well developed collaterals

405. Commonest cause of cardiogenic embolism is

(a) RHD with atrial fibrillation
(b) Non-rheumatic atrial fibrillation
(c) Acute myocardial infarction
(d) Cardiomyopathy

406. Antihypertensive drug of choice in renal parenchymal reformatory hypertension

(a) Ca-blockers (b) Methyldropa
(c) Minoxidil (d) None of the above

407. All are cardiac vascular causes of DVT except

(a) RHF
(b) Deep venous aneurysm
(c) Myocardial infection
(d) None of the above

408. In adrenocortical adenoma the most predictive list is

(a) Adrenal venography
(b) Adrenal venous aldosterone levels
(c) Adrenal 10 to cholesterol scan
(d) Orthostatic fall in plasma aldosterone

409. Most predictive test for adrenal hyperplaria

(a) Adrenal venograpgy
(b) Adrenal 10 do cholesterol scan
(c) Adrenal venous aldosterance level
(d) No orthostatic fall in plasma aldosterone

410. All following statement are correct for myocardial cell death by ischemia except

(a) Myocardial cell death occurs both by necrosis and apoptasis
(b) Necrosis dominates during ischemia
(c) Apoptosis dominates during reperfusion
(d) Corrections of ischemia will present both types of myocardial cell death

411. Acute myocardial infarction in paced patients (RV) may be suspected by all the following except

(a) Marked ST Increase V1-V3
(b) Marked elevation in latency between pace maker stimulus and the onset of QRS
(c) Nofened S in V3-V5
(d) QS Complex in V4-V6

412. Most common symptom of coronary artery disease is

(a) Chest discomfort (b) Palpitations
(c) Dyspnoea (d) Syncope

413. Most common first presentation of coronary artery disease is

(a) Exertional angina (b) Rest angina
(c) Myocardial infarction
(d) Sudden cardiac death

414. Which trial showed no improvement in Survival after myocardial infarction?

(a) Save (b) Trace
(c) Smile (d) Consensus II

415. In which hypertension Beta-blockers are not used?

(a) Portal hypertension
(b) Pulmonary hypertension
(c) Systemic hypertension
(d) Intra vascular hypertension

416. Women with myocardial infarction have all the following except

(a) More mortality than man
(b) More complication than man
(c) More silent myocardial infarction than man
(d) Death is less common than man

417. Women with CAD have following feature compared to man except

(a) Symptoms appear late
(b) Stress test often not occurred
(c) Breast tire may simulate Ischemia on thathim

(d) SCDS are lets fragment

418. Antihypertensive agent of choice in primary aldosteronism

(a) ACE inhibitors
(b) Ca-channel blockers
(c) β-blockers
(d) Spironolachone

419. Most common symptom peripheral arterial occlusion is

(a) Pain (b) Coldness
(c) Pallor (d) Runbness

420. Which of the following reduces cardiovascular events in UA?

(a) Ticlopidine (b) Dipyridomic
(c) Sulfirpyrazone (d) None of the above

421. Aldo sterone antagonist are not useful in hypertension except

(a) Post myocardial infarction
(b) Recurrent stroke prevention
(c) DM
(d) Chronic-kidney disease

422. All are most common cause of HT at age between 6–10 years except

(a) Renal parenchymal disease
(b) Renal artery stenosis
(c) Essential HT
(d) Coarctation of Aorta

423. Which life style modification is associated with least systolic blood pressure reduction

(a) Alcohol intake in moderation
(b) Physical exercise
(c) Sodium restriction
(d) Weight reduction

424. ACE inhibitor are better choice than ARBS in which of the following condition in hypertension

(a) Heart failure
(b) DM
(c) Chronic renal disease
(d) Recurrent stroke prevention

425. All are cortraindication to PTCA except
(a) Unprotected left main stenosis
(b) Long lesion > 20 mm
(c) Old lesions
(d) Mid stenosis in LAD

426. All following finding are found in septal rupture after Acute myocardial infarction except
(a) Increase venous pressure
(b) Coarse systolic murmur (Crescendo–Decrescendo)
(c) Basal crepts
(d) Right sided S3 & S4

427. Acute MI following myocardial infarction has all following feature except
(a) Pan systolic murmur
(b) Increase venous pressure
(c) Pulmonary rales
(d) LVS3 and S4

428. Pathologic Q waves may be absent when infarct location is VS under except
(a) Apical infarct (b) Post infarct
(c) Lateral infarct (d) Septal infarct

429. Normal resting coronary blood flow is
(a) 0.5 ml/GLV mass/min
(b) < 0.5 ml/GLV mass/min
(c) 0.5 to 0.6 ml/GLV mass/min
(d) 0.7 – 0.9 ml/GLV mass/min

430. Which is ECG criteria favourable myocardium in infarct zone?
(a) Early disappearance of Q
(b) Early settling of ST sign
(c) Pseudonormalization of T
(d) None of the above

431. Which is most potent coronary dilator?
(a) Verapamil
(b) Diltiazem
(c) Nifedipine
(d) All the above 3 are similar

432. Anti thrombin deficiency cause commonly

(a) Arterial thrombosis
(b) Deep venus thrombosis
(c) Atrial thrombosis
(d) Ventricular thrombosis

433. All the following statements are correct except

(a) Angina is initial presentation in more in female than male
(b) Short term mortality is higher in female than male
(c) Long term mortality is high in female then male
(d) Initial presentation in myocardial infarction is higher in female than male

434. With all following antihypertensive drugs the cardiac output remains unchanged in pregnancy except

(a) Methyldopa (b) Labetalal
(c) Reserpine (d) Propranalal

435. All following Ca-blockers have myocardial, electrophysiological and vascular effect except

(a) Verapamil (b) Gallopamil
(c) Diltiazem (d) Nifedipine

436. Pedol edema is maximum with which Ca-blockers?

(a) Verapamil (b) Diltiazem
(c) Nitedipine (d) All the above

437. IV NTG is used in all the following situations except

(a) Acute LVF
(b) Variant angina
(c) Preoperative hypertension
(d) Chronic heart failure

438. Which Ca-blocker is powerful coronary dilator?

(a) Verapamil (b) Nifedipine
(c) Amlodipine (d) Diltiazem

439. Which Ca-blocker is most powerful peripheral vasodilator?

(a) Nifedipine (b) Diltiazem
(c) Verapamil (d) All of the above

440. All are physiological causes of hyperlipidemia except

(a) Weight gain after middle age
(b) Pregnancy after 2nd trimester
(c) Sedentery life style
(d) High protein diet

441. All the following drugs produce hyperlipidemia except

(a) Steroids (b) Hormones
(c) Thiazide diuretics (d) Calcium blockers

442. Which valvular lesion causes systolic hypertension?

(a) Mitral regurgitation
(b) Aortic stenosis
(c) Aortic regurgitation
(d) Mitral stenosis

443. Which Ca-antagonist has no effect on AV conduction?

(a) Diltiazem (b) Verapamil
(c) Nifedipine (d) None of the above

444. Abuept with darnel of which anti anginal is avoided in CAD?

(a) Nitrates (b) Nifedipine
(c) β-blocker (d) All of the above

445. Commonest location of free wall rupture is

(a) Left lat wall (b) Post wall
(c) Inferior wall (d) Apical

446. Free wall ruptures occurs more in all following situations except

(a) Advanced age (b) Females
(c) Males (d) Hypertension

447. Most common type of Na-sensitive hypertension is

(a) Non modulating essential hypertension

(b) Hypertension with bitaterial renal artery stenosis
(c) Hypertension with bilateral parenchyma disease
(d) Hypertension with primary aldosteronism

448. Which percentage of hypertension is sodium sensitive?

(a) 10 % (b) 80 %
(c) 20 % (d) 50–60 %

449. Earliest clinical index of cardiac involvement in hypertension is

(a) LVH
(b) Left atrial enlargement
(c) Both (a) and (b)
(d) None of the above

450. All the following cardiac surgical procedure are associated with hypertension except

(a) CABG
(b) Cardiac transplant
(c) Aortic valve replacement
(d) Pericardiectomy

451. Moderately high incidence of phaeochromocytoma may occur in which of the following cardiac disorder?

(a) RHD
(b) Pericardial disease
(c) Heart-muscle disease
(d) Cyanotic congenital heart disease

452. Drug of choice in hypertension associated with pneumoperitoneum for abdominal laproscopic surgery

(a) Diuretics (b) ACE inhibitors
(c) Ca-blockers (d) Clonidine

453. All the following are features of isolated systolic hypertension except

(a) Start after 55 years of age
(b) Due to arterial stiffness
(c) Main complications are stroke/heart failure
(d) β-blockers are the choice for treatment

454. Drug of choice for hypertension with benign prostate hypertrophy is

(a) β-blockers (b) α-blockers
(c) Ca-blocker (d) ACE inhibitors

455. Drug of choice for cyclosporine induced hypertension is

(a) α-blockers (b) β-blockers
(c) ACE inhibitors (d) Ca-blockers

456. Drug of choice for hypertension with myocardial infarction

(a) Diuretics (b) ACE inhibitors
(c) Ca-blockers (d) α-blockers

457. Atherosclerosis is characterized by all except

(a) Disease of intima
(b) Involves medium and large arteries
(c) Accumulation of smooth muscle cells and lipid within vessel wall
(d) Is a disease of media

458. An average expansion rate of abdominal aortic aneurysm is

(a) 0.1 cm/yr (b) 0.2–0.5 cm/yr
(c) 0.6–1 cm/yr (d) > 1 cm/yr

459. Most common cause of aortic dissection is

(a) Hypertension
(b) Genetic abnormality
(c) Ehlers-danlos syndrome
(d) Atherosclerosis

460. Most useful test for diagnosis of dissection of aorta is

(a) Echocardiography
(b) CT
(c) MRI
(d) Aortic angiography

461. Quantification of lower extremity occlusive arterial disease is best done by

(a) Ankle–brachial index
(b) Transcutaneous oximetry
(c) Doppler wave form analysis
(d) Exercise doppler testing

462. Anatomic localization of lower extremity arterial occlusion disease is best done by

(a) Doppler wave form analysis
(b) Trans cutaneous oximetry
(c) Segmental pressure analysis
(d) Pulse volume recording

463. Which arterial diseases cause hypertension?

(a) PAN
(b) Coarctation of aorta
(c) Renal artery stenosis
(d) All the above

464. Best drug out of the following in pregnancy with hypertension

(a) β-blockers (b) Diuretics
(c) Ca-blockers (d) ACE inhibitors

465. Stroke with severe hypertension the blood pressure cautiosly brought down with in few hours to

(a) 150/90 (b) 140/90
(c) 160/100 (d) 170/100

466. How many Indian are hypertensives in rural areas?

(a) 5 % (b) 8 %
(c) 10 % (d) 15 %

467. Stage I hypertension in indian population is

(a) 40 % (b) 50 %
(c) 70 % (d) 80 %

468. Maximum reduction of both systolic & diastolic blood pressure occurs with

(a) Candesartan (b) Irbisartan
(c) Losartan (d) Olmesartan

469. Only proven effective treatment of stent restenosis is

(a) Drug eluting stent
(b) Direct ablation atheroectomy
(c) Brachy therapy
(d) Cutting Balloon

470. Commonest cause of myocardial dysfunction is

(a) Coronary artery disesae
(b) Hypertension
(c) CMP (d) Myocarditis

471. All are mechanism of reduction of blood pressure by thiazolinedone except

(a) Insulin mediated vasodilatation
(b) Decreases intracellular Ca
(c) Decreases myocytes contractility
(d) Decreases endothelin secretion

472. Treatment of hypertension in elderly diabetic causes reduction in CV mortality by

(a) 30% (b) 40%
(c) 50% (d) > 75%

473. Diabetic macro complication are better prevented by

(a) Blood pressure control
(b) Glycemic control
(c) Similar by both
(d) All of the above

474. Insulin sensitizors in type II diabetes mellitus causes all lipid alterations except

(a) Decreases triglycerides
(b) Increases HDL
(c) Decreases LDL-C
(d) Decreases LDL-C oxidation

475. Insulin sensitizors in type II diabetes mellitus cause all the following except

(a) Decreases PAI-1
(b) Decreases fibrinogen
(c) Both of the above (d) None of the above

476. FACET and ABCT trials conclude which anti-hypertensive agent should not be used as first line therapy in diabetic hypertension patients

(a) β-blockers
(b) Thiazides
(c) Verapamil
(d) Dihydropyridines calcium channel blockers

477. Which of the following triggers lipid abnormalities in diabetic patients?

(a) Insulin deficiency (b) Insulin resistance
(c) Hyperglycemia (d) All the above

478. Small dense LDL particles cause enhanced atherosclerosis by all following mechanism except

(a) Bind to intimal proteoglycans more vividly
(b) More susceptable to oxidation and glycation
(c) Have impaired binding to LDL receptor
(d) May modify neutrophils

479. Maximum decrease in TG is obtained by

(a) Niacin
(b) Statins
(c) Bile acid sequestrants
(d) Ezitimibe

480. HDL-C is maximally increased by

(a) Niacin (b) Statins
(c) Fibrates (d) Ezitimibe

481. LDL-C is maximally decreased by

(a) Statins (b) Fibrates
(c) Ezitimibe (d) Niacin

482. Re infarct should be suspected in all except

(a) Prolonged ischemic pain
(b) ST increase and or normal
(c) Enzyme CK or troponin elevation of 100 % of the previous value
(d) > 150 % of the previous value

483. Modest consumption of alcohol (up to 30 G/day) is protective in coronary artery disease because of following except

(a) Increases HDL
(b) Decreases LDL
(c) Decreases fibrinogen
(d) Increases Apo lipoprotein A1

484. Which is compelling contraindication to Beta-blocker in hypertension?

(a) Advanced heart block
(b) Dyslipidemia
(c) Athletes
(d) Peripheral vascular disease

485. Low dose aspirin in hypertension in HOT study showed all the following

(a) 15% reduction in major cardiovascular events
(b) Stroke rate was not altered
(c) All cause mortality was not altered
(d) The benefits are seen in all hypertensives (Low risk & high risk)

486. Ambulatory blood pressure monitoring should be considered in all the following except

(a) Variability in blood pressure
(b) High cardiovascular risk
(c) Symptoms of hypotension
(d) Resistant hypertension

487. All the following are effective drug combinations in hypertension except

(a) Diuretics + Beta-blocker
(b) Diuretics + ACE inhibitors
(c) Calcium antagonists + ACE inhibitors
(d) Calcium antagonists + Diuretics

488. Compelling contra indication to diuretic use in hypertension is

(a) Dyslipidemia
(b) Electrolyte disturbances
(c) Gout
(d) All of the above

489. All are local complications of cardiopulmonary by pass except

(a) Thrombosis (b) Embolism
(c) Hemorrhage (d) Heart failure

490. To prevent death the best drug for 5 weeks in acute myocardial infarction is

(a) Aspirin (b) Streptokinin
(c) A + B (d) All Similar

491. Which is commonest complication of PTCA?

(a) Death
(b) Acute myocardial infarction
(c) Abrupt closure
(d) Re stenosis (clinical)

492. All following conditions increases risk from cardiopulmonary by pass except

(a) Previous stroke (b) Renal disease
(c) COPD (d) Hypertension

493. Which is the commonest complication of streptokinin therapy in acute myocardial infarction?

(a) Hemorrhagic stroke
(b) Major bleed
(c) Allergic reaction (d) Hypertension

494. DVT most commonly occurs in which vein?

(a) Calf vein
(b) Any vein of leg
(c) Veins of upper extremity
(d) All of the above

495. All the following are complications of DVT except

(a) Pulmonary embolism
(b) Post thrombotic syndrome
(c) Pulmonary hypertension
(d) Systemic embolism

496. All following are at high risk for venous thromboembolism except

(a) Upper limb amputation
(b) Major surgery in patients with previous DVT
(c) Major pelvic or abdominal surgery for malignancy
(d) Major orthopedic surgery of pelvis

497. 4S study riveted all the following except

(a) Was done in CAD with hyperlipidemia
(b) Included 4444 cases
(c) Simvastatin was used 20–40 mg /day
(d) No effect on progression of atherosclerosis through out the vascular system

498. Most frequent presentation of acute myocardial infarction in elderly is

(a) Acute LVF
(b) CVA
(c) Peripheral embolism
(d) Atypical chest pain

499. U shaped tortuous retinal arterioles are found in hypertension associated with

(a) Phaechromocytoma
(b) Hyperthyroidism
(c) Coarctation of aorta
(d) Reno vascular disease

500. Stabilization of plaque in coronary artery disease occurs by statins were LDL-C in reduced by

(a) 5% (b) 10%
(c) 15% (d) 20%

501. HDL level are increased by all except

(a) Almonds
(b) Exercise
(c) Moderate alcohol intake
(d) None of the above

502. All of the following drugs increases HDL-C levels except

(a) Nicotinic acid
(b) Fibrates
(c) Ezetimibe
(d) Inhibitors of cholesterol ester transfer protein (CETP)

503. Which of the following drugs maximally increase HDL-C?

(a) Inhibitors of CETP
(b) Nicotinic Acid
(c) Statins
(d) Fibrates

504. Which is best ACE inhibitor for protection in stable CAD?

(a) Ramipril (b) Perindopril
(c) Trandolapril (d) None of the above

505. All are cardioprotective Beta-blockers in post myocardial infarction causes except

(a) Propranolol (b) Bisoprolol
(c) Atenolol (d) Metoprolol

506. Smoking causes loss of cardio protection effect of which β-blockers?

(a) Atenolol (b) Metaprolol
(c) Propranolol (d) Bisoprolol

507. Calcium scoring is not valuable in all the following except

(a) Young with or without risk factors
(b) In high risk for coronary events
(c) Add both to the TMT
(d) In equivocal TMT

508. Most important test for detection of peripheral pulmonary embolism is

(a) Echo
(b) Lung scan
(c) Pulmonary angiography
(d) Spiral CT screening

509. Most common causes of reversible hypertension is

(a) Pregnancy endeared HT
(b) Pheachromacytoma
(c) Alcohol abase > 3 drink/day
(d) Porphyria

510. Most commonly used treatment of pulmonary embolism is

(a) Heparin
(b) Thrombolysis
(c) Surgical embolecting
(d) Catheter thrombosis fragmentation

511. Elderly hypertensive patients derive most benefit from therapy because of the following except

(a) At high risk
(b) Higher systolic blood pressure
(c) Lowering of systolic blood pressure crucial
(d) More responsive to treatment

512. Which antihypertensive agent produces hemolytic anemia?

(a) β-blockers (b) Ca-blocker
(c) Methyldopa (d) ACE inhibitors

513. Eruptive xanthomas are usually present in

(a) Increased TG
(b) Increased TC
(c) Increased TG + TC
(d) Decreased HDLC

514. Symptomatic CAD with diffuse atherosclerosis not amenable for revascularization the preferred treatment is

(a) Enhanced external comter pulsation
(b) Spinal cord stimulation
(c) Gene therapy
(d) Metabolic modulators of myocardial ischemia

515. Refractory cases of microvascular angina are best treated by

(a) Aminophylline (b) Imipramine
(c) Estrogen (d) All of the above

516. Microvascular angina is characterized by all the following except

(a) Atypical chest pain
(b) More in females
(c) Spasm of coronary arteries play dominant role
(d) Positive stress test

517. Abdominal aortic aneurysm needs surgery if

(a) 3 cm in diameter
(b) 4 cm in diameter
(c) 5 cm in diameter
(d) > 5.5 cm in diameter with symptoms

518. Postural tachycardia syndrome is caused by all the following except

(a) Post viral
(b) Diabetes mellitus
(c) Amyloidosis
(d) Coronary artery disease

519. Takayasu's arterits has all the following features except

(a) Predominantly occurs in asian females > 40 years
(b) Evidence of diffuse vascular disease
(c) Vascular aneurysm are found
(d) Renovascular hypertension

520. Commonest risk factor for myocardial infarction with normal coronary arteries

(a) Diabetes mellitus (b) Hypertension
(c) Hyperlipidemia (d) Smoking

521. All the following are the features of myocardial infarction with normal coronary arteries except

(a) Occurs often in young
(b) Spasm may be a factor
(c) Hyperlipidemia is often found
(d) None of the above

522. Most specific electrocardiographic sign of atrial infarction is

(a) PR segment elevation
(b) Bifid P in L2
(c) Increase P in V1
(d) Atrial arrhythmia

523. Commonest cardiovascular feature of polyarteritis nodosa is

(a) Hypertension
(b) Myocardial infarction
(c) Valvular heart disease
(d) Pericardial disease

524. Post prandial angina typically indicates all the following except

(a) Extensive disease
(b) Proximal occlusion
(c) Impaired LV function
(d) Mild disease

525. Which precipitator of angina indicates severe coronary artery disease

(a) Effort (b) Emotion
(c) Cold weather (d) Post meals

526. Least common arrhythmia in acute myocardial infarction is

(a) Atrial fibrillation
(b) Atrial flutter
(c) Ventricular fibrillation
(d) Accelerated idioventricular rhythm

527. All the following statements are true except in myocardial bridging

(a) External compressive epicardial artery
(b) Can lead to myocardial infarction
(c) Is common in normal hearts
(d) Bridged arterial segments are prone to atherosclerosis

528. Which of the following plaque is most vulnerable to produce thrombosis?

(a) Thin cap fibroatheroma
(b) Erosion
(c) Calcified nodule
(d) All of the above

529. Which is best biomarker to predict mortality in non ST elevation acute myocardial infarction?

(a) Troponin-T
(b) Troponin-I
(c) NT-Pro BNP
(d) C-Reactive proteins

530. Which biomarker has strongest relationship with development of subsequent myocardial infarction?

(a) Troponin-T
(b) BNP
(c) C-Reactive protein
(d) All the above

531. All the following situations favour ACE inhibitors as first choice in hypertension except

(a) Type 2 DM
(b) Gout
(c) Hyperlipidemia
(d) Perioperative hypertension

532. All the following situations favour use of diuretics as first choice in hypertension except

(a) With high salt intake
(b) Renal disease with Na retention
(c) Blacks
(d) Gout

533. All the following situations favour initial use of calcium antagonists in hypertension except

(a) Blacks
(b) High salt intake
(c) Associated vasospastic angina
(d) Perioperative hypertension

534. All the following situations favour initial use of Beta-blockers in hypertension except

(a) Associated coronary artery disease
(b) Bilateral renal artery stenosis
(c) Migraine
(d) Variant angina

535. Antihypertensive drug of choice in elderly is

(a) Diuretics (b) ACE Inhibitors
(c) Ca-blockers (d) β-blockers

536. ST elevation in unstable angina usually indicates

(a) Small vessel disease
(b) Double vessel disease
(c) Triple vessel disease
(d) Normal coronary arteries

537. Protective effect of moderate alcohol consumption is related to all the following mechanism except

(a) Increase HDL-C
(b) Improvement of haemostatic factors
(c) Reduction in insulin resistance
(d) Decrease in LDL-C

538. Least reduction of blood pressure is achieved by which life style modification

(a) Regular exercise
(b) Limited alcohol intake
(c) Na restriction (d) DASH eating plan

539. Which dietary changes maximally decreases LDL cholesterol?

(a) Saturated Fat < 7 % of calories
(b) Dietary cholesterol < 200 mg/day
(c) Weigh loss (10 pound)
(d) Total LDL cholesterol decrease

540. Both CABG and AVR is needed in AS in which coronary artery involvement

(a) RCA lesion (b) LAD lesion
(c) Cx lesion (d) Left main lesion

541. In inferior myocardial infarction AV conduction defect has all the following features except

(a) Site of block is AV node
(b) Artery involved is RCA
(c) Narrow QRS complex
(d) Often permanent

542. In anterior myocardial infarction AV conduction defect has all the following features except

(a) Wide QRS
(b) Ventricular rate < 40/min
(c) 4 time more mortality vs compared to without block
(d) Permanent

543. Which statement is incorrect regarding lower extremity blood pressure in normal person?

(a) Systolic blood pressure is same as upper extremity
(b) Systolic blood pressure is higher in lower extremity than upper extremity
(c) DBP is lower in lower extremity than upper extremity
(d) All of the above

544. Ambulatory blood pressure measurement is helpful all the following except

(a) Excluding white coat hypertension
(b) Hypertension with out target organ damage
(c) To ascertain prognosis
(d) To identify nocturnal dipping status

545. Family history is positive in essential hypertension in what percentage of patients

(a) < 20% (b) 40%
(c) 60% (d) > 80%

546. Arterial stiffness is reduced by all the following in hypertension except

(a) Salt decrease (b) Weight decrease
(c) Physical activity (d) Diuretics

547. Which of the following is convenient method for settling the issue of pseudo hypertension?

(a) Finger blood pressure measurement
(b) Wrist blood pressure
(c) Direct recording (intravascular)
(d) All of the above

548. All the following factors are associated with nocturnal nondipping in hypertension except

(a) DM (b) Old age
(c) LVH (d) Hyperlipidemia

549. When measuring the blood pressure which is Better?

(a) Bell of stethoscope
(b) Diaphragm of stethoscope
(c) Either of the above
(d) Finger palpatron

550. All the following are causes of low renin hypertension except

(a) Hyperaldosteronism
(b) Essential hypertension
(c) Phaeochromocytoma
(d) Parenchymal renal disease

551. All the following are causes of normal rennin hypertension except

(a) Essential hypertension
(b) Cushing's syndrome
(c) Coarctation of aorta
(d) Adrenal carcinoma

552. Most common arrhythmia in acute anterior myocardial infarction is

(a) VT (b) CHB
(c) VF (d) AF

553. Most common complication of PTCA is

(a) Prolonged angina
(b) Myocardial infarction
(c) Coronary dissection
(d) Coronary spasm

554. All the following ischemia syndromes are associated with coronary artery spasm except

(a) Prinzmetal's angina
(b) MVP
(c) Monday morning angina in nitroglycerin workers
(d) Aortic stenosis

555. Most common arrhythmia in acute myocardial infarction is

(a) PVC (b) VT
(c) Sinus brady cardia (d) CHB

556. All following metals are related to hypertension development except

(a) Lead (b) Arsenic
(c) Carbon disulphide (d) Copper

557. All following blood components are related to hypertension except

(a) RBC count (b) WBC count
(c) Fibrinogen level (d) Platelets count

558. Following coronary risk factors is internal have been proved to lower risk except

(a) Smokning (b) Elevated LDL-C
(c) Hypertension (d) DM

559. All following risk factors if internal am likely to lower risk except

(a) DM
(b) Decrease HDL-C
(c) Increase TG
(d) Thrombogenic with risk factures

560. Nitrates are indicated in acute myocardial infarction in all the following situations except

(a) Ongoing ischemia in acute myocardial infarction
(b) Hypertension

(c) LVF
(d) Right ventricular infarction

561. Less regression of LVH in hypertensive occurs with which of the following?

(a) ACE Inhibitors (b) ARBs
(c) Ca-blocker (d) β-blockers

562. In hypertensive pilots which drug is avoided?

(a) ACE Inhibitors (b) ARBs
(c) Ca-blockers (d) Clonidine

563. Which antihypertensive drug can causes increased bleeding during surgery?

(a) β-blockers (b) Ca-blockers
(c) ACE inhibitors (d) Clonidine

564. Phentolamine is specifically indicated in which hypertension?

(a) Essential hypertension
(b) Pregnancy related HT
(c) Hypertension in phaeochromocytoma
(d) Hypertension related to increased intracranial hypertension

565. ARBs are potentially better than ACE inhibitors in which following situation?

(a) Hypertension
(b) Proteinuric renal disease
(c) Heart failure
(d) Neuroprotection

566. ACE inhibitors are superior to ARB's in which of the following situation?

(a) Hypertension
(b) Proteinuric renal disease
(c) Heart failure
(d) Reduction of heart attacks in high risk patients

567. Combination of ACE inhibitors and ARBs is particularly useful in which condition?

(a) Hypertension
(b) Heart failure
(c) Proteinuric patients
(d) Neuroprotection

568. All the following antihypertensive drugs are primary vasodilators except

(a) Ca-blockers
(b) α-blockers
(c) ACE inhibitors/ARBS
(d) Diuretics

569. All the following are clinical characteristics of accelerated malignant hypertension except

(a) Diastolic blood pressure usually > 140 mm Hg
(b) LVH
(c) Fundus shows hemorrhage, exudates, papilloedema
(d) Renal dysfunction

570. Which of the following antihypertensive drug initialty reduces cardiac output?

(a) ACE inhibitors (b) ARB's
(c) β-blockers (d) Ca-blockers

571. All the following antihypertensives require no dose modification in CRF except

(a) Ca-blockers (b) ARBs
(c) Clonidine (d) ACE inhibitors

572. All the following antihypertensive require dose modification in CRF except

(a) ACE inhibitors (b) Atenolol
(c) Nadolol (d) α-blockers

573. All the following antilipidemic drugs require dose modification except

(a) Statins (b) Fenofibrates
(c) Benofibrates (d) Ezetimibe

574. Which antilipidemic agent reduces proteinuria and slow the progression of CRD?

(a) Simvastatin (b) Fenofibrate
(c) Atorvastatin (d) Lovastatin

575. Which ARB causes abdominal pain?

(a) Losartan (b) Valsartan
(c) Irbesartan (d) Telmesartan

576. Maximum reduction of blood pressure occurs with which ARB?

(a) Olmesartan (b) Valsartan
(c) Telmesartan (d) Losartan

577. Aerobic excercise reduces blood pressure by all the following mechanisms except

(a) Increase NO production
(b) Decreases sympathetic activity
(c) Decreases arterial stiffness
(d) Decreases stroke volume

578. Which insect bite may causes hypertension?

(a) Spider (b) Scorpion
(c) Both of the above (d) None of the above

579. Clonidine may be particularly useful in hypertensive with following conditions except

(a) Restless leg syndrome
(b) Menopausal hot flushes
(c) Diarrhoea due to diabetic nephropathy
(d) To prevent recurrent stroke

580. α-blockers are particularly useful in hypertension with all the fancus except

(a) BPH (b) Impotence
(c) Increase lipids
(d) Postural hypertension

581. Hypertension in hypothyriodsm in has all following features except

(a) More often diastolic hypertension
(b) Have highest SNS activity
(c) Is a volume dependent hypertension
(d) Have low cardiac output

582. Hypertension in hyperthyroid is has all following features except

(a) Both systolic and diastolic hypertension
(b) Only stolic hypertension
(c) Diastolic blood pressure normal
(d) Only systolic hypertension

583 Only prover effective means of treating in-restenosis is

(a) PTCA
(b) Cutting balloon angioplasty
(c) Rotablation drug (d) Brachy therapy

584. All following are mechanism of hypertension in obstructive sleep apnea except

(a) Increase SNS activity
(b) Increase enothelon 1
(c) Blunted vasodilating response
(d) Increased cardiac output

585. Persestant severe hypertension of head injury is best trcuted by

(a) IV nitroprusside (b) Hydralazine
(c) IV Esmolal (d) IV Nitroglyerone

586. Which antihypertensive agent causes rebound hypertension on withdrawal?

(a) Thiazides (b) β-blockers
(c) Clonidine (d) Amlodipine

587. Best drug for hypertensive in post menopausal women is

(a) Ca-blocker (b) β-blockers
(c) ACE inhibitor (d) Thiazide divretrcy

588. Which life style modification reduces blood pressure maximally?

(a) Weight reduction
(b) DASH eating plan
(c) Sodium reduction
(d) Moderate alcohol consumption

589. P Fox inhibitors are used as

(a) Anti arrhythmic (b) Anti ischemic
(c) Anti congestive (d) All of the above

590. Silent ischemia occurs least frequently in

(a) LAD lesion
(b) Cx lesion
(c) RcA lesion
(d) Extensive coronary artery disease

591. Pathological hallmark of pulmonary arterial hypertension is

(a) Proliferation of endothelial cells
(b) Proliferation of smooth muscle cells
(c) Myofibroblast (d) Macrophages

592. Most commonly used treatment of pulmonary embolism in community hospital is

(a) Heparin
(b) Thrombolytics
(c) Embolectomy
(d) Catheter thrombus fragmentation

593. All the following lipoprotien classes have ApoB100 except

(a) VLDL (b) HDL
(c) IDL (d) LDL

594. All the following statins are lipophyllic except

(a) Simvastatin (b) Pravastatin
(c) Atorvastatin (d) Rosuva statin

595. All the following are more common in females than males in ACS except

(a) Mortality (b) Pulmonary edema
(c) Cardigenic shock (d) VF

596. Maximum risk reduction occurs with which strategy in patients with established cardiovascular disease

(a) Lipid lowering (b) Beta-blockers
(c) ACE inhibitors (d) Aspirin

597. Which of the following drug is most proven to reduce mortality in acute myocardial infarction both in early phase and at long-term

(a) Verapamil (b) Magnesium
(c) Nitrates (d) β-blockers

598. Oral drug in hypertension emergencies is

(a) β-blockers (b) Diuretic
(c) Captopul (d) Losartan

599. All the following are correct for step I diet except

(a) Total fat < 40%
(b) Saturated fat < 10%
(c) Chotesteriol < 300 / day
(d) All of the above

600. All the following are correct for step II diet

(a) Total fat < 30%
(b) Saturated fat < 7%
(c) Cholesterol 250 mg / day
(d) None of the above

601. TG is Increased by which Hypolipidemic Agent?

(a) Atorvastatin (b) Gemofibrozil
(c) Cholestyramine (d) Nicotnic acid

602. HDL–C increased by all except

(a) Nicotenic acid (b) Cremfibiozil
(c) Probucal (d) Atorvastatin

603. Which histological changes pulmonary vascular tree indicates irreversible pulmonary vascular obstruction?

(a) Medial thickening (b) Intimal thickening
(c) Both (a) and (b) (d) Plexi form lesion

604. Which of the following indicates good myocardial function in heart disease?

(a) Sinus bradycardia (b) Sinus tachycardia
(c) Sinus arrhythmia (d) None of the above

605. Which secondary systemic hypertensives usually do not exhibit fundal changes?

(a) Renal
(b) Coarctation of sorta
(c) Hyperaldsteronism
(d) Pregnancy telated hypertension

606. First line drug for treatment of uncomplicated hypertension in patients < 55 years age is

(a) β-blocker (b) Thiazides
(c) ACE inhibitors (d) Any of the above

607. Sphygmonometer is a instrument to measure which one of the following?

(a) Femoral artery pressure
(b) Brachial artery pressure
(c) Aortic pressure
(d) None of the above

608. Which of the following location for blood pressure measurement is ideal?

(a) Aortic pressure
(b) Brachial artery pressure
(c) Femoral artery pressure
(d) All the above

609. Best drug to reduce central aortic pressure is

(a) ACE inhibitors (b) β-blockers
(c) Diuretics (d) Methyldopa

610. Most common cause of chest pain at rest

(a) Unstable angina
(b) Variant angina
(c) Non cardiac chest pain
(d) Acute myocardial infarction

611. Pumpkin heart is found in

(a) Large pericardial effusion
(b) Severe congestive heart failure
(c) Ebstein's anomaly
(d) Transposition of great arteries

612. Acute apical VSD following acute myocardial infarction has all following feature except

(a) Often occurs in acute anterior myocardial infarction
(b) Often occurs during first myocardial infarction
(c) Often occurs with associated hypertension
(d) Often occurs in young

613. Most common risk factor for development of ascending aortic aneurysm is

(a) Smoking (b) Hyperlipidemia
(c) Hypertension (d) Age over 65 years

614. Best initial screening test for ascending aortic aneurysm is

(a) Ultrasound (b) CT
(c) Angiography (d) All the above

615. Microvascular angina does not occurs at which time of the day?

(a) Morning hours (b) Afternoon
(c) Evening (d) Night

616. Drug of choice for refractory microvascular angina

(a) Antiplatelet (b) Nitrates
(c) Ca-blockers (d) Imipramine

617. Which of the following drug is avoided in cocaine induced increase acute coronary syndrome?

(a) Nitrates
(b) Aspirin
(c) Thrombolytics agents
(d) β-blockers

618. LV aneurysm occur commonly with

(a) Single vessel disease
(b) Small vessel disease
(c) Double vessel disease
(d) Multi vessel disease

619. Rupture of free wall of which chamber is most common in acute myocardial infarction

(a) Left ventricle (b) Right ventricle
(c) Right atrium (d) Left atrium

620. Which therapy has reduced the frequency of LV free wall rupture in acute myocardial infarction?

(a) Antiplatelet (b) Thrombolytics
(c) Anticoagulants (d) Nitrates

621. In which anginal syndrome aspirin increase severity of ischemia?

(a) S4
(b) Minimal effort angina of recent onset
(c) Acute myocardial infarction
(d) Variant angina

622. Variant angina is common in

(a) India (b) China
(c) Japan (d) Pakistan

623. Which syndrome of myocardial ischemia presents with severe chest pain

(a) SA
(b) Progressive SA
(c) Acute myocardial infarction
(d) Variant angina

624. Which is best drug to reduce silent myocardial ischemia?

(a) Nitrates (b) β-blockers
(c) Ca-blockers (d) Antiplatelet agent

625. All following Beta-blockers are best studied in post infarct protection except

(a) Atenolol (b) Propranolol
(c) Metoprolol (d) Carvedilol

626. Which of the following cholesterol reduction correlate best with cardiovascular risk reduction?

(a) Decrease total cholesterol
(b) Decrease LDL cholesterol
(c) Decrease TG
(d) Increase HDL-C

627. Maximum efficacy of lipid lowering treatment is achieved in

(a) I week's time (b) 2 week's time
(c) 3 week's time (d) 4 week's time

628. At what age systolic BP is most important risk factor than diastolic blood pressure?

(a) Age 10 – 20 years (b) Age 20 – 25 years
(c) Age 26 – 40 years (d) Age > 50 years

629. Single most effective therapy in uncomplicated hypertension is

(a) Low dose thiazide diuretics
(b) Calcium blocker
(c) β-blockers
(d) ACE inhibitors

630. Which β-blockers might not increase the risk of stroke in treatment of hypertension?

(a) Atenolol (b) Propanolol
(c) Metoprolol (d) Nebivolol

631. Addition of ezetimibe to statins causes addsional reduction LDL-C by

(a) 10% (b) 20%
(c) 15% (d) 25%

632. Beneficial effects of statins are related to

(a) Age
(b) Gender
(c) Base line serum cholesterol
(d) All the above

633. Which of the following antianginal agents has no haemodynamic effect?

(a) Nitrates (b) Nicorandil
(c) Trimetazidine (d) Beta-blockers

634. In middle aged and elderly total and vascular mortality is strongly and directly correlated with blood pressure beyond

(a) 120/80 (b) 115/75
(c) 130/90 (d) 140/89

635. Which blood pressure is better indication of cardiovascular risk?

(a) Systolic blood pressure
(b) Diastolic blood pressure
(c) Both (a) and (b)
(d) Mean arterial pressure

636. How frequent is LVH in severe hypertension on echo?

(a) 20% (b) 30%
(c) 40% (d) 50%

637. Which antihypertensive does not reduce LVH in hypertension?

(a) ACE inhibitor (b) Diuretics
(c) Beta-blockers (d) Minoxidil

638. Significant reduction of blood pressure occurs with how much reduction in weight

(a) 2 kg (b) 3 kg
(c) 4 kg (d) ≥ 4.5 kg

639. In practice what level of salt intake is recommended?

(a) 2 g/day (b) 3 g/day
(c) 4 g/day (d) 6 g/day

640. In posterior myocardial infarction direct changes are seen in which leads?

(a) V1 – V2 (b) V5 – V6
(c) L1 – aVR (d) V8 – V9

641. All following antihypertensives cause sinus node dysfunction except

(a) Clonidine (b) β-blockers
(c) Methyldopa (d) Losartan

642. Use of β-blocker in STEMI benefits in all the following except

(a) Recurrent ischemia reduction
(b) Reduction in ventricular ectopics
(c) Reduction progression threatened infarction to completed infarction
(d) Reduces development AV block

643. On predischarge exercise ECG in acute myocardial infarction which of the parameter has highest sensitivity of cardiac death?

(a) ST depression
(b) Impaired systolic blood pressure
(c) Exercise duration (d) Angina

644. On predischarge exercise ECG in acute myocardial infarction which of the following parameter has highest specificity for cardiac death?

(a) ST depression
(b) Impaired systolic blood pressure
(c) Exercise duration (d) Angina

645. For late detection (22 hours after chest pain) of acute myocardial infarction which test is most sensitive and specific?

(a) Trop-T
(b) Trop-I
(c) Total CK-MB activity
(d) Total CK-MB mass

646. Which test more sensitive marker of acute myocardial infarction at 2 hours after chest pain?

(a) Total CK-MB activity
(b) Myoglobin
(c) Troponin T
(d) Troponin I

647. Which test is most specific marker of acute myocardial infarction at 2 hours after chest pain?

(a) Total CK-MB activity
(b) Troponin T
(c) Troponin I (d) Myoglobin

648. Hibernating myocardium has all following feature except

(a) Reduced coronary flow
(b) Typical histological charges
(c) No lactate production
(d) Recovers spontaneously

649. All following factors are thrombogenic except

(a) Hypercholesteremia
(b) DM
(c) Hypertension
(d) Smoking

650. All the following conditions may be associated with coronary vasculitis except

(a) Buerger's disease
(b) Marfan's syndrome
(c) Infective endocarditis
(d) Polyarterites nodosa

651. Spontaneous coronary artery dissection may occur in all the following condition except

(a) Pericardium
(b) Hypertension
(c) Aortic root dissection
(d) Diabetes mellitus

652. HDL-C is maximally increased by

(a) Status
(b) Niacin
(c) Omega-3 fatty acids
(d) Resins

653. TG is maximally decreased by

(a) Fibrates
(b) Statins
(c) Omega-3 fatty acids
(d) Ezetimibe

654. All following drugs if used with statins are risk factors for development of myopathy except

(a) Cyclosporins
(b) Azoles antifungale
(c) Macrolide antibiotics
(d) β-blockers

655. LDL-C is maximally reduced by

(a) Statins (b) Niacin
(c) Fibrates (d) Ezetimibe

656. Which drug produces coronary vasospasm?

(a) Doxorubicin (b) 5-Fluorouracil
(c) Cyclophosphamide
(d) Interluekin-2

657. Which vascular ulcer has most severe pain?

(a) Venous (b) Arterial
(c) Neuropathic (d) Arteriolar

658. Wet vascular ulcer is found in

(a) Venous (b) Neuropathic
(c) Arterial (d) Arteriolar

659. Which antihypertensive drug produces neonatal meconium ileus during pregnancy?

(a) Diureties (b) β-blockers
(c) Methydopa
(d) Ganglionic blockers

660. Which antihypertensive drug in pregnancy produces neonatal thrombocytopenia?

(a) Thiazides (b) Methyldopa
(c) Clonidine (d) Reserpine

661. Systemic vascular resistance is deceased most by

(a) Nitrous oxide (b) Fentanyl
(c) Enflurane (d) Morphine

662. Most sensitive method for detection of dissection of descending aorta is

(a) TTE (b) TEE
(c) PT (d) MRI

663. Most specific method for detection of dissection of arch aorta is

(a) TTE (b) TEE
(c) CT (d) MRI

664. Most specific method for detection of dissection ascending aorta

(a) TTE (b) TEE
(c) CT (d) MRI

665. Which is most sensitive method for detection of dissection of aorta?

(a) Trans thoracic echo
(b) Trans esophagcal echo
(c) CT
(d) MRI

666. Increased activity of lipoprotein liprase occurs with which drug

(a) Nicotinic acid (b) Statins
(c) Fibrates (d) Ezetimibe

667. Increased activity of LDL receptors occurs with

(a) Nicotinic acid
(b) Statins
(c) Bile acid segnestrants
(d) Fibrates

668. Following are the common cardiac manifestation of hypertension except

(a) Heart failure
(b) Arrhythmia
(c) Ischemic syndrome
(d) Valvular lesion

669. All following vascular alteration in hypertension except

(a) Endothelial dysfunction
(b) Vascular remodeling
(c) Reduced compliance
(d) Reduced reactivity

670. All following drugs decrease digoxin plasma level except

(a) Neomycin
(b) Erythroycin
(c) Sulfasalazine
(d) P-Amino salicylic acid

671. Which is the rarest coronary artery anomaly?

(a) Separate ostia for LAD & LX
(b) RCA from left CA
(c) Circumflex from right CA
(d) Single coronary artery

672. Most common complication with 24 hours of coronary angiography is

(a) Death
(b) Myocardial infarction
(c) VT
(d) Acute renal failure

673. Which is the common coronary artery anomaly?

(a) Separate ostia for LAD & LX
(b) Coronary-Pulmonary artery fistula
(c) RCA from left coronary sinus
(d) Single coronary artery

674. Most specific method for predicting cardiac CV event after myocardial infarction

(a) Rest ejection fraction
(b) Killip class
(c) Positive exercise test
(d) Anterior myocardial infarction

675. All following Ca-blockers have active metabolic except

(a) Verapamil (b) Diltiazem
(c) Nifedipine (d) All of the above

676. All following antihypertensive drugs may cause pericardial disease except

(a) Hydralazime (b) Caplopril
(c) Minoxidial (d) Diuretics

677. All following parasitic disease may involve pericardium except

(a) Amoebiasis (b) Filariasis
(c) Hydatid disease (d) None of these

678. All following fungal organism may involve pericardium except

(a) Actinomycosis (b) Aspergillosis
(c) Candidiasis (d) None of these

679. All following agents cause vasculitis except

(a) Gold (b) Arsenic
(c) Lead (d) DDT

680. Aortitis does not occurs in all following connective disorders except

(a) Rheumatoid arthritis
(b) Systemic lupus erythromatosis
(c) Scleroderm
(d) Ankylosing spondylitis

681. Which hematological disorder may cause hypertension?

(a) Anaemia (b) CML
(c) Acute leukemia (d) Sickle cell crisis

682. Which G1 disorder may cause hypertension?

(a) Pancreatitis
(b) Cholecystitis
(c) Acid peptic disease
(d) IBS

683. All are cause of systolic hypertension except?

(a) Aortic regurgitation
(b) In elderly
(c) Thyroloxicosis
(d) Increased intravascular volume

684. Which metal poisoning may cause hypertension?

(a) Copper (b) Zinc
(c) Lead (d) Arsenic

685. All following are intra arterial sources of embolic material except

(a) Thrombus (b) AIR
(c) Cholesterol (d) Tumor

686. All are cardiac sources of embolic material except

(a) Thrombus (b) Vegetation
(c) Calcium (d) Cholesterol

687. All following are gastrointestinal manifestation of atheroembolism except

(a) Mesenteric ischemia
(b) Splenic enlargement
(c) Pancreatitis
(d) Intestinal bleeding

688. All are neurological manifestation of atheroembolism except

(a) TIA
(b) Stroke
(c) Amaurosis fungax
(d) Subarachnoid hemorrhage

689. All are renal manifestation of atheroembolism except

(a) Renal failure
(b) Renal abscess
(c) Uncontrolled hypertension
(d) None of above

690. Statins interact with all the following drugs except

(a) Erythromycin (b) Neomycin
(c) Antifungal (d) Cyclosporin

691. All following natural agents are used in hypertension except

(a) Aconite (b) Garlic
(c) Co QIW (d) Ginkgobiloba

692. All are indication of nitrates in acute myocardial infarction except

(a) Persistent and recurrent chest pain
(b) Sustained hypertension
(c) Acute pulmonary edema
(d) Right ventricular infarction

693. Which nitrate preparation has longest duration of action?

(a) Oral isosorbide dinitrate
(b) Oral NTG
(c) NTG ointment
(d) NTG discs patch

694. Which Ca antagonist is vasculoselective?

(a) Flunarizine (b) Nifedipine
(c) Nimodipine (d) Diltiazem

695. Which Ca antagonist has complex pharmacological profile?

(a) Verapamil (b) Nifedipine
(c) Beperiail (d) Felodipine

696. Which Ca antagonist has fastest onset of action when given orally?

(a) Diltiazem (b) Nifedipine
(c) Verapamil (d) None of these

697. Which Ca antagonist interacts maximally with digoxin?

(a) Verapamil (b) Nifedipine
(c) Diltiazem (d) None of these

698. Which antianginal increases cardiac contractility?

(a) Nitrates (b) Verapamil
(c) Diltiazem (d) β-blockers

699. Which anti anginal does not dilate coronary arteries?

(a) Nitrate (b) β-blocker
(c) Ca-blocker (d) All of the above

700. Which anti anginal does not reduce silent ischemia?

(a) Verapamil (b) Diltiazem
(c) β-blocker (d) Nitrates

701. Tolerance develops to which antianginal?

(a) Nitrate (b) Verapamil
(c) Diltiazem (d) β-blocker

702. Which drug is not used in variant angina?

(a) Nitrate (b) β-blockers
(c) Verapamil (d) Diltiazem

703. Tinnitus occurs with which Ca antagonists

(a) Verapamil (b) Nifedipine
(c) Diltiazem (d) All of the above

704. Which drug prevents sudden death and reinfarction?

(a) Nitrate (b) Nifedipine
(c) β-blockers (d) Verapamil

705. Which drugs present sudden cardiac death in coronary artery disease?

(a) β-blockers (b) Aspirin
(c) Statins (d) Ca-blockers

706. Which lipid lowering agent prolongs QT interval?

(a) Pravastatin (b) Resins
(c) Fibrates (d) Probucal

707. Statins have which of the following properties?

(a) Antihypertensive (b) Cardioprotective
(c) Antiischaemic (d) All of them

708. ACE inhibitor don't have which of the following property

(a) Anti ischamic
(b) Antihypertension
(c) Cardiovascular protective
(d) All of them

709. Aspirin has which of the following action

(a) Antihypertension
(b) Antiischaemic
(c) Cardiovascular protective
(d) All of the above

710. Which of the following properties is handeted by β-blocker?

(a) Antiischamic (b) Antihypertensive
(c) Cardioprotective (d) Cardioprotective

711. DBP maximally rass with which of the following activity compased to relaxing line

(a) Mecting (b) Corking
(c) Entary (d) Dressing

712. Non dippring is associated with all the following except

(a) LVH
(b) Normal renal function
(c) DM
(d) Obesity

713. Low blood pressure is recorded if it is measured in following situation except

(a) Arm above heart level
(b) Too rapid deflation
(c) Excess bell pressure
(d) During talking

714. Maximum rise of SBP occurs complamed to relaxating stage all which activity

(a) Meetings (b) Telephone
(c) Cature (d) Walking

715. All following factors don't blood pressure accruing except

(a) Menstrual phase
(b) Chronic cafferise ingestion
(c) Thin shiot undercut
(d) Recent meal

716. High blood pressure recorded if measured in following situations except

(a) Cuff too narrow
(b) Arm below heart level
(c) Arm unsupported (d) Low mercury level

717. In children which type of fibromusclar dysplasia of renal artery is most common?

(a) Intimal (b) Medial
(c) Adventitial (d) None of these

718. Which renal artery disease involves the ostia of renal artery?

(a) Atherosclerosis
(b) Fibromuscular dysplasia
(c) Arterio venous malformation
(d) Arteritis

719. All following are the clues for renovascular hypertension except?

(a) Worsening of hypertension
(b) Severe resistant hypertension
(c) Abdominal bruits
(d) Normal plasma renin

720. All following are indicators of renovascular hypertension except

(a) High renin level
(b) Normal resistance level
(c) Low serum K^+ (d) Low serum Na

721. Which antihypertensive if given IV has no effect on after load?

(a) Labetalol (b) Hydralazine
(c) Methyldopa (d) Esmolol

722. Which IV antihypertensive increase renal perfusion?

(a) IV methyldopa
(b) IV hydralazine
(c) IV sodium nitroprosside
(d) IV fenoldopam

723. Lactic acidosis occurs with which antihypertensive?

(a) IV sodium nitroprosside
(b) Hydralazine
(c) Methyldopa
(d) Labetalol

724. All following cardiac condition are associated with platypnaea orthodeoxia syndrome except

(a) ASD
(b) Atrial septal aneurysm
(c) Mitral stenosis
(d) Persistaent foramen ovale

725. All following disorder cause pulmonary hypertension except

(a) Schistosomiasis (b) Sarcoidosis
(c) Histocytosis (d) Trypanosomiasis

726. All following condition are associated with pulmonary hypertension with hypoxia except

(a) Interstitial lung disease
(b) Sleep disordered breathing
(c) Chronic exposure to high altitude
(d) Pleural effusion

727. All following are platelet dysfunction DM except

(a) Increased are chronic acid metabolism
(b) Increased are tyaz synthesis
(c) Decreased antioxidant levels
(d) Increased nitric oxide production

728. All following antihypertension have no effect on preload when given IV except

(a) IV methyldopa
(b) IV hydralazine
(c) IV sodium nitroprosside
(d) IV labetalol

729. Prevention of cardiovascular disease is accomplished by all in DM except
(a) Statin
(b) ACE inhibitors
(c) AT1 blockers
(d) Hormone replacement therapy

730. Endothelial function is improved in DM by
(a) Statins (b) ACE inhibitors
(c) Antioxidant (d) All the above

731. All following are acute benefits of insulin and glucose therapy in acute myocardial infarction except
(a) Improve glucose oxidation
(b) Decrease TXA2 levels
(c) Vasodiltation
(d) Arrhythmogenic

732. Post CABG stenosis is most common in
(a) RCA stenosis (b) LMCA stenosis
(c) Lx stenosis (d) LAD stenosis

733. All following are effects of hyperglycemia in acute myocardial infarction except
(a) Endothelial dysfunction
(b) Impaired ischemic preconditioning
(c) Reduced glucose oxidation
(d) Decrease cytosis oxidation

734. HDL-C is maximally increased by
(a) Statins (b) Fibrates
(c) Niacin (d) Ezetimibe

735. All following are clinical criteria for metabolic syndrome except
(a) DM (b) Hypertension
(c) Obesity (d) Increased LDL-C

736. All following are used for endothelial dysfunction except
(a) Life style modification
(b) β-blockers
(c) Statins
(d) Decrease ACE

737. Drug of choice for coronary spasm
(a) Aspirin (b) β-blocker

(c) Ca-blockers (d) All of the above

738. Drug of choice for myocardial bridging

(a) β-blockers (b) Ca-blockers
(c) Nitrate (d) None of above

739. Which parameter is of least predictive valve for HOV associated myocarditis?

(a) VES
(b) ST increase
(c) Increase troponin I
(d) CKMB

740. Which is commonest secondary form of hypertension?

(a) Renovascular
(b) Coarctation of aorta
(c) Hypothyroidism
(d) Phaeochromocytoma

741. Annuloectasic atresia has all following feature except

(a) Dilatation of aortic sinuses
(b) Dilatation of ascending aorta
(c) Dilatation of valve ring
(d) Deformity of aortic cusps

742. All following antihypertensive drugs produces edema except

(a) Nifedipine (b) Reserpine
(c) Hydralazine (d) β-blockers

743. ST elevation in ventricular aneurysm is due to all except

(a) Reinfarction
(b) Subepicardial
(c) Trammission of ventricular activity potentials
(d) None of the above

744. Commonest sign of LV aneurysm is

(a) Double apical impulse
(b) Large area of apical impulse
(c) Normal apical impulse
(d) All the above

745. Paroxysmal and postural hypertension suggest

(a) Renal hypertension
(b) Essential hypertension
(c) Phaeochromocytoma
(d) Thyrotoxicosis

746. Most common site ventricular aneurysm in myocardial infarction

(a) Apex (b) Inferior wall
(c) Posterior wall (d) All the above

747. All are clinical features of cardiac rupture except

(a) Occurs commonly in LV
(b) Severe in anterior and lateral wall
(c) Usually with long myocardial infarction
(d) Occurs after a week of myocardial infarction

748. Which one is pure arterial dilator?

(a) Prazosin
(b) Hydralazine
(c) Phentolomine
(d) Phenoxybenzamine

749. Which is the most potent lipid lowering agent in raising HDL-C levels?

(a) Statins (b) Fibrates
(c) Cholestyramine (d) Niacin

750. All following improve survival in acute myocardial infarction except

(a) Thrombolysis (b) Antiplatelets
(c) β-blockers (d) Nitrates

751. Which Ca-blocker causes reflex tachycardia?

(a) Amlodipine (b) Nifedipine
(c) Diltiazem (d) Verapamil

752. Which antihypertensive is not recommended as first line drug?

(a) Diuretic (b) Ca-blocker
(c) α-blocker (d) ACE inhibitor

753. All are renal haemodynamic effects of felodipine except

(a) Increase NA and water excretion

(b) Decrease vascular resistance
(c) Decrease ischaemic damage
(d) Increase filtration fraction

754. Which is the drug of choice in first line of treatment in acute myocardial infarction?

(a) Morphine (b) Aspirin
(c) Thrombolysis (d) Pentazocin

755. 30 Days mortality after successful reperfusion is lowest in which location of coronary occlusion?

(a) Left circumflex
(b) Right coronary artery
(c) Proximal LAD
(d) Mid LAD

756. All discontinuation intervals before surgery of antiplatelets are correct except

(a) Aspirin-5 – 10 days
(b) Clopidogrel-7 – 10 days
(c) Dipyrimadole-2 days
(d) Ticlopidine-3 days

757. Withdrawal syndromes are associated with all the following except

(a) Clonidine (b) β-blockers
(c) Sertraline (d) ACE inhibitors

758. All the following genetic disorders causes low HDL-C except

(a) LCAT deficiency
(b) CETP excess
(c) Tangier's disease
(d) Familial hypercholestrolemia

759. HDL-C reduced in all the following except

(a) Poorly controlled DM
(b) β-blockers
(c) Metabolic syndrome
(d) Nephrotic syndrome

760. Ezetimibe affects chiefly which lipid fraction?

(a) TG (b) LDL-C
(c) HDL-C (d) All the above

761. Omega 3 fatty acids act on

(a) TG (b) LDL-C
(c) HDL-C (d) All the above

762. Which level of HDL-C level is protective against CAD?

(a) < 45 mg % (b) 45–50 mg %
(c) 50–55 mg % (d) > 60 mg %

763. All following cardiac disorder occurs in obesity except

(a) Hyperlipidemia
(b) Hypertension
(c) Coronary artery disease
(d) Pericardial effusion

764. Which lipid abnormality is found in pancreatic disease?

(a) Increase TC (b) Increase LDL-C
(c) Increase TG (d) Decrease HDL-C

765. Intestinal angina has all of following features except

(a) Atherosclerosis of 2, 3 major arteries of gut
(b) Mid abdominal pain
(c) Worsesing of symptoms during eating
(d) Relieved by NTG

766. All following factors modulate LVH in HT except

(a) Genetic factor
(b) Dietary sodium
(c) Sympathetic nervous system activation
(d) Reduced angiotension II

767. All are structural changes in angina heart except

(a) Cardiac weight decrease
(b) LV mass increase
(c) LVH is present (d) LA dilatation

768. All following are the mechanism sinus of accelerated atherosclerosis is diabetes

(a) Endothelial dysfunction
(b) Dyslipidemia
(c) Impaired fibrinolysis
(d) All the above

769. HDL-C reduced by all the drugs except

(a) Probucal (b) β-blockers
(c) Aspirin (d) Methyldopa

770. Most beneficial antihypertensive therapy in term of years of life saved is

(a) β-blockers (b) Thiazides
(c) ACE inhibitors (d) Ca-blockers

771. In NIDDM all following lipid abnormalities occurs except

(a) Increase TG (b) Increase LDL
(c) Increase TC (d) Decrease HDL

772. Which size of aortic atheroma is likely to embolise to brain with high rate of recurrence?

(a) 1 mm (b) 2 mm
(c) 3 mm (d) > 4 mm

773. Which is commonest sign in pulmonary embolism?

(a) Rales (b) S4
(c) Loud P2 (d) S3

774. Drug of choice for resistant hypertension

(a) Ca-blocker (b) Furosemide
(c) Reserpine (d) Minoxidil

775. Drug of choice in hypertensive subarchnoid hemorrhage

(a) Amlodipine (b) Nifedipine
(c) β-blockers (d) Nimodipine

776. All following antihypertensives decrease microalbuminuria

(a) ACE inhibitors (b) Amlodipine
(c) Diuretics (d) β-blocker

777. All of following antihypertensives have no effect on microalbuminuria

(a) Methyldopa (b) Clonidine
(c) β-blocker (d) Diltiazem

778. All following antihypertensive increase microalbuminuria except

(a) Minoxidil (b) Nifedipine
(c) Amlodipine (d) Verapamil

779. Drug of choice for hypertensive crisis in pheochromocytoma

(a) Nitroprusside (b) β-blocker
(c) Phentolamine (d) Nitroglycerine

780. Which thrombolytic agent has low clot selectivity?

(a) Streptokinase (b) Reteplase
(c) Tenecteplase (d) tPA

781. Which thrombolytic agent causes hypotension?

(a) PA (b) Streptokinase
(c) Reteplase (d) Tenecteplase

782. Allergic reaction occurs with which thrombolytic agent?

(a) Streptokinase (b) Reteplase
(c) Tenecteplase (d) tPA

783. Papilledema occurs in which cardiac vascular disorder?

(a) Malignant hypertension
(b) Pulmonary hypertension
(c) AV disease
(d) Thyrotoxic heart disease

784. PTCA affects most which of the event in coronary artery disease?

(a) Increase in coronary flow reserve
(b) Reduction in stenosis
(c) Increase in exercise tolerance
(d) Reduction in mortality

785. CABG affects most which event in coronary artery disease?

(a) Increase in coronary flow reserve
(b) Increase in exercise tolerance
(c) Reduction in mortality
(d) Reduction in non fatal cardiovascular events

786. How much cholesterol is recommended in step II dietary management of lipids?

(a) 200 – 300 mg% (b) > 300 mg%
(c) < 200 mg% (d) 350 – 400 mg%

787. Mode of action all following thrombolytic agents is direct except

(a) Streptokinase (b) Urokinase
(c) Alteplase (d) Reteplase

788. Which of the following effects is most affected by lipid management in CAD?

(a) Reduction in stenosis
(b) Increase in exercise tolerance
(c) Reduction in cardiovascular events
(d) Reduction in mortality

789. Gastro intenstinal symptoms maximally occurs with

(a) Verapamil (b) Diltiazem
(c) Nifedipine (d) β-Blockers

790. Which calcium blocker is maximal myocardial depresiant?

(a) Verapamil (b) Nifedipine
(c) Diltazem (d) None of above

791. Maximal LV dysfunction occurs with which drug

(a) Diltazem (b) Nifedipine
(c) Verapamil (d) Nitrates

792. Headache/flushing maximally occurs with

(a) Nifedipine (b) Verapamil
(c) Diltiazem (d) β-blockers

793. Best antianginal agent when patient has concomitant peripheral vascular disease

(a) Amlodipine (b) β-blockers
(c) Nitrates (d) Verapamil

794. All are causes of disturbed coronary microcirculation except

(a) Anaemia (b) Hypertension
(c) Hyperlipidemia
(d) Endothelial dysfunction

795. All following physiological conditions are associated with venous thrombo-embolism except

(a) Young (b) Elderly
(c) Obesity (d) Post partem

796. All following orthopedic surgery require prophylaxis of deep vein thrombosis except

(a) Total hypreplacement
(b) Total base replacement
(c) Hip fracture
(d) Upper extremity fraction

797. Which activity require maximum energy cost (METS)?

(a) Walking 3 MPH (b) Sexual activity
(c) Cycling (d) Swimming

798. In acute myocardial infarction which of the following is most common

(a) Single vessel disease
(b) Double vessel disease
(c) Triple vessel disease
(d) Left main disease

799. Preferred antihypersive drug in cyclosporine induced hypertension is

(a) α-blocker (b) β-blocker
(c) Diuretic (d) Ca-blocker

800. Most commonly used drug for presention and treatment of eelamporia

(a) Nifedipine
(b) Methyldopa
(c) β-blocker
(d) Magnesium sulphate

801. All following hypertensive emergencies with acute myocardial infarction except

(a) Acute left ventricular failure
(b) Aortic dissection
(c) Microangiopathic haemolytic anaemia
(d) Rupture of papillay muscle

802. Most specific and sensitive test for diagnosis of renovascular hypertension is

(a) Renal arteriography
(b) Rapid sequence IVP
(c) Captopril renal scan
(d) MRI

803. Preferred antihypertensive drug in liddle's syndrome is?

(a) ACE inhibitors (b) β-blockers
(c) Amiloride (d) α-blockers

804. LV aneurysm after myocardial infarction has all following features except

(a) Occurs with in 3 months post myocardial infraction
(b) ECG shows ST increase
(c) Seen with large Q infarct with LVH
(d) Causes severe heart failure

805. In postural hypotension all following are found except

(a) Increase HR
(b) Decrease HR
(c) SBP decrease
(d) DBP increase or constant

806. Parasympathetic stimulation in ACS is indicated by all except

(a) Vomiting (b) Bradycardia
(c) Hypertension (d) Hypotension

807. Vomiting in acute myocardial infarction usually occurs

(a) Acute inferior wall infarction
(b) Acute anterior wall infarction
(c) Cardiac rupture
(d) Morphine

808. What is adequate β-blockade in IHD?

(a) HR < 50/m (b) HR 60 – 70/m
(c) HR 70 – 80/m (d) HR > 80/m

809. Antihypertensive of choice is pregnancy

(a) Methyldopa (b) β-blocker
(c) Ca-blocker (d) Diuretics

810. Which antihypertensive is contraindicated in pregnancy?

(a) Diuretics (b) ACE inhibitors
(c) Ca-blocker (d) β-blocker

811. Drug of choice for perioperative hypertensive emergency

(a) IV Labetalol (b) IV Hydralazine
(c) IV Nitroprusside (d) IV Nitroglycerine

812. Which Ca-antagonist has most marked decreased PVR?

(a) Amlodepine (b) Nifedipine
(c) Verapamil (d) Diltiazem

813. Which Ca-blockers should not be combined with Beta-blocker?

(a) Amlodipine (b) Nifedipine
(c) Verapamil (d) Diltiazem

814. Which Ca-antagonist does not depresses sinus node function?

(a) Amlodipine (b) Nifedipine
(c) Diltazem (d) Verapamil

815. Which antihypertensive increase bone mass?

(a) Ca-blocker (b) Thiazides
(c) β-blockers (d) Methyldopa

816. Which is the maximum antihypertensive dose of ramipril?

(a) 2.5 mg/Day (b) 5 mg/Day
(c) 10 mg/Day (d) 20 mg/Day

817. Which life style change may regress LVH in hypertension?

(a) Weight reduction (b) Exercise
(c) Alcohol reduction (d) Smoking cessation

818. Diuretic are the drug of choice in ISH in which group?

(a) Black > 65 Y (b) Black < 65 Y
(c) White < 65 Y (d) In all above

819. Which drug in chronic stable angina is more effective?

(a) Nitrates (b) β-blocker
(c) Nitrate + BR (d) None of above

820. Angina and bradycardia which antianginal is best

(a) β-blocker
(b) Nitrates
(c) Amlodipine
(d) Short acting nipedipine

821. Patients who exhibits persistantly raised CRP levels after coronary stenting should be given which of the following agent?

(a) IV heparin (b) IV β-blocks
(c) Steroids (d) Antibiotic

822. Which is commonest cause of LV dysfunction (systolic)?

(a) IHD (b) CMI
(c) Valvular HD (d) Hypertension

823. Drug of choice of coronary artery disesae with aortic stenosis is

(a) Nitrates
(b) Short acting nifedipine
(c) β-blocker
(d) Diltiazem

824. Which Ca-blocker does not cause bradycardia?

(a) Nifedipine (b) Diltiazem
(c) Verapamil (d) All of the above

825. Palpitation occurs with which Ca-blocker

(a) Nifedipine (b) Diltiazem
(c) Verapamil (d) All of the above

826. All following antihypertensive drugs cause pericarditis except

(a) Reserpine (b) Procauegimide
(c) Hypialazenes (d) β-blockers

827. All are indications for nitratès in acute myocardial infarction except

(a) Persistent and recurrent pain
(b) Sustained hypertension
(c) Major left ventricular dysfunction
(d) Right ventricular infarction

828. Which Ca-blockers is vasculoselective?

(a) Vimodipine (b) Nifedipine
(c) Felodipine (d) Flunarizine

829. Which antianginal does not dilate coronary artery?

(a) Nitrates (b) β-blockers
(c) Nifedipine (d) Diltiazem

830. Which antianginal does not reduce silent ischaemia?

(a) Nitrates (b) Verapamil
(c) β-blockers (d) Diltiazem

831. Tolerance develops with which antianginal agent?

(a) Verapamil (b) Diltiazem
(c) Nitrates (d) β-blockers

832. Left anterior descending coronary artery stenotic murmur has all following features except

(a) Diastolic
(b) Systolic
(c) High pitched
(d) Crescendo decrescendo

833. Increased CK MB is found in

(a) Acute myocarditis
(b) Chronic myocarditis
(c) Inflammatory cardiomyopathy
(d) None of the above

834. All are common symptoms of acute myocarditis except

(a) Reduced physical efficiency
(b) Palpitation
(c) Arrhythmia
(d) Angina

835. All are non modifiable risk factors for IHD except

(a) Age (b) Sex
(c) Family history (d) Social class

836. All are major modifiable risk factors for IHD except

(a) Smoking (b) Hyperlipidemia
(c) Hypertension (d) DM

837. How much alcohol consumption is beneficial in IHD?

(a) < 10 G of absolute alcohol/day
(b) 10–20 G of absolute alcohol/day
(c) 20–30 G of absolute alcohol/day
(d) > 30 G of absolute alcohol/day

838. Which is the least common cardiac complication of hypertension?

(a) Valvular heart disease
(b) LVH
(c) Heart failure
(d) Arrhythmias

839. Most visible manifestation of hypertensive target organ damage is

(a) Coronary artery disease
(b) LVH
(c) PVD
(d) Nephropathy

840. ECG diagnosis of LVH in hypertension

(a) Less specific
(b) Less sensitive
(c) More sensitive
(d) More specific and less sensitive

841. Most common and earliest ventricular dysfunction in hypertension is

(a) Diastolic artery
(b) Systolic artery
(c) Combined
(d) All of the above

842. Re-do CABG is associated with more complication then primary CABG except

(a) Mortality
(b) Bleeding
(c) Perioperative myocardial infarction
(d) Wound complications

843. Which of the following has maximum systolic and diastolic pressure?

(a) Aorta
(b) Left ventricle
(c) Pulmonary artery
(d) Right ventricle

844. Most specific clinical sign of hypercholestrolemia is

(a) Corneal arcus
(b) Xanthelasma
(c) Tendon X anthoma
(d) None of above

845. Most commonly vascular calcification occurs in which of the following?

(a) Aortic arch
(b) Coronary artery
(c) Pulmonary artery
(d) Ascending aorta

846. Syndrome X is characterised by all except

(a) Ischemic pain
(b) Ischaemic ECG changes
(c) Normal ceronmes
(d) Good Responseto sublingual nitrates

847. All are features of myocardial ischemia except

(a) Inadequate perfusion
(b) No lactate production
(c) Lactate production
(d) Impairs contractility function

848. All are features of myocardial stunning except

(a) Develops after ischemia/reperfusion
(b) Regional blood flow is preserved
(c) Transient function
(d) Lactate impaired contractile function production

849. All are features of myocardial hibernation except

(a) Develop after repeated episodes of ischaemia/reperfusion
(b) Preserved regional blood flow
(c) Contraction is preserved
(d) No lactate production

850. Most common cause of renal failure is

(a) Hypertension
(b) Polycystic kidney
(c) Glomerulonephritis
(d) Pyelonephritis

851. Which is most useful diagnostic test in pulmonary embolism?

(a) ECG (b) X-ray chest
(c) ABG analysis (d) Lung V/Q scan

852. All are risk factor for development of HT except

(a) Sedentary lifestyle
(b) Obesity
(c) Increased salt intake
(d) Type A personality

853. All are logical combination of antihypertensive drugs except

(a) Diuretic + β1-blocker / ACE inhibitor
(b) β-blocker + ACE inhibitor
(c) β-blocker + Ca-blocker
(d) ACE inhibitor + Ca-blocker

854. β-blockers should be availed in all following condition existing with hypertension except

(a) Heart failure (b) PVD
(c) Heart block
(d) Raynaud's phenomenon

855. Foam cells are cholesterol iaden

(a) Macrophage (b) Lymphycytes
(c) Fibriblus (d) Neurophills

856. Foam cells first appear in

(a) Aorta (b) Coronary Vs
(c) Cerebral Vs (d) Renal Vs

857. Which immunosuppressive drug produces hypertension?

(a) Azathioprine (b) Methotrexate
(c) Cyclosporine (d) Tacrolimus

858. Calcified assending aortic aneurysm with aortic regurgitation is highly suggestive of

(a) Atherosclerosis
(b) Hypertension
(c) Marfan's syndrome
(d) Syphillis

859. Drug of choice for cyclosporine induced hypertension

(a) β-blocker (b) Ca-blocker
(c) Thiazide (d) ACE inhibitors

860. Most common was precipitating factor for angina is

(a) Emotion (b) Exertion physical
(c) Eating (d) Coldweather

861. All are non ischemic cardiac vascular causes of chest pain except

(a) Aortic dissection (b) MVP
(c) Pericarditis (d) Hypertension

862. All following may be present in raynaud's phenomena

(a) Primary pulmonary hypertension
(b) Systemic hypertension
(c) Corpulmonale
(d) Aortic stenosis

863. What happens to systolic blood pressure by palpation or auscultation?

(a) Systolic blood pressure is higher by auscultation than palpation
(b) Systolic blood pressure same by both auscultation and palpation
(c) Systolic blood pressure higher by palpation than auscultation
(d) All of the above

864. Where should you place the chest piece of stethoscope while measuring BP normally?

(a) Adjacent to lower edge of cuff
(b) Under the cuff
(c) Edge of stethoscope should be under the cuff
(d) 1 cm away from lower edge of cuff

865. All following procedure made korotkoff sound louder if they are soft except

(a) Opening and closing of fist
(b) Elevate the arm before you inflate the cuff
(c) Inflate the cuff quickly
(d) Inflate The cuff slowly

866. Highest blood pressure recorded with severe aortic stenosis

(a) 160/100 (b) 180/100
(c) 200/90 (d) 280/140

867. In all the following situations korotkoff sounds are difficult to hear except

(a) Narrow pulse pressure
(b) Aortic stenosis
(c) Poor blood flow to limbs
(d) Mitral regurgitation

868. All following endocrinal disorders produce hypertension

(a) Hyperparathyroid

(b) Primary aldosteronism
(c) Pheochromocytoma
(d) DM

869. What is mechanism for renal hypertension?
(a) Volume dependent
(b) Renin angiotensin
(c) Both (a) and (b)
(d) None of the above

870. All following are used for smoking cessation except
(a) Clonidine
(b) α-methyl dopa
(c) Vicinal against nicotine
(d) Rimonabent

871. Which statin lowers maximal LDL-C reduction?
(a) 10 mg/day of atorvastatin
(b) 20 mg/day of simvastatin
(c) 20 mg/day of fluvastatin
(d) 20 mg/day of pravastatin

872. All are feature volume expanded mechanism of renal hypertension except
(a) Edema
(b) Plasma rennin low
(c) Plasma angiotensis low
(d) Dyspnoea

873. All are features of high rennin angiotensin dependent renal hypertension except
(a) Plasma rennin high
(b) Excessive thirst
(c) Plasma angiotens in high
(d) Edema is present

874. All are causes of transient hypertension except
(a) Acute CVA
(b) Acute myocardial infarction
(c) Acute glomerulonephritis
(d) Over infusion of fluids

875. Commonest secondary causes of hypertension is

(a) Renal
(b) Endocrinal
(c) Drug induced
(d) Coarctation of aorta

876. Which antihypertensive agent does not causes sexual dysfunction?

(a) ACE inhibitor (b) Reserpine
(c) Methyldopa (d) Clonidine

877. How frequent is S4 in hypertension (DBP) 100 mm Hg?

(a) 10% (b) 20%
(c) 40% (d) 50%

878. All are ECG manifestation of atrial infarction except

(a) PR segment deviation
(b) Atrial flutter
(c) Atrial tachycardia
(d) Junctional tachycardia

879. Angina in elderly usually present as

(a) Pain (b) Dyspnoea
(c) Fatigue (d) Arrhythmias

880. Myocardial infarction in elderly is characterized by all except

(a) Pain less
(b) Atypical
(c) Pulmonary edema
(d) Commonly occurs in the morning

881. Which antiarrhythmic agent can produce macrocytic anemia?

(a) Quinidine (b) Phenyloin
(c) Lidocaine (d) Bretyllium

882. All are indication for surgical therapy for dissecting aortic aneurysm except

(a) Severe aortic regurgitation
(b) Heart failure
(c) Recurrent ventricular arrhythmia
(d) 1° AV block

883. Which antihypertensive drug may produce hemolytic anemia?

(a) Clonidine (b) Methyldopa
(c) β-blocker (d) Ca-blockers

884. Which antihypertensive drug produces hypertrichosis?

(a) Hydralazine (b) Minoxidil
(c) Captopril (d) Prazosin

885. All following antihypertensive drugs may produce edema except

(a) Ca-antagonists
(b) Minoxidil
(c) Sodium nitroprusside
(d) Hydralazine

886. Which antihypertensive agent may produce agranulocytosis?

(a) Ca-blocker (b) Reserpine
(c) β-blocker (d) Captopril

887. Which secondary hypertension may present as Café-AU-Lait spots?

(a) Renal artery stenosis
(b) Hemochromocytoma
(c) Primary aldosteronism
(d) Cushing's syndrome

888. Incidences of toxemia of pregnancy is lowest in which type of hypertension?

(a) Essential hypertension
(b) Renal hypertension
(c) Endocrinal hypertension
(d) Co-arctation of aorta

889. Which of the following is most sensitive test for diagnosis of CAD?

(a) ECG resting (b) Exercise ECG
(c) Spect (d) PET

890. Which is most specific test for diagnosis of coronary artery disease?

(a) Resting ECG (b) Exercise ECG
(c) SPECT (d) PET

891. All following therapeutic modalities are found to be useful in end stage coronary disease except?

(a) Spinal cord stimulation
(b) Trans myocardial laser revascularisation
(c) Enhanced external counted pulsation
(d) Oxyfedrial

892. Common initial presentation of coronary artery disease in females is

(a) Sudden cardiac death
(b) Unstable angina
(c) Silent myocardial infarction
(d) Stable angina

893. Most common initial presentation of coronary artery disease in males

(a) Acute myocardial infarction
(b) Silent myocardial infarction
(c) Sudden cardiac death
(d) Unstable angina

894. Best drug for treatment of hypertension in elderly

(a) Diuretic (b) Ca-blocker
(c) ACE inhibitor (d) β-blocker

895. Best drug for treatment as hypertension in elderly diabetic is

(a) ACE inhibitor (b) Diuretic
(c) Beta-blocker (d) Ca-blockers

896. Which antihypertensive decrease insulin resistance?

(a) Diuretic (b) β-blocker
(c) ACE inhibitor (d) AT II antagonists

897. CAD risk is not there with all lipid abnormalities except

(a) High HDL
(b) Polygenic hypercholestrolemia
(c) Lipoprotein lipase defect
(d) Familial hypercholestrolemia

898. Corticosteroids causes all following lipid changes except

(a) Increase total cholesterol
(b) Increase TG
(c) Increase LDL-C (d) Decrease HDL-C

899. Heparin decrease which Lipid?
(a) Total cholesterol (b) TG
(c) LDL-C (d) HDL-C

900. Cyclosporin increase all following lipids except
(a) TC (b) TG
(c) LDL-C (d) HDL-C

901. Valporate increase which lipid fraction?
(a) LDL-C (b) HDL-C
(c) Apo A1 (d) Apo B

902. Estrogen increases all lipid fraction except
(a) TG (b) HDL-C
(c) Apo-A1 (d) LDL-C

903. Phenytoin increase all lipid fraction except
(a) HDL-C (b) Apo A1
(c) Apo B (d) LDL-C

904. Phenobarbitone increase all lipid fraction except
(a) TG (b) LDL-C
(c) HDL-C (d) Apo A1

905. Micro unsaturated fat decrease all lipid fraction except
(a) HDL-C (b) TC
(c) LDL-C (d) LP

906. β-Agonist increase which lipid fraction?
(a) Total cholesterol (b) TG
(c) LDL-C (d) HDL-C

907. Which statin decrease LDL-C & TG maximally?
(a) Atorvastatin (b) Simvastatin
(c) Lovastatin (d) Pravastatin

908. Trans unsaturated fats cause increase in all following lipid fraction except?
(a) VLDL (b) HDL-C
(c) LDL-C (d) LP

909. Earliest serum marker to rise in acute myocardial infarction

(a) Troponin-T (b) Troponin-I
(c) CKMB (d) Myoglobin

910. Ca-blockers block which types of channels?

(a) L-Type (b) T-Type
(c) N-Type (d) All the above

911. Cystic medial necrosis of aorta occurs in all except

(a) Marfan's syndrome
(b) Hypertension
(c) Atherosclerosis
(d) Pregnancy

912. Syphilitic aortic aneurysm in valves

(a) Ascending aorta
(b) Thoracic descending aorta
(c) Abdominal descending aorta
(d) All the above

913. Most common causes of aortic arch aneurysm is

(a) Hypertension (b) Atherosclerosis
(c) Pregnancy (d) Marfan's syndrome

914. Which is antihypertensive of choice in osteoporosis?

(a) β-blocker (b) Ca-blocker
(c) Diuretics (d) ACE inhibitors

915. Which antihypertensive drug may produce pericardial effusion?

(a) Diuretics (b) Ca-blocker
(c) Minoxidil (d) ARBS

916. Hypertension in children is commonly due to

(a) Renovascular
(b) Coarctation of aorta
(c) Essential
(d) Primary hyperaldosteronism

917. Which is the commonest visceral artery aneurysm?

(a) Hepatic
(b) Splenic

(c) Superior mesentric
(d) Celiac

918. All antihypertensive are lipid neutral except

(a) Ca-blocker (b) β-blocker
(c) ACE inhibitor (d) ARBS

919. All antihypertensive are lipid neutral except

(a) Ca-blocker (b) β-blocker
(c) ACE inhibitor (d) ARBS

920. Reduction in infarct size is best accomplished by

(a) Nitartes (b) β-blocker
(c) ACE inhibitors (d) Ca-blockers

921. Which drug reduces blood viscosity?

(a) Aspirin (b) Anticoagulant
(c) Thrombolytics (d) Pentoxy phylline

922. Facial flushing is maximum with

(a) Diltiazem (b) Verapamil
(c) Amlodipine (d) Nifedipine

923. Headache is not a features of all following Ca-blockers except

(a) Verapamil
(b) Diltizem sustained release
(c) Amlodipine
(d) Nifedipine

924. All following Ca-blocker do not cause constipation except

(a) Amlodipine (b) Verapamil
(c) Felodipine (d) Nifedipine

925. Which Ca-blocker usually does not causes ankle edema?

(a) Verapamil (b) Amlodipine
(c) Dilitiazem (d) Nifedipine

926. In which myocardial ischaemic syndrome β-blockers are avoided?

(a) SA
(b) UA
(c) Acute myocardial infarction
(d) Prinzmetal's angina

927. Allergic reaction occurs with which thrombolytics?

(a) SK (b) UK
(c) rtPA (d) All the above

928. Thrombolytics efficacy is maximum with

(a) SK (b) rtPA
(c) UK (d) Alteplase

929. Variant angina has all the features except

(a) On rest
(b) ECG shows ST elevation
(c) Typical ischemic pain
(d) Angiography reveals significant CAD

930. Severe coronary artery disease is normally found in which type of angina

(a) Stable (b) Unstable
(c) Variant (d) All the above

931. ST increase in coronary artery disease is found in all except

(a) STEMI
(b) Variant angina
(c) During stress testing
(d) SA

932. All are indications of anticoagulation in acute myocardial infarction except

(a) Post thrombolytics
(b) Post PTCA
(c) Atrial fibrillation
(d) CHB

933. Haemostatic breakdown occurs maximally with which thrombolytics

(a) Streptokinase (b) tPA
(c) UK (d) None of above

934. Hypotension occurs with which thrombolytics

(a) SK (b) t PA
(c) UK (d) All the above

935. Hyperglycemia occurs in all lipid disorder except

(a) Familial combined hyperlipidemia
(b) Familial type V hyperlipoproteinemia

(c) Type III hyperlipoproteinemia
(d) APOC II deficiency

936. Peripheral vascular disease occurs in which type lipid disorder?

(a) Familial hyperglycemia
(b) Familial type V hyperlipoproteinemia
(c) Apoc II deficiency
(d) Type III hyperlipoproteinemia

937. Obesity is a feature of all following lipid disorder except

(a) Familial combined hyperlipidemia
(b) Familial hypertriglyceridemia
(c) Familial type V hyperlipoproteinemia
(d) Apoc II deficiency

938. Tendon xanthelasma occurs in which lipid disorder?

(a) Familial hypercholestrolemia
(b) Familial combined hyperlipidemia
(c) Polygenic hypercholestrolemia
(d) All the above

939. Coronary heart disease is unknown in which lipid disorder?

(a) Familial type V hyperlipoproteinemia
(b) Familial hypercholestrolemia
(c) Familial combined hyperlipidemia
(d) Polygenic hypercholestrolemia

940. All following lipid disorders have TG (order) 500 mg except

(a) Type V hyperlipoproteinemia
(b) LPL deficiency
(c) Apoc II deficiency
(d) Familial hypercholestrolemia

941. Which is the least site of radiation of anginal pain?

(a) Medial aspect of left arm
(b) Left shoulder
(c) Groin
(d) Right arm

942. Papillary muscle rupture following acute myocardial infarction has all following features except

(a) Peak incidence 3.5 days after infarction
(b) More frequent in infero posterior infarction
(c) Flail or prolapsed leaflet
(d) Occurs in 5% of all infarct

943. Which antihypertensive drug does not cause pericarditis?

(a) Captopril (b) Minioxidil
(c) Hydralazine (d) Ca-blockers

944. Which disease of aorta dose not cause myocardial infarction?

(a) Aortic dissection (b) Marfans syndrome
(c) Aortic stenosis
(d) Aortic regurgitation

945. All following are normal plasma renin hypertension except

(a) Essential hypertension
(b) coarctation of aorta
(c) Pheochromocytoma
(d) Liddle's syndrome

946. In following situations the arbitrary blood pressure monitoring is helpful except

(a) Assessing 24 hours control
(b) Nocturnal dip status
(c) White coat hypertension
(d) During treatment of hypertensive emergency

947. All following metals are implicated in Hypertension except

(a) Lead (b) Arsenic
(c) Carbon disulfide (d) Copper

948. Combined systolic and diastolic hypertension has all the features except

(a) Age of Onset 30–50 years
(b) Multifactorial
(c) Renin angiotension blockers
(d) More effectic CAD is less common

949. Isolated systolic hypertension has all following features except

(a) Age > 55 years
(b) Stroke is more common
(c) Diuretics are effective
(d) Progression is slow

950. All following features occurs in aortic dissection except

(a) Hypertension occurs in < 50%
(b) Type-A requiring surgery
(c) Type-B usually treated medically
(d) Mechanism of dissection involve both high pulsatile wave strets and accelerated atherosclerosis

951. Conduction defect is more with

(a) Verapamil (b) Diltiazem
(c) Nifedipine (d) None of the above

952. Most common cause of age related pulmonary stenosis is

(a) Rheumatic
(b) Connective tissue disease
(c) Sclerodema (d) Carcinoid

953. Tendon xanthelasma occurs in which lipid disorder?

(a) Familial hypercholestrolemia
(b) Familial combined hyperlipidemia
(c) Polygenic hypercholestrolemia
(d) All the above

954. Coronary heart disease is unknown in which lipid disorder?

(a) Familial type-V hyperlipoproteinemia
(b) Familial hypercholestrolemia
(c) Familial combined hyperlipidemia
(d) Polygenic hypercholestrolemia

955. All following lipid disorders have TG (order) 500 mg except

(a) Type-V hyperlipoproteinemia
(b) LPL deficiency
(c) Apoc II deficiency
(d) Familial hypercholestrolemia

956. Which is the least site of radiation of anginal pain?

(a) Medial aspect of left arm
(b) Left shoulder
(c) Groin
(d) Right arm

957. Papillary muscle rupture following acute myocardial infarction has all following features except

(a) Peak incidence 3.5 days after infarction
(b) More frequent in infero posterior infarction
(c) Flail or prolapsed leaflet
(d) Occurs in 5% of all infarct

958. Nitrates are contraindicated is which infarction?

(a) Anterior infarction
(b) Inferior infarction
(c) RV infarction
(d) Atrial infarction

959. ST increase occurs in prinzmetal angina

(a) Before pain (b) During pain
(c) After pain (d) All the above

960. Patients of coronary artery disease with mitral regurgitation the drug of choice is

(a) Slow release DHP
(b) Nitrates
(c) β-blockers
(d) All the above

961. Drug of choice patients of coronary artery disease with mitral stenosis

(a) β-blockers (b) Amlodipine
(c) Nitrates (d) None of the above

962. Smoking causes loss of cardioprotictive effect of which β-blocker?

(a) Atenolol (b) Propenolol
(c) Metoprolol (d) All the above

963. Which cation is increased by β-blockers?

(a) Na (b) K
(c) Ca (d) Mg

964. In elderly patients of angina which is better?

(a) β-blockers (b) Nitrates
(c) Verapamil (d) All of the above

965. Anticoagulation in coronary artery disease is done in all following except

(a) Associated AF
(b) Associated LV dysfunction
(c) Ventricular aneurysm
(d) Chronic stable angina

966. Which is the rare SVT in acute myocardial infarction?

(a) Atrial fibrillation
(b) Atrial flutter
(c) Ectopic atrial tachycardia
(d) AV nodal re-entrant tachycardia

967. Which antianginal agent prevents sudden cardiac death in CAD?

(a) β-blocker (b) Verapamil
(c) Diltiazem (d) Nitrates

968. Rupture of thoracic aortic aneurysm is most common at which aortic site?

(a) 3.5 cm (b) 4.5 cm
(c) 5.5 cm (d) > 6 cm

969. To which drug in angina with normal coronaries respond?

(a) Nitrates (b) β-blockers
(c) Ca-blockers (d) None of the above

970. All are containdications of IABP in acute MI except

(a) Severe peripheral vascular disease
(b) Aortic anurysm
(c) Contraindication to anticoagulation
(d) Sinus bradycardia

971. All following are indications of IABP in acute MI except

(a) Cardiogenic shock
(b) Post infarct angina
(c) Early mechanical complication of acute MI
(d) Uncomplicated RV infarction

972. All are early mechanical complication of MI except

(a) Free wall rapture
(b) IVS rapture
(c) Aneuoysis fornolis
(d) Mitral regurgitation

973. Which of the following agent increases preload and after load in myocardial infarction?

(a) Dopamine (b) Dobutamine
(c) Nitroprosside (d) ACE inhibitors

974. Which of the following statement is coronary in ageing heart?

(a) Large arteries dilate
(b) Intima thickness
(c) Callagen decrease
(d) SN pacemaker cells decrease

975. Highest mortality in 1st year of acute myocardial infarction is in

(a) MI with EF < 30%
(b) Previous infarct
(c) Post infarct angina
(d) Acute MI in young

976. Highest mortality in 2nd years of acute MI is in

(a) MI with EF < 30%
(b) Previous infarct
(c) Anterior MI
(d) Inferior MI

977. ST increase in lead avR occurs in all the following except

(a) LMCA lesion
(b) Cx lesion
(c) Right ventricular overload
(d) LAD lesion

978. Highest mortality in acute MI in hospital is in which situarion?

(a) Cardiogenic shock
(b) MI in prior MI
(c) Large acute infarct
(d) MI with EF < 30%

ANSWERS

1. (*c*)	2. (*a*)	3. (*b*)	4. (**d**)	5. (*c*)
6. (*a*)	7. (*c*)	8. (*a*)	9. (*a*)	10. (*d*)
11. (*c*)	12. (*a*)	13. (*a*)	14. (**b**)	15. (*d*)
16. (*d*)	17. (*c*)	18. (*d*)	19. (*c*)	20. (*c*)
21. (*b*)	22. (*a*)	23. (*c*)	24. (*c*)	25. (*a*)
26. (*a*)	27. (*d*)	28. (*d*)	29. (*a*)	30. (*d*)
31. (*d*)	32. (*d*)	33. (*d*)	34. (*d*)	35. (*b*)
36. (*d*)	37. (*c*)	38. (*d*)	39. (*d*)	40. (*d*)
41. (*d*)	42. (*b*)	43. (*b*)	44. (*d*)	45. (*d*)
46. (*d*)	47. (*d*)	48. (*d*)	49. (*b*)	50. (*c*)
51. (*c*)	52. (*c*)	53. (*d*)	54. (*c*)	55. (*d*)
56. (*d*)	57. (*a*)	58. (*c*)	59. (*d*)	60. (*d*)
61. (*c*)	62. (*d*)	63. (*d*)	64. (*d*)	65. (*c*)
66. (*d*)	67. (*d*)	68. (*d*)	69. (*d*)	70. (*b*)
71. (*a*)	72. (*b*)	73. (*b*)	74. (*b*)	75. (*b*)
76. (*d*)	77. (*d*)	78. (*d*)	79. (*b*)	80. (*b*)
81. (*d*)	82. (*d*)	83. (*d*)	84. (*d*)	85. (*a*)
86. (*d*)	87. (*d*)	88. (*a*)	89. (*a*)	90. (*d*)
91. (*a*)	92. (*a*)	93. (*a*)	94. (*a*)	95. (*d*)
96. (*d*)	97. (*d*)	98. (*c*)	99. (*c*)	100. (*c*)
101. (*b*)	102. (*c*)	103. (*d*)	104. (*b*)	105. (*d*)
106. (*d*)	107. (*d*)	108. (*b*)	109. (*a*)	110. (*c*)
111. (*d*)	112. (*d*)	113. (*d*)	114. (*a*)	115. (*a*)
116. (*a*)	117. (*a*)	118. (*d*)	119. (*d*)	120. (*d*)
121. (*d*)	122. (*c*)	123. (*b*)	124. (*b*)	125. (*d*)
126. (*c*)	127. (*d*)	128. (*d*)	129. (*g*)	130. (*c*)
131. (*c*)	132. (*c*)	133. (*a*)	134. (*c*)	135. (*b*)
136. (*b*)	137. (*a*)	138. (*b*)	139. (*d*)	140. (*a*)
141. (*d*)	142. (*c*)	143. (*d*)	144. (*c*)	145. (*b*)
146. (*b*)	147. (*c*)	148. (*b*)	149. (*a*)	150. (*e*)
151. (*e*)	152. (*a*)	153. (*b*)	154. (*c*)	155. (*b*)
156. (*b*)	157. (*c*)	158. (*d*)	159. (*a*)	160. (*d*)

161. (c)	162. (d)	163. (c)	164. (a)	165. (d)
166. (b)	167. (c)	168. (b)	169. (c)	170. (b)
171. (c)	172. (d)	173. (c)	174. (c)	175. (a)
176. (a)	177. (b)	178. (c)	179. (b)	180. (d)
181. (a)	182. (d)	183. (b)	184. (a)	185. (d)
186. (a)	187. (a)	188. (c)	189. (d)	190. (b)
191. (d)	192. (d)	193. (d)	194. (c)	195. (d)
196. (d)	197. (d)	198. (d)	199. (c)	200. (a)
201. (d)	202. (a)	203. (d)	204. (a)	205. (a)
206. (b)	207. (d)	208. (a)	209. (d)	210. (b)
211. (a)	212. (d)	213. (a)	214. (b)	215. (d)
216. (d)	217. (d)	218. (d)	219. (c)	220. (a)
221. (a)	222. (a)	223. (b)	224. (b)	225. (b)
226. (d)	227. (b)	228. (a)	229. (c)	230. (d)
231. (c)	232. (c)	233. (a)	234. (d)	235. (a)
236. (a)	237. (a)	238. (a)	239. (d)	240. (d)
241. (a)	242. (c)	243. (a)	244. (a)	245. (d)
246. (b)	247. (c)	248. (d)	249. (d)	250. (d)
251. (c)	252. (d)	253. (d)	254. (d)	255. (c)
256. (c)	257. (d)	258. (a)	259. (d)	260. (d)
261. (b)	262. (d)	263. (d)	264. (a)	265. (d)
266. (a)	267. (b)	268. (b)	269. (a)	270. (a)
271. (a)	272. (d)	273. (d)	274. (a)	275. (d)
276. (b)	277. (b)	278. (a)	279. (d)	280. (d)
281. (d)	282. (d)	283. (a)	284. (d)	285. (d)
286. (b)	287. (c)	288. (d)	289. (c)	290. (d)
291. (d)	292. (a)	293. (d)	294. (d)	295. (c)
296. (a)	297. (d)	298. (d)	299. (d)	300. (c)
301. (b)	302. (c)	303. (a)	304. (b)	305. (a)
306. (a)	307. (c)	308. (d)	309. (d)	310. (d)
311. (a)	312. (b)	313. (a)	314. (a)	315. (a)
316. (d)	317. (d)	318. (d)	319. (d)	320. (a)
321. (d)	322. (a)	323. (d)	324. (d)	325. (d)
326. (d)	327. (d)	328. (b)	329. (d)	330. (b)
331. (b)	332. (d)	333. (d)	334. (d)	335. (d)

336. (*d*)	337. (*b*)	338. (*c*)	339. (*b*)	340. (*c*)
341. (*d*)	342. (*c*)	343. (*c*)	344. (*b*)	345. (*a*)
346. (*c*)	347. (*a*)	348. (*a*)	349. (*a*)	350. (*c*)
351. (*d*)	352. (*d*)	353. (*c*)	354. (*c*)	355. (*b*)
356. (*d*)	357. (*d*)	358. (*d*)	359. (*b*)	360. (*b*)
361. (*b*)	362. (*d*)	363. (*b*)	364. (*a*)	365. (*d*)
366. (*b*)	367. (*d*)	368. (*a*)	369. (*d*)	370. (*c*)
371. (*b*)	372. (*d*)	373. (*a*)	374. (*c*)	375. (*a*)
376. (*a*)	377. (*a*)	378. (*b*)	379. (*a*)	380. (*d*)
381. (*a*)	382. (*b*)	383. (*c*)	384. (*a*)	385. (*d*)
386. (*b*)	387. (*c*)	388. (*a*)	389. (*c*)	390. (*a*)
391. (*a*)	392. (*c*)	393. (*c*)	394. (*a*)	395. (*d*)
396. (*c*)	397. (*d*)	398. (*d*)	399. (*a*)	400. (*d*)
401. (*a*)	402. (*a*)	403. (*d*)	404. (*d*)	405. (*b*)
406. (*c*)	407. (*d*)	408. (*b*)	409. (*d*)	410. (*a*)
411. (*d*)	412. (*a*)	413. (*a*)	414. (*d*)	415. (*b*)
416. (*d*)	417. (*d*)	418. (*d*)	419. (*a*)	420. (*a*)
421. (*a*)	422. (*d*)	423. (*a*)	424. (*d*)	425. (*d*)
426. (*c*)	427. (*b*)	428. (*d*)	429. (*d*)	330. (*c*)
431. (*c*)	432. (*b*)	433. (*d*)	434. (*d*)	435. (*d*)
436. (*c*)	437. (*d*)	438. (*d*)	439. (*a*)	440. (*d*)
441. (*d*)	442. (*c*)	443. (*d*)	444. (*b*)	445. (*a*)
446. (*c*)	447. (*a*)	448. (*d*)	449. (*b*)	450. (*d*)
451. (*d*)	452. (*d*)	453. (*d*)	454. (*b*)	455. (*d*)
456. (*b*)	457. (*d*)	458. (*b*)	459. (*a*)	460. (*d*)
461. (*d*)	462. (*a*)	463. (*d*)	464. (*a*)	465. (*d*)
466. (*c*)	467. (*c*)	468. (*d*)	469. (*c*)	470. (*a*)
471. (*d*)	472. (*d*)	473. (*a*)	474. (*c*)	475. (*c*)
476. (*d*)	477. (*d*)	478. (*d*)	479. (*a*)	480. (*a*)
481. (*a*)	482. (*c*)	483. (*b*)	484. (*a*)	485. (*d*)
486. (*b*)	487. (*d*)	488. (*c*)	489. (*d*)	490. (*c*)
491. (*d*)	492. (*d*)	493. (*d*)	494. (*a*)	495. (*d*)
496. (*a*)	497. (*d*)	498. (*a*)	499. (*c*)	500. (*c*)
501. (*d*)	502. (*c*)	503. (*a*)	504. (*a*)	505. (*c*)
506. (*c*)	507. (*d*)	508. (*c*)	509. (*c*)	510. (*a*)

511. (*d*) 512. (*c*) 513. (*a*) 514. (*a*) 515. (*b*)
516. (*c*) 517. (*d*) 518. (*d*) 519. (*a*) 520. (*d*)
521. (*c*) 522. (*a*) 523. (*a*) 524. (*d*) 525. (*d*)
526. (*b*) 527. (*d*) 528. (*a*) 529. (*d*) 530. (*a*)
531. (*d*) 532. (*d*) 533. (*d*) 534. (*d*) 535. (*a*)
536. (*a*) 537. (*d*) 538. (*b*) 539. (*d*) 540. (*d*)
541. (*d*) 542. (*d*) 543. (*a*) 544. (*c*) 545. (*c*)
546. (*d*) 547. (*a*) 548. (*d*) 549. (*a*) 550. (*c*)
551. (*d*) 552. (*a*) 553. (*a*) 554. (*d*) 555. (*c*)
556. (*d*) 557. (*d*) 558. (*d*) 559. (*d*) 560. (*d*)
561. (*d*) 562. (*d*) 563. (*b*) 564. (*c*) 565. (*d*)
566. (*d*) 567. (*c*) 568. (*d*) 569. (*b*) 570. (*c*)
571. (*d*) 572. (*d*) 573. (*d*) 574. (*c*) 575. (*c*)
576. (*a*) 577. (*d*) 578. (*c*) 579. (*d*) 580. (*d*)
581. (*c*) 582. (*c*) 583. (*d*) 584. (*d*) 585. (*c*)
586. (*c*) 587. (*d*) 588. (*b*) 589. (*b*) 590. (*d*)
591. (*a*) 592. (*a*) 593. (*b*) 594. (*b*) 595. (*d*)
596. (*a*) 597. (*d*) 598. (*c*) 599. (*a*) 600. (*d*)
601. (*c*) 602. (*c*) 603. (*d*) 604. (*c*) 605. (*b*)
606. (*c*) 607. (*c*) 608. (*a*) 609. (*a*) 610. (*a*)
611. (*c*) 612. (*d*) 613. (*d*) 614. (*a*) 615. (*d*)
616. (*d*) 617. (*d*) 618. (*d*) 619. (*a*) 620. (*b*)
621. (*d*) 622. (*c*) 623. (*d*) 624. (*b*) 625. (*a*)
626. (*b*) 627. (*d*) 628. (*d*) 629. (*a*) 630. (*d*)
631. (*d*) 632. (*d*) 633. (*c*) 634. (*b*) 635. (*a*)
636. (*d*) 637. (*d*) 638. (*d*) 639. (*d*) 640. (*d*)
641. (*d*) 642. (*d*) 643. (*c*) 644. (*b*) 645. (*d*)
646. (*b*) 647. (*a*) 648. (*d*) 649. (*c*) 650. (*b*)
651. (*d*) 652. (*b*) 653. (*a*) 654. (*d*) 655. (*a*)
656. (*b*) 657. (*d*) 658. (*a*) 659. (*d*) 660. (*a*)
661. (*c*) 662. (*d*) 663. (*d*) 664. (*c*) 665. (*d*)
666. (*c*) 667. (*b*) 668. (*d*) 669. (*d*) 670. (*b*)
671. (*d*) 672. (*c*) 673. (*a*) 674. (*a*) 675. (*c*)
676. (*d*) 677. (*d*) 678. (*d*) 679. (*c*) 680. (*d*)
681. (*d*) 682. (*a*) 683. (*d*) 684. (*c*) 685. (*d*)

686. (*d*)	687. (*b*)	688. (*d*)	689. (*b*)	690. (*b*)
691. (*d*)	692. (*d*)	693. (*d*)	694. (*a*)	695. (*c*)
696. (*a*)	697. (*a*)	698. (*a*)	699. (*b*)	700. (*c*)
701. (*a*)	702. (*b*)	703. (*b*)	704. (*c*)	705. (*d*)
706. (*d*)	707. (*b*)	708. (*a*)	709. (*c*)	710. (*a*)
711. (*a*)	712. (*b*)	713. (*d*)	714. (*a*)	715. (*d*)
716. (*d*)	717. (*d*)	718. (*a*)	719. (*d*)	720. (*b*)
721. (*d*)	722. (*d*)	723. (*a*)	724. (*c*)	725. (*d*)
726. (*d*)	727. (*d*)	728. (*c*)	729. (*d*)	730. (*d*)
731. (*d*)	732. (*a*)	733. (*d*)	734. (*c*)	735. (*d*)
736. (*b*)	737. (*c*)	738. (*a*)	739. (*a*)	740. (*a*)
741. (*d*)	742. (*d*)	743. (*a*)	744. (*b*)	745. (*c*)
746. (*a*)	747. (*d*)	748. (*b*)	749. (*b*)	750. (*d*)
751. (*b*)	752. (*c*)	753. (*d*)	754. (*a*)	755. (*a*)
756. (*d*)	757. (*d*)	758. (*d*)	759. (*d*)	760. (*b*)
761. (*a*)	762. (*d*)	763. (*d*)	764. (*c*)	765. (*d*)
766. (*d*)	767. (*a*)	768. (*d*)	769. (*c*)	770. (*a*)
771. (*d*)	772. (*d*)	773. (*a*)	774. (*d*)	775. (*d*)
776. (*b*)	777. (*d*)	778. (*d*)	779. (*c*)	780. (*a*)
781. (*b*)	782. (*a*)	783. (*a*)	784. (*a*)	785. (*a*)
786. (*c*)	787. (*a*)	788. (*d*)	789. (*a*)	790. (*a*)
791. (*c*)	792. (*a*)	793. (*a*)	794. (*a*)	795. (*a*)
796. (*d*)	797. (*d*)	798. (*a*)	799. (*d*)	800. (*d*)
801. (*d*)	802. (*a*)	803. (*c*)	804. (*c*)	805. (*b*)
806. (*c*)	807. (*b*)	808. (*b*)	809. (*a*)	810. (*b*)
811. (*a*)	812. (*b*)	813. (*c*)	814. (*b*)	815. (*b*)
816. (*d*)	817. (*a*)	818. (*a*)	819. (*c*)	820. (*c*)
821. (*c*)	822. (*a*)	823. (*c*)	824. (*a*)	825. (*a*)
826. (*d*)	827. (*d*)	828. (*d*)	829. (*b*)	830. (*c*)
831. (*c*)	832. (*b*)	833. (*a*)	834. (*d*)	835. (*d*)
836. (*d*)	837. (*b*)	838. (*a*)	839. (*b*)	840. (*d*)
841. (*a*)	842. (*d*)	843. (*a*)	844. (*c*)	845. (*a*)
846. (*d*)	847. (*b*)	848. (*d*)	849. (*c*)	850. (*a*)
851. (*d*)	852. (*d*)	853. (*b*)	854. (*a*)	855. (*a*)
856. (*a*)	857. (*c*)	858. (*d*)	859. (*b*)	860. (*b*)

861. (*d*)	862. (*d*)	863. (*a*)	864. (*c*)	865. (*d*)
866. (*d*)	867. (*d*)	868. (*d*)	869. (*c*)	870. (*b*)
871. (*a*)	872. (*c*)	873. (*d*)	874. (*d*)	875. (*a*)
876. (*a*)	877. (*d*)	878. (*d*)	879. (*a*)	880. (*d*)
881. (*b*)	882. (*d*)	883. (*b*)	884. (*b*)	885. (*d*)
886. (*d*)	887. (*b*)	888. (*d*)	889. (*d*)	890. (*d*)
891. (*d*)	892. (*d*)	893. (*a*)	894. (*a*)	895. (*a*)
896. (*c*)	897. (*d*)	898. (*d*)	899. (*b*)	900. (*d*)
901. (*a*)	902. (*d*)	903. (*d*)	904. (*a*)	905. (*d*)
906. (*d*)	907. (*a*)	908. (*b*)	909. (*d*)	910. (*a*)
911. (*c*)	912. (*a*)	913. (*b*)	914. (*c*)	915. (*c*)
916. (*a*)	917. (*a*)	918. (*b*)	919. (*b*)	920. (*b*)
921. (*d*)	922. (*d*)	923. (*d*)	924. (*b*)	925. (*a*)
926. (*d*)	927. (*a*)	928. (*b*)	929. (*d*)	930. (*b*)
931. (*d*)	932. (*d*)	933. (*a*)	934. (*a*)	935. (*d*)
936. (*d*)	937. (*d*)	938. (*a*)	939. (*a*)	940. (*d*)
941. (*d*)	942. (*d*)	943. (*d*)	944. (*d*)	945. (*d*)
946. (*d*)	947. (*d*)	948. (*d*)	949. (*d*)	950. (*d*)
951. (*a*)	952. (*d*)	953. (*a*)	954. (*a*)	955. (*d*)
956. (*d*)	957. (*d*)	958. (*c*)	959. (*b*)	960. (*a*)
961. (*a*)	962. (*b*)	963. (*b*)	964. (*c*)	965. (*d*)
966. (*d*)	967. (*a*)	968. (*d*)	969. (*d*)	970. (*d*)
971. (*d*)	972. (*c*)	973. (*a*)	974. (*c*)	975. (*a*)
976. (*a*)	977. (*d*)	978. (*a*)		

SECTION–5

Valvulular Heart Disease, Infective Endocarditis Congenital Heart Disease and Pericardial Disease

1. **Commonest type of congenital heart disease seen in adults**
   (a) Atrial septal defect
   (b) Ventricular septal defect
   (c) Tetralogy of fallot
   (d) Patent ductus arteriosus
   (e) Bicuspid aortic valve
2. **In atrial septal defect the aorta is**
   (a) Small (b) Normal
   (c) Enlarged (d) Aneurysmal
3. **The following is true of tetralogy of fallot except**
   (a) Squatting
   (b) Clubbing
   (c) Cyanosis
   (d) Increased lung vascularity
4. **Hilar dance is seen in**
   (a) Ventricular septal defect
   (b) Atrial septal defect
   (c) Patent ductus arteriosus
   (d) Transposition of great vessels
5. **Rheumatic disease commonly involves which of the following?**
   (a) Aortic and tricuspid
   (b) Aortic and pulmonary
   (c) Mitral and tricuspid
   (d) Mitral and aortic

6. Which of the following statement regarding rheumatic nodules is false?

(a) Found over extensor surface
(b) Tender on palpation
(c) Associated with severe carditis
(d) Pea size nodules

7. Sudden death is common in

(a) Mitral stenosis
(b) Ventricular septal defect
(c) Aortic stenosis
(d) Patent ductus arteriosus

8. Hemoptysis is commonly seen in

(a) Aortic stenosis
(b) Pulmonary stenosis
(c) Mitral stenosis
(d) Tricuspid stenosis

9. The area of mitral valve orifice in mitral stenosis not compatible with life is

(a) $< 0.5 \text{ cm}^2$ (b) 1.0 cm^2
(c) 1.5 cm^2 (d) 3.0 cm^2

10. ST Segment elevation in pericarditis occurs in all leads except

(a) V2.6 (b) Lead III
(c) aVF (d) aVR

11. In rheumatic heart disease most common cause of embolism is

(a) Tight mitral stenosis with atrial fibrillation
(b) Aortic stenosis
(c) Tricuspid regurgitation
(d) Atrial septal defect

12. All the following are seen in tricuspid atresia except

(a) Right axis deviation
(b) Left axis deviation
(c) Left atrial hypertrophy
(d) Cyanosis

13. Patent foramen ovule in adult is found

(a) None of the adults (b) 10% of adults
(c) 1/3 of adults (d) 1/2 of adults

14. Mitral valve prolapse has all the following features except

(a) Thickened and redundant leaflets
(b) Annular dilatation
(c) Short & thick chordae tendineae
(d) Posterior leaflet prolapse more common than anterior

15. The phrase 'A disease that licks in joints but bites the heart' is used for

(a) Acute infective endocarditis
(b) Acute rheumatic fever
(c) Rheumatoid arthritis
(d) None of the above

16. The term angina means

(a) Chest pain
(b) Burning in chest
(c) Strangling
(d) None of the above

17. Most common cause of chronic mitral regurgitation in our country is

(a) Rheumatic
(b) Dilated cardiomyopathy
(c) Restrictive cardiomyopathy
(d) Ischemia

18. Secondary mitral regurgitation is characterized by all except

(a) Enlarged left ventricular
(b) Reduced cardiac output
(c) Pulmonary venous hypertension
(d) Regurgitant fraction is usually > 0.4

19. Mitral facies in mitral stenosis is characterized by all except

(a) High cardiac output
(b) Low cardiac output
(c) Systolic vasoconstriction
(d) Severe mitral stenosis

20. All of the following statements regarding atrial fibrillation in mitral stenosis are correct except

(a) Its development is related to left atrial size
(b) It is present in 40% of cases
(c) Its development is related to age
(d) Its development is related to severity of mitral stenosis

21. Symptoms in mitral stenosis appears at which valve area?

(a) 3.5 cm^2 (b) 3 cm^2
(c) 2.5 cm^2 (d) < 2.5 cm^2

22. Non critical mitral stenosis may result in acute pulmonary edema in following conditions except

(a) Atrial fibrillation with fast ventricular rate
(b) Pregnancy
(c) Surgery
(d) Thromboembolism

23. Reactive pulmonary hypertension in mitral stenosis occurs because of all of the following except

(a) Atrial fibrillation
(b) Increased pulmonary capillary pressure
(c) Hypoxia
(d) Alvcolar fibrosis

24. Prime symptom in mitral stenosis occurs because of

(a) Pulmonary arterial hypertension
(b) Pulmonary venous hypertension
(c) Right ventricular failure
(d) Arrhythmia

25. Mitral stenosis is caused by all except

(a) Rheumatic myocarditis
(b) Infective endocarditis
(c) Viral myocarditis
(d) Congenital

26. Normal mitral valve shape is

(a) Tubular (b) Ellipsoid
(c) Funnel (d) Oval

27. Which of the following statement is correct regarding cortriatration?

(a) Presence of systolic murmur
(b) Presence of diastolic murmur
(c) Presence of opening Snap
(d) Common in adults

28. Congenital mitral stenosis is associated with all except

(a) Mitral regurgitation
(b) Patent ductus arteriosus
(c) Coarctation of aorta
(d) None of the above

29. Which of the following is usually absent in the mitral stenosis?

(a) Opening snap
(b) Middiastolic murmur
(c) S3
(d) Right ventricular enlargement

30. Which of the following feature is uncommon in acquired aortic stenosis?

(a) Murmur is best heard in right 2nd intercostal space
(b) Aortic ejection sound is common
(c) A2 decreased or absent
(d) Aortic regurgitant murmur

31. Which valve is not involved in CREST syndrome?

(a) Mitral (b) Aortic
(c) Pulmonary (d) Tricuspid

32. Most common cardiac abnormality in klippel feil syndrome is

(a) Fallot's tetralogy
(b) Patent ductus arteriosus
(c) Atrial septal defect (ostium secundum)
(d) Ventricular septal defect

33. Teratogenic congenital heart disease are not related to

(a) Alcohol (b) Lithium
(c) Phenytoin (d) Erythromycin

34. Most common congenital heart disease as ellis vencreveld syndromes

(a) Singh atrium/large aortic stenosis defect
(b) Ventricular septal defect
(c) Singh ventricle
(d) Auto pulmonary window

35. Acute mitral regurgitation is characterized by all except

(a) Abrupt onset of symptoms
(b) S4 gallop
(c) Apical systolic murmur
(d) Cardiac enlargement

36. Most common ECG abnormality in mitral valve prolapse is

(a) T-wave inversion in inferior leads
(b) T-wave inversion in lateral leads
(c) QT prolongation
(d) None of the above

37. Bacterial endocarditis most commonly occurs in

(a) Mitral stenosis
(b) Mitral regurgitation
(c) Aortic regurgitation
(d) Aortic stenosis

38. Most uncommon symptom in chronic severe mitral regurgitation is

(a) Fatigue (b) Angina
(c) Dyspnea (d) None of the above

39. Which NSAID is the drug of choice in acute viral pericarditis?

(a) Aspirin (b) Indomethacin
(c) Ibuprofen (d) Naproxen

40. Least commonly encountered physical sign in pulmonary arterial hypertension is

(a) Loud P2
(b) Tricuspid regurgitation
(c) Right sided S4
(d) Graham steel murmur

41. Which atrial arrhythmia is most common in heart failure?

(a) Atrial tachycardia
(b) AVN reentrant tachycardia
(c) Atrial flutter
(d) Atrial fibrillation

42. Which component of pericardial fluid acts as a lubricant?

(a) Prostaglandins (b) Phospholipids
(c) Proteins (d) None of the above

43. Most common cause of acute pericarditis is

(a) Bacterial
(b) Post myocardial infarction
(c) Viral
(d) Uremic

44. Parietal pericardium entirely cover all the following structures except

(a) Right ventricle (b) Left ventricle
(c) Right atrium (d) Left atrium

45. Normal volume of pericardial fluid is

(a) 100 ml (b) Up to 50 ml
(c) Up to 150 ml (d) More than 150 ml

46. Most common cause of tricuspid stenosis is

(a) SLE
(b) Carcinoid syndromes
(c) Rheumatic
(d) Infective endocarditis

47. Which is not found in ECG of tricuspid stenosis?

(a) Right ventricular hypertrophy
(b) Atrial fibrillation
(c) P pulmonale
(d) RA enlargement

48. Tricuspid valve area in severe tricuspid stenosis is

(a) $< 1\ cm^2$ (b) $1.2\ cm^2$
(c) $1.5\ cm^2$ (d) None of the above

49. Which valvular lesion is most common?

(a) Mitral stenosis
(b) Tricuspid regurgitation
(c) Mitral regurgitation
(d) None of the above

50. Most common organism causing infective endocarditis is

(a) Streptococcus (b) Staphylococcus
(c) Gram negative bacilli
(d) Fungal infection

51. Most common organism causing native valve endocarditis is

(a) Streptococci
(b) Fungal infection
(c) Staphylococcus
(d) Gram negative bacilli

52. Prolongation of PR interval in infective endocarditis indicates all except

(a) Ring abscess
(b) Generalized myocarditis
(c) Focal myocarditis
(d) Extension of infection

53. Most important complication of infective endocarditis is

(a) Arrhythmias (b) Heart failure
(c) Embolization (d) Mycotic aneurysm

54. Syncope at rest in aortic stenosis is due to

(a) Bradycardia
(b) Ventricular arrhythmias
(c) Hypotension
(d) Complete heart block

55. Acute severe aortic regurgitation is caused by all except

(a) Infective endocarditis
(b) Rheumatic carditis
(c) Chest trauma
(d) Aortic dissection

56. Holt-oram syndrome has all the features except

(a) Ostium primum ASD
(b) VSD
(c) Upper limb dysplasias
(d) AVN conduction defect

57. All drugs are associated with hypersensitive myocarditis except

(a) Methyldopa (b) Streptomycin
(c) Tetracycline (d) Chloromycetin

58. All drugs causes toxic myocarditis except

(a) Emetine (b) Lithium
(c) Theophylline (d) Procanamide

59. Earliest ECG change in mitral stenosis is

(a) Right axis deviation
(b) Left atrial enlargement
(c) R/S > 1 in V_1
(d) Right atrial enlargement

60. Constrictive pericarditis has all features except

(a) Pulsus paradoxes (b) Kussmaul's sign
(c) S3 (d) Murmurs

61. Culture negative infective endocarditis occurs in

(a) 20% (b) 25%
(c) < 5% (d) 5.10%

62. Which of the following is a feature of active endocarditis?

(a) Increse ESR (b) Leukocytosis
(c) Proteinuria
(d) Increased polyclonal immunoglobulin

63. Which of the following condition has highest maternal mortality during pregnancy?

(a) VSD left to right shunt
(b) Pulmonary stenosis
(c) Pulmonary hypertension
(d) ASD left to right shunt

64. Aortic stenosis patients are fit for pregnancy with all the following factors except

(a) Moderate aortic stenosis
(b) Negative exercise test
(c) Left ventricle dysfunction
(d) Normal ECG

65. Higher INR (3-5-4) is recommended for which prosthetic valve?

(a) Bileaflet (b) Tilting discs
(c) Caged ball (d) All of the above

66. Long term anticoagulation is done in all patients with bioprosthetic valve except

(a) With atrial fibrillation
(b) With atrial thrombus on echo cardiography
(c) Previous history of embolism
(d) None of the above

67. Optimum duration of antibiotic therapy in majority of patients with infective endocarditis is

(a) 2 weeks (b) 10 days
(c) 4 weeks (d) 6 weeks

68. Strong indication for surgical intervention in infective endocarditis includes all except

(a) Resistant heart failure
(b) Endocarditis caused by filamentous fungi
(c) Occlusion of valve by large vegetation
(d) Late onset prosthetic valve endocarditis

69. Average over all survival in severe aortic stenosis is

(a) < 2 years (b) 5 years
(c) 2 years (d) 3 years

70. Chronic severe aortic regurgitation is characterized by all except

(a) Increased systolic blood pressure
(b) Increased peripheral vascular resistance
(c) Increase pulse pressure
(d) Increase ejection fraction

71. Acute severe aortic regurgitation is characterized by all except

(a) Increase ejection fraction
(b) Increase heart rate
(c) Increase peripheral vascular resistance
(d) Increase left ventricle end diastolic pressure

72. Classic and characteristic electrocardiography finding in congenitally corrected transposition of great vessels is

(a) Advanced AV block
(b) I degree AV block
(c) Voltages of precordial leads reflect hemodynamic situation
(d) Loss of normal Q wave in V_6

73. Congenital mitral stenosis has all of the features except

(a) Loud S_1 (M_1)
(b) Middiastolic murmur

(c) Presystolic murmur
(d) Pulmonary hypertension

74. Commonest cause of aortic regurgitation is
(a) Rheumatic
(b) Aortic root dilatation
(c) Bicuspid aortic valve
(d) Infective endocarditis

75. All following abnormalities of pulse are found in aortic regurgitation except
(a) Corrigan's pulse
(b) Water hammer pulse
(c) Bisferiens
(d) Pulses alternans

76. Linear calcification in ascending aorta is characteristic of which etiological type of aortic regurgitation?
(a) Bicuspid aortic valve
(b) Syphilis
(c) Rheumatic
(d) Degenerative disease

77. Which is least common complication of atrial regurgitation?
(a) LVF
(b) Atrial arrhythmias
(c) Infective endocarditis
(d) Ventricular arrhythmias

78. Which of the following complication of mitral stenosis is not related to its severity?
(a) Infective endocarditis
(b) Thromboembolism
(c) Atrial fibrillation
(d) All of the above

79. Which of the following is potential intracardiac shunt?
(a) Patent foramen ovale
(b) Atrial septal defect
(c) Ventricular septal defect
(d) None of the above

80. Neonatal marfan syndromes has all the following cardiac lesion except

(a) Mitral regurgitation
(b) TR
(c) PR
(d) Dilatation of aorta/AR

81. Aortic regurgitation in hypertension is found in

(a) Isolated systolic hypertension
(b) Combined systolic and diastolic hypertension
(c) Severe diastolic hypertension
(d) None of the above

82. All the following cardiac disorders are associated with pericarditis except

(a) Acute myocardial infarction
(b) Post myocardial infarction syndromes
(c) Atrial septal defects
(d) Aortic regurgitation

83. Which metabolic disorder does not produce pericarditis?

(a) Uremia
(b) Ketoacidosis (diabetic)
(c) Cholesterol (d) Gout

84. Which component of pericardial rub is usually loudest?

(a) Ventricular systole component
(b) Atrial component
(c) Early diastolic
(d) All component

85. Pericardial rub is loudest at

(a) Apex of heart
(b) Pulmonary area
(c) Aortic area
(d) Left mid to lower sternal border

86. All following leads show ST depression in acute pericarditis except

(a) aVR (b) V_4 R
(c) V_1 (d) L_1

87. Most common virus causing human myocarditis is

(a) Coxsackie virus A (b) Coxsackie virus B
(c) Echo virus (d) Viral hepatitis

88. Which of the following lesion is not associated with infective endocarditis?

(a) Ostium secundum ASD
(b) Ostium primum ASD
(c) VSD
(d) PDA

89. Right ventricle is enlarged in all the following except

(a) Pulmonary stenosis
(b) Tricuspid atresia
(c) Complete TGA
(d) Eisenmenger syndromes

90. Pulmonary conus is concave in all the following except

(a) Complete TGA (b) TOF
(c) Ebsteins anomaly (d) Common atrium

91. Abnormal LAD of 'P' wave is found in

(a) OP ASD (b) OS ASD
(c) SV ASD (d) PFD

92. Which arrhythmia particularly occurs in operated VSD patients?

(a) LBBB
(b) LAFB
(c) RBBB
(d) Left post hemiblock

93. All the following have no or low risk of infective endocarditis except

(a) Ostium secundum ASD
(b) MVP without mitral regurgitation
(c) Pulmonary stenosis
(d) Bicuspid aortic valve

94. Commonest neurological complication of infective endocarditis is

(a) Ischamic cerebral infarct
(b) Brain abscess
(c) Intracranial haemorrhage
(d) Meningoencephalitis

95. Anatomic closure of ductus arteriosus is caused by

(a) Shortening of ductal wall
(b) Thickening of ductal wall
(c) Both (a) and (b)
(d) None of the above

96. Which is the commonest associated condition with coaretation of aorta?

(a) PDA
(b) Common veulricle
(c) ASD
(d) Hypo plastic left heart syndromes

97. What is abnormal pericardial thickness?

(a) 1 mm (b) 1.2 mm
(c) 2.4 mm (d) > 4 mm

98. Murmur of tricuspid stenosis is characterized by all the features except

(a) Usually heard in xiphoid area
(b) It is diamond shaped
(c) Increases during inspiration
(d) Large 'V' waves in Jugular venous pulse

99. Predominant congenital cardiac disease for arrhythmic SCD are all except

(a) PS (b) TOF
(c) TGA (d) AS

100. Which congenital cardiac malformation is consistently associated with pre-excitation (WPW)?

(a) Endocardial cushion defect
(b) Ebsteins anomaly
(c) Arrhythmogenic right ventricular cardiomyopathy
(d) Complete transposition of great vessels

101. All are characteristic features of ECG in ebsteins anomaly except

(a) Tall 'P' wave
(b) Short PR interval
(c) RBBB
(d) Deep Q in inferior and V1-V3

102. VSD is essential element of all except

(a) TOF
(b) Persistent truncus arteriosus
(c) A-V canal defect (d) TAPVC

103. Beck's traid in acute cardiac tamponade include all except

(a) Rising venous pressure
(b) Falling arterial pressure
(c) Small quiet heart
(d) Tachycardia

104. ASD with significant pulmonary hypertension is characterized by all except

(a) Narrow split S2 which widens on inspiration
(b) Graham steell murmur
(c) Prominent 'a' wave in neck
(d) The murmur of relative TS present

105. Which of the following ECG finding is most common in Ebsteins disease?

(a) Increase PR
(b) RAD
(c) Multiphasic QRS complex
(d) Low voltage QRS

106. Aortic stenosis is featured by all the following except

(a) Occurs after age 65 years
(b) High prevalence in patients with hypertension and LVH
(c) Increased risk of cardiovascular events
(d) May lead to significant grater increase

107. Aortic dissection is common during all the following except

(a) Pregnancy
(b) Coarctation of aorta
(c) Aortic stenosis (d) Exercise

108. Young patients of aortic stenosis having atrial fibrillation usually suggest

(a) Associated hypertension
(b) Associated coronary artery disease
(c) Associated MV disease
(d) Associated thyroioxicesis

109. Which hemodynamic component decreases during exercise in severe mitral stenosis?

(a) Pulmonary vein pressure
(b) Left atrial pressure
(c) Pulmonary artery pressure
(d) Cardiac output

110. Chorea in rheumatic fever has all of the features except

(a) Late manifestation
(b) Self limited
(c) Associated with increased ESR
(d) Chronic rheumatic heart disease may occur

111. Pericardiocentesis is usually done in all except

(a) Pericardial effusion suspected
(b) Cardiac tamponade
(c) Purulent effusion
(d) Small effusion which are hemodynamically insignificant

112. Which of the following is test of choice for diagnosis of pericardial effusion?

(a) X-ray chest (b) Echocardiography
(c) CT (d) MRI

113. All the ECG finding are suggestive of cardiac tamponade except

(a) Low voltage complexes
(b) Electrical alternans
(c) Both (a) and (b)
(d) Right axis deviation

114. Peripheral pulmonary artery stenosis is commonly associated with

(a) Patent ductus arteriosus
(b) ASD
(c) Single atrium
(d) VSD

115. Tetralogy of fallot has all the following features except

(a) Cyanotic spells (b) Squatting
(c) Prominent 'a' wave
(d) Aortic ejection click

116. Common cause of rupture of sinus of valsalva

(a) Spontaneous (b) Hypertension
(c) Exercise (d) Emotion

117. Which side most commonly ruptures in sinus of valsalva ruptures?

(a) Right (b) Left
(c) None coronary (d) All of the above

118. In which chamber sinus of valsalva rupture most commonly?

(a) RA (b) LA
(c) RV (d) LV

119. Fallots trilogy has all the features except

(a) Heart failure
(b) Cardiomegly
(c) S4 Gallop
(d) Pulmonary bay on X-ray

120. Which of the following are the acronyms for percutaneous Transmyocardial revascularization?

(a) PTMR (b) PMR
(c) DMR (d) PMLR
(e) TMR (f) None of these
(g) All of these

121. Micromitral operation means

(a) Operation in small mitral valve
(b) It denotes small atrial incision and cardiac instrument manipulation using video guidance
(c) Mitral valve surgery under microscope
(d) All the above

122. The world's first video assisted mitral valve operation was done by

(a) Calafiore (b) Subramanian
(c) Carepentier (d) All the above

123. The first video assisted mitral valve operation done on

(a) Arrested heart (b) Fibrillating heart
(c) Beating heart (d) All the above

124. World's first robotic assisted mitral valve operation was performed on

(a) September 21, 1997
(b) February 21, 1996
(c) May 21, 1998
(d) All the above

125. World's first robotic assisted mitral valve operation was done by

(a) Professor fredrich Mohr
(b) Dr. Carpentier
(c) Dr. Venermin
(d) None of the above

126. All the following are typical symptoms of mitral stenosis except

(a) Exertional dyspnoea
(b) Chest pain
(c) Paroxysmal nocturnal dyspnoea
(d) Hemoptysis

127. Mitral valve area can be estimated echocardiographically by the following

(a) Planimetry
(b) Pressure half-time method
(c) Continuity method
(d) All of the above

128. Current indications of intervention in mitral stenosis include all of the following except

(a) Symptoms exceeding NYHA class II
(b) Thromboembolism
(c) Pulmonary hypertension
(d) Hemoptysis

129. All of the following are only relative contraindications for balloon mitral valvuloplasty except

(a) Calcification of mitral leaflets
(b) Left atrium thrombus
(c) Subvavular crowding
(d) Mitral regurgitation [Grade > 3]

130. Forward stroke volume is increased or normal in

(a) Acute mitral regurgitation (MR)

(b) Chronic compensated mitral regurgitation
(c) Chronic decompensated mitral regurgitation
(d) All of the above

131. Severe mitral regurgitation is denoted echocardiographically by all of the following except
(a) Colour flow jet area > 7.0 cm^2 with TTE
(b) Colour jet occupying > 50% of LA
(c) Colour flow jet area > 8.0 cm^2 with TEE
(d) Systolic reversal of flow in pulmonary veins

132. Indications of mitral valve replacement in chronic mitral regurgitation include all except the following
(a) NYHA class III symptoms
(b) LV ejection fraction < 60%
(c) LV end systolic dimension >45 mm
(d) LV end systolic volume > 30 m^l/m^2

133. Mitral valve repair is preferable to mitral valve replacement because of
(a) Superior post operative left ventricular function
(b) Better survival
(c) Obviation of need for anticoagulation
(d) All of the above

134. Commonest cyanotic congenital heart disease at birth is
(a) Fallots tetralogy
(b) TAPVD
(c) Eisenmenger syndrome
(d) D-TGA

135. Commonest cyanotic congenital heart disease at 2 years is
(a) TGA (b) TOF
(c) Fallots triology (d) TAPVD

136. Absence of fever in infective endocarditis is found in all the following except
(a) Young (b) CHF
(c) Severe sepsis (d) Renal failure

137. Which murmur in acute rheumatic fever is of no significance?

(a) Mitral regurgitation
(b) Carrey coombs murmur
(c) Aortic ejection murmur
(d) Early diastolic murmur of AR

138. Snowmans heart is found in

(a) Supradiaphragmatic type of TAPVD
(b) Infra-diaphragmatic type of TAPVD
(c) Both of the above
(d) None of the above

139. Cyanotic spells are managed by all except

(a) Lying position (Supine)
(b) IV morphine
(c) IV Sodabicarb
(d) Propranolol

140. Which block commonly occurs postoperatively in TOF?

(a) 1 degree AVB (b) CHB
(c) LBBB (d) RBBB

141. Pericarditis is associated with all except

(a) Hydralazine (b) Procainamide
(c) Amiodarone (d) Emetine

142. All following cyanotic heart disease are mild BVH except

(a) DORV with out PS
(b) TGA with out PS
(c) Truncus arteriosus
(d) Fallot's tetralogy

143. Pouring pulmonary regurgitation occurs commonly in

(a) Complete absence of pulmonary valve
(b) Idiopathic dilation of PA
(c) Post surgical in PS
(d) All the above

144. Which is commonest cause of severe atrial regurgitation in young child?

(a) VSD with aortic valve
(b) Rheumatic

(c) Bicuspid valve (d) Dissection of aorta

145. Commonest cause of mild aortic regurgitation in adults

(a) Hypertension
(b) Rheumatoid arthritis
(c) Osteogenesis imperfecta
(d) Marfans syndrome

146. All are causes of non pansystolic murmur in TR except

(a) Pulmonary hypertensive TR
(b) Carcinoid syndromes
(c) Tricuspid valve prolapse
(d) Acute Tricuspid regurgitation

147. Acute tricuspid regurgitation is found in all except

(a) Infective endocarditis
(b) Pacemaker ulcer
(c) blunt trauma in chest
(d) Tricuspid valve prolapse

148. All are causes of MVP without myxomatous degeneration except

(a) Coronary artery disease
(b) RHD
(c) Flail AML
(d) Marfan's syndrome

149. VSD is associated with all the following except

(a) A-V canal defect (b) TOF
(c) Tricuspid atresia (d) Fallot's triology

150. Small ventricular sepal defect has all the following features except

(a) Left to right shunt < 1.5 : 1
(b) No cardiac enlargement
(c) Pansystolic murmur
(d) MDM flow murmur at apex

151. AR is caused by aortic root dissection occurs in all the following except

(a) Ankylosing spondylitis
(b) Syphilis
(c) Rheumatoid
(d) Marfan's syndromes

152. AR due to aortic root dilation occurs in all the following except

(a) Marfan's syndrome
(b) Ehlers Danlos
(c) Pseudoxanthicum elasticum
(d) Behcets disease

153. Mild atrial regurgitation has none of the following features except

(a) Murmur
(b) Peripheral signs
(c) Left ventricular enlargement
(d) Left ventricular failure

154. Moderate mitral regurgitation has all the following features except

(a) Murmur
(b) Peripheral sign
(c) Left ventricular enlargement
(d) Left ventricular failure

155. All the following cyanotic congenital heart diseases causes pulmonary venous engorgement except

(a) Aortic atresia
(b) Aortic and mitral atresia
(c) TAPVD with obstruction
(d) Ebstein's anomaly

156. Unusually loud A2 in VSD indicates all the following except

(a) Associated coarctation of aorta
(b) Systemic hypertension
(c) Bicuspid aortic valve
(d) Associated anemia

157. Single S2 in pulmonary atresia suspect all the following except

(a) Severe PS
(b) TOF
(c) Dysplastic pulmonary valve
(d) Mild PS

158. Wide fixed splitting in eisenmenger syndrome is found in all the following underlying diseases except

(a) ASD (b) TAPVD
(c) VSD of AV canal type
(d) PDA

159. Diminished A2 in aortic regurgitation is found in all except

(a) Rheumatic
(b) Associated aortic stenosis
(c) Infective endocarditis
(d) VSD with aortic regurgitation

160. Which organism is most commonly causing infective endocarditis?

(a) Staphylococcus aureus
(b) Enterococci
(c) Gram –ve bacilli (d) Pneumococcal

161. Recurrent pericarditis drug of choice is

(a) Steroids
(b) NSAIDS
(c) Both above in combination
(d) Colchicine

162. All following is correct in pulmonary arterio-venous fistula except

(a) Right to left shunt
(b) Cardiomyopathy is found in all the cases
(c) Continuous murmur becomes loud with inspiration
(d) Telangiectasia on skin and mucous membranes

163. All following are causes of generalized pericardial rub except

(a) Viral
(b) Disseminated disease
(c) Uremia
(d) Acute myocardial infarction

164. Most common associated disease with ebsteins anamoly is

(a) ASD
(b) VSD
(c) Accessory pathway with ventricular excitation
(d) Ventricular arrhythmia

165. Most common ECG finding in tricuspid atresia is

(a) Marked LAD
(b) LVH
(c) P congenitale
(d) All of the above

166. In which type of left ventricular out-flow obstruction AR is rare?

(a) Valvular congenital aortic stenosis
(b) Acute aquired valvular aortic stenosis
(c) HOCM
(d) Supravalvular aortic stenosis (Cong)

167. Commonest finding in ventricular septal defect is

(a) LVH
(b) Katz-Watchzel phenomenon
(c) RBBB
(d) RVH (A)

168. All following cyanotic heart disease associated with no cardiac enlargement except

(a) Pulmonary A-V fistula
(b) SVC draining in to LA
(c) IVC draining in to LA
(d) Tricuspid atresia

169. 3rd Heart sound is found in all following cyanotic congenital heart diseases except

(a) TAPVD
(b) DORV with out PS
(c) Truncus arteriosus
(d) Fallot's tetralogy

170. Which is the most reliable sign in heart in infective endocarditis?

(a) Changing cardiac murmur
(b) Heart failure
(c) New early diastolic murmur of aortic regurgitation
(d) Pericardial rub

171. Aortic regurgitation and conduction defect is found in all except

(a) Ankylosing spondylitis

(b) Infective endocarditis
(c) Rheumatoid arthritis
(d) Syphilitic

172. Following renal lesions occur in infective endocarditis except

(a) Renal infarct
(b) Diffuse glomerulonephritis
(c) Pyelonephritis
(d) Focal embolic nephritis

173. Cooing-dove murmur of aortic regurgitation is due to all except

(a) Laceration of cusps
(b) Perforation of cusps
(c) Eversion of cusps
(d) Calcification of cusps

174. Which ECG finding is highly characteristic of organic tricuspid regurgitation?

(a) RAE (b) AF
(c) RBBB (d) qR in V1

175. Which is the most uncommon finding in organic mitral regurgitation?

(a) LAE (b) LVH
(c) Atrial fibrillation (d) Left axis deviation

176. Which of the ECG finding in Mitral regurgitation indicates it to be functional?

(a) LAE (b) LVH
(c) RAD (d) LAD

177. Which ECG finding is included in criteria for diagnosis of acuté rheumatic fever?

(a) Prolonged QT interval
(b) Prolonged PR interval
(c) ST/T wave changes
(d) CHB

178. Commonest arrhythmia in mitral stenosis is

(a) VE (b) AE
(c) Atrial fibrillation (d) 1 degree AV block

179. Which of the following is indicative of severe rheumatic carditis?

(a) Mitral regurgitation
(b) Aortic regurgitation
(c) Pericarditis
(d) Heart failure

180. Which of the following peripheral sign is most specific for aortic regurgitation?

(a) Corrigan's pulse
(b) Water hammer pulse
(c) Pistol shot sounds
(d) Duroziez's murmur

181. Which manifestation of acute rheumatic fever is most common?

(a) Chorea
(b) Arthritis
(c) Carditis
(d) Sub cutaneous nodule

182. Which valve is most frequently involved in acute rheumatic fever?

(a) Aortic (b) Mitral
(c) Tricuspid (d) Pulmonary

183. Ortner's syndrome is due to dilation of

(a) RA (b) LA
(c) RV (d) None of the above

184. Which manifestation of aortic stenosis has highest mortality rate?

(a) Palpitation
(b) Chest pain (Angina)
(c) Syncope
(d) Dyspnea (heart failure)

185. Atrial fibrillation in AS indicates all except

(a) Infective endocarditis
(b) Associated coronary artery disease
(c) Associated MV disease
(d) Associated heart failure

186. Which of the following feature is found in acute aortic regurgitation?

(a) Wide pulse pressure
(b) Austin flint murmur

(c) Acute LVF
(d) Significant left ventricular dilatation

187. Most important complication of infective endocarditis is

(a) Embolism (b) Mycotic aneurysm
(c) Heart failure (d) Hematuria

188. How many patients of acute rheumatic carditis develop chronic rheumatic valvular heart disease?

(a) 10% (b) 25%
(c) 50% (d) 90%

189. Pathological hallmark of rheumatic carditis is

(a) Myocarditis
(b) Valvulitis
(c) Commissural fusion
(d) Aschoff's nodule

190. Which complication is related to severity of mitral stenosis?

(a) Atrial fibrillation
(b) Thrombo embolism
(c) Infective endocarditis
(d) RVF

191. Most common organism of right sided endocarditis is

(a) Staphylococcus aureas
(b) Staphylococcus epidermidis
(c) Pseudomonas
(d) Serratia

192. All the following drugs are avoided in treatment of acute pericarditis following acute myocardial infarction except

(a) Aspirin (b) Heparin
(c) Indomethacin (d) Steroids

193. All the following congenital heart disease may be associated congenital coronary artery anomaly except

(a) Bicuspid aortic valve
(b) TOF
(c) Coarctation of aorta
(d) PDA

194. Growth retardation in congenital heart disease is due to all except

(a) Recurrent infection
(b) CHF
(c) Hypoxia
(d) Poor intake

195. All are cerebral complications of congenital heart disease except

(a) Embolic episodes
(b) Cerebral abscess
(c) Venous thrombosis
(d) Aneurysmal rupture

196. All following viruses commonly cause pericarditis except

(a) Coxsackie Group 'B'
(b) Mumps
(c) Ebstein-barr
(d) Herpes-simplex

197. All following parasites can cause pericarditis except

(a) E-histolytica
(b) Echinococcus
(c) Toxoplasma
(d) Tapeworm

198. All the following antihypertensive drugs may cause pericarditis except

(a) Reserpine
(b) Methyldopa
(c) hydralazine
(d) α-blockers

199. Which pericardial disease particularly occurs in mulibrey namison?

(a) Lax pericardial effusion
(b) Cardiac tamponade
(c) Constrictive pericarditis
(d) None of the above

200. All the following statement for infective endocarditis are correct except

(a) Left sided valves more commonly involved than right side
(b) Regurgitant lesions more prone than stenotic lesions
(c) Right sided vegetations are larger than left sided

(d) Fungal endocarditis the vegetation is smaller than streptococcal viridians

201. Petechial in infective endocarditis occur in all following places except

(a) Conjunctiva
(b) Buccal mucosa
(c) Skin above the clavicle
(d) Hands

202. Multiple small potency infiltrate in X-ray chest suggest endocarditis of which value.

(a) Aortic (b) Pulmonary
(c) Mitral (d) Tricuspid

203. All are common location for mycotic aneurysm in infective endocarditis except

(a) Proximal aorta
(b) Intracranial arteries
(c) Visceral arteries
(d) Carotids

204. Weight-loss medication causes commonly which valve lesion?

(a) Aortic stenosis
(b) Mitral regurgitation
(c) T regurgitation
(d) Aortic regurgitation

205. The major cause of mitral regurgitation in mitral valve prolapse is

(a) Chordal abnormality
(b) Infective endocarditis
(c) Prolapse of leaflet
(d) Annular dilatation

206. Mitral valve calcification correlate with which of the following features?

(a) LA-LV gradient
(b) Atrial fibrillation
(c) Pulmonary hypertension
(d) Right ventricular failure (RVF)

207. Most common congenital heart disease is

(a) Aortic stenosis (b) MVP
(c) Bicuspid valve (d) Fallot's tetralogy

208. Annular calcification of mitral valve (MV) occurs in all the following except

(a) Hypertension
(b) Hyperlipidemia
(c) DM
(d) Marfan's syndrome

209. Which congenital valve lesion is associated with G1 bleeding?

(a) Pulmonary stenosis (PS)
(b) Aortic stenosis
(c) Mitral stenosis
(d) Tricuspid stenosis

210. Most common hematological finding in infective endocarditis is

(a) Anemia
(b) Increased ESR
(c) Leukocytosis
(d) Thrombocytopenia

211. Most common serological finding in infective endocarditis is

(a) Immune complexes
(b) Hyper gammaglobinemia
(c) Rheumatoid factor
(d) Hypercomplementemia

212. Most common urinary finding infective endocarditis is

(a) Proteinuria
(b) Microscopic hematuria
(c) WBC cast
(d) RBC cast

213. Clot formation in LA most commonly occurs in

(a) Appendage (b) Inter atrial septum
(c) Body of LA (d) Near MV

214. Endocarditis prophylaxis is not indicated in all except

(a) ASD (OS)
(b) MVP with mitral regurgitation
(c) Cardiac pacemakers
(d) Implanted defibrillators

215. All are medication for surgery in IE except

(a) Heart failure
(b) Acute severe regurgitation
(c) Large vegetation
(d) Severe acidemia

216. Mild aortic stenosis is characterized by all except

(a) Slow rising pulse
(b) Normal apex beat
(c) Absent S4
(d) Early diastolic murmur

217. Severe aortic stenosis with normal left ventricular function has all following features except

(a) Slow rising low volume pulse
(b) Apex beat sustained
(c) S4 is absent
(d) Late peaking ESM

218. Severe aortic stenosis with heart failure has all the following feature except

(a) Heaving apex beat
(b) S3 is present
(c) S4 is present
(d) No thrill with murmur

219. Most common cause of acquired PS is

(a) Rheumatic
(b) Infective endocarditis
(c) Carcinoid syndrome
(d) Collagen diseases

220. Normal amount of pericardial fluid is

(a) < 5 ml (b) 5.10 ml
(c) 11.14 ml (d) 15.50 ml

221. Most common etiology of isolated tricuspid regurgitation is

(a) Infective endocarditis in drug addicts
(b) Carcinoid syndrome
(c) TVP
(d) Myocardial infarction

222. Most common cause of tricuspid stenosis is

(a) Rheumatic (b) Carcinoid
(c) Infective endocarditis
(d) SLE

223. Most common cause of pulmonary regurgitation is

(a) Pulmonary hypertension
(b) Rheumatic
(c) Infective endocarditis
(d) Tuberculosis

224. Commonest cause of death in ASD (OS) is

(a) Heart failure
(b) Eisenmengers syndrome
(c) Paradoxical embolism
(d) Brain abscess

225. Most common defect associated with fallot's tetralogy

(a) ASD
(b) Absent ductus arteriosus
(c) Persistent left superior venacava
(d) Right sided aortic arch

226. Most common cyanotic congenital heart disease in adult is

(a) Transposition of great arteries
(b) Double outlet right ventricle
(c) Eisenmenger syndrome
(d) Fallot's tetralogy

227. Atrial fibrillation in mitral stenosis appears to be related to all the following except

(a) Atriomegaly (b) Fibrosis of LA
(c) Duration of atriomegaly
(d) Pulmonary hypertension

228. Which is commonest anatomical abnormality in mitral stenosis?

(a) Commissural (b) Chordal
(c) Cuspal (d) Combined

229. Calcification of aortic valve most commonly occurs in

(a) Bicuspid aortic valve
(b) Rheumatic aortic valve disease

(c) Degenerative aortic valve disease
(d) Aortic valve disease in rheumatoid arthritis

230. Mitral valve calcification is more common in which of the following?

(a) Mitral stenosis
(b) Mitral regurgitation
(c) Mitral stenosis + Mitral regurgitation
(d) Mitral stenosis with pulmonary regurgitation

231. Rheumatic etiology of mitral valve disease is confirmed by presence of calcification at which site?

(a) Leaflet calcification
(b) Annular calcification
(c) Chordal calcification
(d) LA wall calcification

232. Which statin is known to increase fibrinogen level?

(a) Revastatins (b) Atorvastatins
(c) Simvastatins (d) Pravastatins

233. Which drug commonly produces pericarditis?

(a) Procamiamide
(b) Methyldopa
(c) Diphenyl-hydantion
(d) Isoniazid

234. Which electrocardiographic abnormality indicated severe rheumatic mitral stenosis?

(a) LA enlargement (b) RAD
(c) Atrial fibrillation (d) Sinus tachycardia

235. β-blockers in mitral stenosis with VSR cause all the following except

(a) HR decrease (b) Cardiac out put
(c) Decrease gradient (d) Harm full

236. Organic pulmonary regurgitation is caused by all except

(a) IE
(b) Following pulmonary valvotomy
(c) Rheumatic
(d) Rheumatoid arthritis

237. Rupture of sinuses of valsalva causes couetichous murmur except

(a) Rupture into RA (b) Rupture into RV
(c) Rupture into LA (d) Rupture into LV

238. Acute aortre regurgitation occurs in all the following except

(a) Infective endocarditis
(b) Trauma
(c) Acute aortic dissection
(d) Marfan syndrome

239. Right stornal border murmur of AR occurs in all the following except

(a) Hartains syndrome
(b) Reiter's syndrome
(c) Ankylosing spondylitis
(d) Infective endocarditis

240. Presystolic murmur is absent in mitral stenosis in following except

(a) Atrial fibrillation
(b) Mild mitral stenosis
(c) 1 degree AVB
(d) Tachycardia

241. Aortic sclerosis has all the following except

(a) Short murmur
(b) Aortic regurgitation absent
(c) No LVH (d) S4 present

242. Which is commonest cardiac lesion in ellis van cravald syndrome?

(a) ASD (OS) (b) ASD (OP)
(c) VSD (d) Snyteatrium

243. Webbing of neck is associated with all following cardiac lesion except

(a) Coorctation of aorta
(b) PS
(c) HCM (d) ASD

244. All the following cardiac lesion occur in velocardial facial syndrome except

(a) VSD
(b) ASD

(c) Fallotes tetralogy
(d) Right sided aortic arch

245. Most common complication of BMV is

(a) Death
(b) Cardiac perforation
(c) Mitral regurgitation
(d) ASD

246. ASD following BMV had all the feature except

(a) Usually Small 1–2 mm
(b) Haemodynamically insignificant
(c) Enounce of paradoxical comboliesm
(d) Often persist for more than one years

247. Pericardium is most commonly involved in

(a) Scleroderma
(b) Poly arteritis nodosa
(c) SLE
(d) Ankylosing spondylitis

248. Myocardium is most commonly involved in

(a) SLE
(b) Seleroderma
(c) Rheumatoid arthritis
(d) Ankylosing spondylitis

249. Valves are most commonly involved in

(a) SLE
(b) Seleroderma
(c) Poly arteritis nodosa
(d) Rheumatic arthritis

250. The most characteristic cardiovascular finding in williams syndrome is

(a) Supravalvular aortic stenosis
(b) Peripheral arterial stenosis
(c) Pulmonary valve stenosis
(d) ASD

251. Bolloon aortic valvuloplaty result in all the following except

(a) Initial haemodynamic improvement
(b) Initial symptomatic improvement
(c) Early restenosis
(d) Improvement of large torn sorceries

252. All are indications of bolloon valvuloplasty except

(a) Bridge for value replacement
(b) Price to agent non cardiac surgery
(c) Critical symptomatic aortic stenosis
(d) Critical symptomatic aortic stenosis with comorbid condition

253. Staphyll occurs coagulase position is most common organism involved which IE

(a) NVE (b) IV drug user
(c) Early PVE (d) Late PVE

254. Streptococcus viridian is commonest agent for 1E in

(a) NVE (b) IV drug user
(c) Early PVE (d) Late PVE

255. Streptococcus viridian is least commonly invalved in IE of

(a) NVE (b) IV drug user
(c) Early PVE (d) Late PVE

256. Highest morbidity and mortality in chronic aortic regurgitation is related to

(a) LVESD $\geq$ 50 mm
(b) LVESD $\geq$ 70 mm
(c) LVESD $<$ 70 mm
(d) LVESD $<$ 50 mm

257. Value replacement in chronic aortic regurgitation causes all the following except

(a) Increase survival
(b) Improve LV function irrespective of duration of dysfunction
(c) Improve functional class
(d) Regression of LVH

258. Which of the following is associated with culture negative endocarditis?

(a) NVE (b) IV drug user
(c) Early PVE (d) Late PVE

259. Thrombus in LA is a contraindication to bolloon valvuloplasty (intone) in following situations except

(a) Thrombus along the septum
(b) Free in the cavity
(c) On the surface of valve
(d) Organized clot in LA appendage

260. Staphylococcus IE occur most commonly in which of the following

(a) Early PVE (b) Late PVE
(c) IV drug user (d) NVE

261. When aspirin is combined to oral anti coagulant in mechanical prosthetic valve?

(a) Prileaflet (b) Tilting
(c) Caged ball/disc (d) Systemic embolism

262. Which of the following is commonest laboratory finding in IE?

(a) Increase ESR
(b) Microscopic hematuria
(c) Preliminaries
(d) Positive rheumatoid factor

263. All are immunologic phenomena of IE except

(a) Thievedo Glumeruleneptritrs
(b) Osler node
(c) Roth spot
(d) Mycotic aneurysms

264. All following congenital heart disease can cause abnormal LAD except

(a) ASD (OP)
(b) Tricuspid artesia
(c) Single ventricle
(d) TOF

265. Most common cause of death in unoperated ASD (OS) is

(a) Heart failure
(b) Pulmonary embolism
(c) Brain abscess
(d) Atrial arrhythmia

266. Most common and diagnostic feature in ECG of A-V canal defect is

(a) Superior mean QRS axis in frontal plane
(b) Short PR interval
(c) RVH (d) LVH

267. Superior QRS frontal axis is found in (OS) ASD in all following situations except

(a) Single coronary artery
(b) MVPS
(c) HOCM
(d) ASD (OS) with MS

268. Cholesterol pericarditis is associated with all except

(a) Hypothyroidism
(b) Rheumatoid arthritis
(c) TB
(d) Malignancy

269. Pericardiocentesis is indicated in all except

(a) Cardiac tamponade
(b) Purulent pericarditis
(c) Progressive effusion
(d) Mild pericardial effusion

270. Which valve has prediction for gonococcal endocarditis?

(a) Aortic (b) Mitral
(c) Tricuspid (d) Pulmonary

271. Anemia in normal heart causes heart failure at which level of Hb?

(a) 9 G% (b) 7 G%
(c) 5 G% (d) 4 G%

272. All the following changes may occur in anemia except

(a) Cardiomegaly
(b) Systolic flow murmur
(c) S3
(d) S4

273. Balloon mitral valvotomy may be done if required which trimester of pregnancy

(a) 1st (b) 2nd
(c) 3rd (d) any

274. Which type of congenital aortic stenosis is not associated with post stenotic dilation of aorta?

(a) Unicuspid valve
(b) Bicuspid valve

(c) Hypoplastic aortic valve
(d) Dysplatic aortic valve

275. Which vascular malformation is associated with cyanosis with normal ECG and normal cardiac size?

(a) Fallot's
(b) Eissenemnger
(c) Pulmonary aterio venous fistula
(d) Ebstein disease

276. Congenital corrected TGA is characterized by all except (No coexisting lesion)

(a) Loud S2 in PA
(b) PR elevation
(c) LAD
(d) Prominent Q in left precordial leads

277. Common atria has all following features except

(a) Left axis deviation 'P'
(b) Cyanosis
(c) Significant PH
(d) Left axis deviation of QRS

278. Lutembacher syndrome has all following features except

(a) Reduced signs of mitral stenosis
(b) Prominent pulmonary systolic murmur
(c) RA/RV dilated (d) PVH is usual

279. Accelerated atrial rhythm is found in which of the following

(a) PS (b) ASD (OS)
(c) Mitral stenosis (d) VSD

280. PR interval is prolonged in all the following ASD except

(a) Holt oran syndrome
(b) Ostium prime defect (APD)
(c) familial OS ASD
(d) Sinus venosus defect

281. Ebsteins anomaly is particularly found in which maternal disorder

(a) Alcohol use (b) Lithium
(c) Rubella (d) α^2-blocker

282. In common variety of tricuspid atresia all the following may be found except

(a) Cyanosis from birth
(b) Palpable right ventricle
(c) Murmur of VSD restrictive
(d) Left axis deviation

283. ECG in anomalous origin of left coronary artery from pulmonary track exhibits all the following except

(a) Infect pattern
(b) LVH
(c) Normal frontal plan QRS axis
(d) Persistent ST elevation

284. Paradoxical embolism are rare in which type of ASD?

(a) OSASD (b) SVASD
(c) PFO (d) OPASD

285. Angina with aortic stenosis the choice of antianginal is

(a) α^2-blockers
(b) Ca-blockers
(c) Nitrate
(d) Metabolic modulator

286. Angina with mitral stenosis which is drug of choice as antianginal agent

(a) Nitrate
(b) α^2-blockers
(c) Dihydropyridine Ca-blockers
(d) Metabolic modulator

287. Hilar dance is found in which of the following condition?

(a) ASD (b) VSD
(c) PH (d) Ebsteins

288. Most common ECG finding in constrictive pericarditis is

(a) Generalized T wave inversion
(b) Generalized ST depression
(c) Low voltage
(d) Abnormal Q

289. Commonest cause of primary acute pericarditis is

(a) Acute idiopathic
(b) Neoplastic
(c) Tuberculosis
(d) Collagen vascular disease

290. Least common finding in constractive pericarditis is

(a) Hepatomegaly
(b) Increase jugular venous pressure
(c) Ascites
(d) Pericardial knock

291. Which is the commonest complication in female with eisenmenger syndrome?

(a) Premature delivery
(b) Maternal mortality
(c) Spontaneous abortion
(d) Intrauterine growth retardation

292. All are the associated conditions with coarctation of aorta except

(a) PDA
(b) VSD
(c) ASD
(d) Cong. mitral stenosis

293. Which ASD repair is most common associated with sick sinus syndrome?

(a) ASD (OS) (b) ASD (OP)
(c) Siuns venous ASD (d) All of the above

294. Most common congenital heart disease associated with post operative VT

(a) Tricuspid atresia (b) TOF
(c) Aortic stenosis (d) TAPVD

295. Mitral annular calcification occurs in all the following except

(a) Marfans syndrome
(b) Mitral valve prolapse
(c) Secondary hyperparathyroidism
(d) Diabetes mellitus

296. Aschoff nodule consist of all the following except

(a) Fibrinoid necrosis (b) Lymphocyte
(c) Macrophages (d) Platelets

297. Most frequent clinical manifestation of chronic rheumatic heart disease is

(a) Mitral stenosis
(b) Mitral stenosis + Mitral regurgitation
(c) Mitral regurgitation
(d) Aortic stenosis + Aortic regurgitation

298. Aschoff nodule are found most commonly in which rheumatic valve lesion

(a) Mitral stenosis
(b) Mitral regurgitation
(c) Aortic stenosis + Mitral regurgitation
(d) Aortic regurgitation + Mitral regurgitation

299. Ebstein's anomaly commonly associated with all the following except

(a) ASD (b) VSD
(c) Pulmonary atresia (d) PDA

300. Healing vegetation of IE contains all the following cells except

(a) Lymphocyte (b) Neutrophils
(c) Macrophages (d) Plasma cells

301. Which joint is mainly involved in acute rheumatic fever?

(a) knee (b) Elbow
(c) Ankle (d) Hip

302. In which situation systemic embolism rarely occur in IE?

(a) Before antibiotic therapy
(b) Within 48 hours of therapy
(c) In patients of uncontrolled infection
(d) Successful antibiotic therapy

303. Embolization in infective endocarditis has all the following feature except

(a) High risk in left sided endocarditis
(b) With large vegetation
(c) Predictor of in hospital mortality
(d) Is related to type of organism

304. Usually heart failure in infective endocarditis is due to

(a) Destruction of valve causing regurgitation
(b) Myocardial abscess
(c) Myocarditis
(d) Rhythm disorders

305. Most common site of embolism in IE is

(a) Cerebral (b) Peripheral
(c) Renal (d) Coronary

306. Endocarditis of which valve is not associated with neurological complication

(a) Aortic (b) Mitral
(c) Tricuspid (d) Pulmonary

307. Bacteremia in IE usually is

(a) Intermittent (b) Transient
(c) Persistent (d) All the above

308. Positive culture (blood) in infective endocarditis occur in

(a) < 50% (b) 60%
(c) 70% (d) > 90%

309. Most common congenital heart disease is

(a) Bicuspid aortic valve
(b) ASD
(c) VSD
(d) MVP

310. Calcification in Mitral stenosis depends on all the following except

(a) Older age
(b) Increase MV gradient
(c) Related to sex
(d) Related to poor nutrition

311. Thrombus formation in body of LA is found in

(a) Mitral stenosis (b) Atrial fibrillation
(c) SSS (d) All the above

312. Avian type of right aortic arch is most commonly associated with

(a) TOF
(b) Truncus anteriorsus
(c) TGA (d) ASD

313. Common type of right aortic arch is commonly associated with

(a) TOF (b) TGA
(c) ASD (d) VSD

314. In a combined lesion of aortic stenosis + Aortic regurgitation the predominant stenosis is favored by all except

(a) Syncope
(b) Angina
(c) Prolonged systolic murmur
(d) LV dilatation

315. In a combined lesion of Aortic stenosis + Aortic regurgitation predominant regurgitation is suggested by all following except

(a) Angina
(b) Prolonged diastolic murmur
(c) LV dilated
(d) Syncope

316. Commonest pathological cause of pulmonary stenosis is

(a) Dane shaped valve
(b) Dysplastic valve
(c) Unicommissural valve
(d) Bicuspid valve

317. Which ECG sign correlates with RV pressure in PS?

(a) R wave height in V1
(b) Degree of RAD
(c) Magnitude of ST depression in right precordial leads
(d) Height of 'P' wave

318. Associated lesions with pulmonary artery stenosis are all except

(a) TOF
(b) PDA
(c) PS
(d) Bicuspid aortic valve

319. Most common cause of pulmonary regurgitation is

(a) Idiopathic dilation of PA

(b) Balloon pulmonary valvuloplasty
(c) Rheumatic
(d) Infective endocarditis

320. All the following signs are found in TS except

(a) MDM
(b) Crescendo presystolic murmur
(c) Large A wave in neck veins
(d) Tricuspid OS

321. Angina in non syphilitic aortic regurgitation has all features except-

(a) Coronary artery disease is usually present
(b) Occurs in paroxysms
(c) Usually nocturnal
(d) Profuse sweating

322. Which of the following cardiac lesion most after complicated by infective endocarditis?

(a) Discrete sub aortic stenosis
(b) Tunnel sub aortic stenosis
(c) HCM
(d) Supravalvular aortic stenosis

323. Which of the pressure may increase compensated Aortic regurgitation?

(a) LA (b) LVEDP
(c) PAP (S) (d) PAP (D)

324. In combined lesion of Mitral stenosis + Mitral regurgitation, predominant mitral stenosis is suggested by all except

(a) Dyspasea
(b) Parasternal heave
(c) Prolonged diastolic murmur
(d) S3

325. In combined lesion of mitral stenosis + mitral regurgitation predominant mitral regurgitation is suggested by all except

(a) Fatigue (b) S3
(c) LV enlargement (d) Dyspnoea

326. In patients of combined lesion of Aortic stenosis + Mitral stenosis the predominant lesion as aortic stenosis is suggested by all except

(a) Syncope
(b) Angina
(c) Low volume slow rising pulse
(d) RVH

327. In combined lesion of Aortic stenosis + Mitral stenosis the predominant mitral stenosis is suggested by all except

(a) Systemic embolism
(b) Dyspnoea
(c) Dilated left atrium
(d) Aortic valve calcitied

328. Vasodilator therapy in chronic mitral regurgitation may be given for treatment in all the following except

(a) Severe
(b) A symptomatic
(c) Normal LV function
(d) Depressed LV function

329. All the following are the causes of acute aortic regurgitation except

(a) IE
(b) Dissection of ascending aorta
(c) Traumatic
(d) Rheumatic

330. Usual organism for infective endo-carditis leading to acute aortic regurgitation is

(a) Streptococcus
(b) Staphylococcus aureus
(c) Pneumococcus
(d) Gram negative

331. In patients of combined Aortic regurgitation + Mitral stenosis, the predominant lesion as aortic regurgitation is suggested by all except

(a) Angina (b) Wide pulse pressure
(c) LV enlargement (d) Loud S1

332. In patients of combined lesion of Aortic regurgitation + Mitral stenosis, mitral stenosis predominant is favoured by all except

(a) Dyspnea (b) Embolism
(c) Atrial fibrillation (d) S4

333. Following agents are avoided or used cautiously in significant aortic stenosis

(a) Proanhythmics antiarrhythmics
(b) Inotropic agent
(c) Vasodilators
(d) All the above

334. Which cardiac chamber is normal in mitral stenosis?

(a) RA (b) LA
(c) LV (d) RV

335. Highest operative mortality of aortic valve replacement is in which of the following?

(a) Aortic stenosis with coronary artery disease
(b) Aortic stenosis with DM
(c) Aortic stenosis older patients
(d) Aortic stenosis NYHA class IV

336. Aortic valve replacement causes all the following except

(a) Improves survival
(b) LVH regression usual
(c) Diastolic dysfunction may persist even after
(d) No LVH

337. All are common cardiac signs in normal pregnancy except

(a) Pedal edema (b) PND
(c) DOE (d) Hemophysis

338. Functional murmurs heard in ASD are all the following except

(a) SM in PA
(b) MDM in TA
(c) Systolic murmur at ASD site
(d) None of the above

339. How many % of mild mitral regurgitation are clinically detectable?

(a) 10% (b) ≤ 20%
(c) 30% (d) 40%

340. All the following are features of fresh vegetation in bacterial endocarditis except

(a) Soft
(b) Friable
(c) Independent motion
(d) Echo dense

341. Severe mitral annular calcification demonstrated on echo in which degree of sclerosis?

(a) 2 mm (b) 5 mm
(c) 10 mm (d) > 10 mm

342. In which aortic valve disease statins are helpful in preventing progression?

(a) Aortic sclerosis
(b) Rheumatic aortic stenosis
(c) Cong. aortic stenosis
(d) Degenerative aortic stenosis

343. Which is the commonest echo finding in constrictive pericarditis?

(a) Abnormal pulmonary venous doppler pattern
(b) Pericardial calcification
(c) Restrictive mitral flow pattern
(d) Pericardial thickening

344. Aortic stenosis has all the following feature except

(a) Pulsars perrvuset lording
(b) Normal AZ
(c) Ejection click absent
(d) Early peaking SM

345. Aortic stenosis has all the following feature except

(a) Thickened Cusp
(b) Peak gradient 20 – 25 mm Hg
(c) Mean gradient < 10 mm Hg
(d) AVH is > 200 cm 2

346. All are renal complication of infective endocarditis except

(a) Renal infarct (b) Renal abscess
(c) Pyelonephritis
(d) Focal embolicglomervionephritis

347. Which size ASD (OS) is likely to close spontaneously?

(a) 5 mm (b) 10 mm
(c) 15 mm (d) 3 mm

348. Which size ASD (OS) unlikely to close spontaneously?

(a) 3 mm (b) 5 mm
(c) 7 mm (d) > 8 mm

349. Cardiac tamponade in renal disease has all the following feature except

(a) Pulses parodoxius after absent
(b) RA pressure = Pericardial pressure
(c) Wedge pressure is high there RAD
(d) JVP is after elevated

350. Which of the ECG indicative of large ASD (OS)?

(a) Atrial arrhythmias
(b) RAD
(c) RV conduction delay
(d) Both B + C

351. Enormous dilatation of main PA and proximal pulmonary artery branches occur in

(a) Idiopathic dilatation of PA
(b) PS
(c) PH
(d) Congenital absence of PV

352. Calcification most commonly invalves which valve?

(a) Mitral (b) Aortic
(c) Pulmonary (d) Tricuspid

353. Hemophysis is usually a feature of

(a) Pulmonary valve stenosis
(b) Sub valvular pulmonary stenosis
(c) Pulmonary artery stenosis
(d) None of the above

354. Following are the features of idiopathic dilatation of PA except

(a) Pulmonary ejection sound
(b) Pulmonary systolic murmur
(c) S2 wide and fixed
(d) No RVH

355. Following are arterial pulse abnormalities in acute severe aortic regurgitation except

(a) PR increase
(b) Rate of rise is increase
(c) Bisferiense contour
(d) Pulse alternans common

356. Following are arterial pulse abnormality in chronic severe aortic regurgitation except

(a) Pulses alternans common
(b) Bisferins contour present
(c) Pulse pressure is increased
(d) Rate of rise is increased

357. All are ECG features of pulmonary vein except

(a) P-pulmonate (b) P-mitral
(c) RAD (d) RVH

358. All are hemodynamic features of severe acute aortic regurgitation except

(a) LVEDP markedly increased
(b) Aortic pressure not increased
(c) Ejection cardiac out put decreased
(d) PVR in Normal

359. All are hemodynamic features of chronic severe aortic regurgitation except

(a) LV compliance is increased
(b) LVEDP is increased
(c) Systolic blood pressure markedly increased
(d) Effective cardiac out put is normal

360. All are physical findings in TR except

(a) Prominent 'v' wave in jugular
(b) Enlarged pulsatile liver
(c) Typical murmur
(d) Absent x & y deicent

361. BVH is eissenmager syndrome found in all the following causes of except

(a) Single verotricle (b) TGA
(c) Truncus arteriesis (d) TAPVD

362. Ebsteins anomaly has all following signs except

(a) Multiple sounds (b) TR murmur
(c) TS murmur (d) RV left

363. Inured movement of precardiac drugs systolic occurs in all except

(a) Pure TR
(b) Constrictive pericarditis
(c) ASD
(d) All of the above

364. All following are complications of PDA except

(a) Pulmonary artery aneurysm
(b) Ductal calcification
(c) Paradoxical embolism
(d) None of the above

365. Which of the following drug is given for prevention and treatment of hypoxic spells?

(a) Ca-blockers (b) Propranolol
(c) Diuretics (d) ACE inhibitors

366. In cardiac tamponade all the following signs are absent except

(a) Pulses paradoxus (b) Kussmaul's sign
(c) Pericardial knock (d) Absent X descent

367. Adult patients with cyanotic congenital heart disease has all the following renal function abnormalities except

(a) Decrease GFR (b) Proteinuria
(c) Hyperuricemia (d) Hematuria

368. In aortic failure of mitral stenosis which strategy is particularly effective?

(a) DC shock (b) Amiodarone
(c) Maze procedure (d) All the above

369. Which is more natural cause of infective endocarditis vegetations?

(a) Appear during therapy
(b) Increase in size during therapy
(c) Unchanged during therapy
(d) Gradually contract during prolonged period with therapy

370. In all the following situations endocarditis occurs comments except

(a) Valvular heart disease
(b) Prosthetic valve
(c) Drug abusers
(d) Intracardiac foreign body

371. Commonest fungus involved in endocarditis

(a) Histoplarma (b) Cryptococeos
(c) Blastomycosis (d) Aspergillosis

372. Commonest cause of multivalvular disease

(a) Rheumatic
(b) Infective endocarditis
(c) Degenerative valve calcification
(d) Marfan's syndrome

373. All the following disorders have definite association with MVP except

(a) Morfan's syndrome
(b) Osteogenesis imperfecta
(c) Ehlers-Danlos syndrome
(d) Psendoxanthoma elasticum

374. Most reliable investigation for assessing volume of aortic regurgitation is

(a) Clinical reliable
(b) X-ray chest
(c) Echo
(d) Supravalvular aortogram

375. Silent or nearly silent severe aortic regurgitation occur in all the following except

(a) Paravalvular leak
(b) Severe aortic regurgitation with severe heart failure
(c) S-Regurgitation occurring due to marked loss of valve substance
(d) Congenital aortic regurgitation

376. Musical aortic regurgitant murmur indicate all the following except

(a) Calcification of aortic valves
(b) Fenestration of aortic valves cusp
(c) Perforation of aortic valves cusp
(d) Aversion of aortic valves cusps

377. The term free aortic regurgitation is used to decrolic which finding

(a) Long early diastolic murmur
(b) LV enlargement
(c) Diastolic blood pressure > 30 mmHg
(d) All the above

378. If ascending aorta is greatly enlarged in aortic stenosis which etiology is likely

(a) Rheumatic
(b) Degenerative
(c) Bicuspid valve
(d) Ankylosing spondylitis

379. Presence of S4 in aortic stenosis in child signifies the gradient at aortic value is

(a) < 40 mmHg (b) 40–50 mmHg
(c) 50–60 mmHg (d) ≥ 70 mmHg

380. Syncope in aortic stenosis may caused by all the following except

(a) VT
(b) Transient electromechanical dissociation
(c) Vasodilatation
(d) CHB

381. Brain abscess as a complication of cyanotic heart most frequently found in

(a) Fallots tetralogy
(b) Eissenmengers syndrome
(c) TAPVD
(d) Tricuspid atresia

382. The peak systolic gradient across PV in ASD without PS usually is

(a) < 10 mmHg (b) 20 mmHg
(c) 30 mmHg (d) 60 mmHg

383. Mean pressure gradient of 3 mmHg or more between two atria with O_2 step up at atrial level except

(a) Left ventricular RA shunt
(b) Partial TAPVD without ASD
(c) Patent foromen ovale with Lt atrial hypertension
(d) All the above

384. P-mitrale suggest what in patients of mitral stenosis

(a) RAE (b) LAE
(c) RVH (d) None of the above

385. Extremely Tall 'P' is seen in

(a) Eissenmenger's (b) Fallot's tetralogy
(c) TGA (d) Ebstein's disease

386. Dyspnoea appears in mitral stenosis at which valve area

(a) < 1 cm^2 (b) < 1.5 cm^2
(c) 2.0 cm^2 (d) 2–2.5 cm^2

387. In aortic stenosis associated CAD is favoured by all the following

(a) ACQMI (b) Remote QMI
(c) Root angina (d) Effort angina

388. Risk of congenital heart disease in offspring if one parent is effected is in all the following except

(a) VSD
(b) Left sided obstruction
(c) Right sided obstruction
(d) Ebstein's disease

389. All the following statements regarding PDA are correct except

(a) Functional closure with in 10–15 hours
(b) Anatomical closure completed within 2–3 weeks
(c) Closure commonly begun at aortic end
(d) Closure most commonly begins at pulmonary end

390. All the following factors influence ductal closure except

(a) Increase O_2 tension

(b) Vasoactive substances
(c) pH
(d) Hypocapnia

391. Negligible risk for infective endocarditis is in all the following except

(a) ASD (OS)
(b) Atherosclerotic plaque
(c) Syphilitic aortitis
(d) Catheter in right heart

392. Culture negative endocarditis is found in all except

(a) If culture taken after 3 months
(b) Uremia
(c) Right sided endocarditis
(d) If patients on antibiotics

393. Least common sign in prosthetic valve endocarditis is

(a) Splenomegaly
(b) Cutaneous lesion
(c) Systemic embolism
(d) Petechioe

394. Commonest laboratory finding in prosthetic valve endocarditis is

(a) Leukocytosis (b) Anemia
(c) Haematuria (d) Leucopoenia

395. Least common physical finding in infective endocarditis is

(a) Clubbing (b) Retinal lesion
(c) Splenomegaly (d) Osler's node

396. Fever in infective endocarditis may be absent in all the following except

(a) Renal failure (b) CHF
(c) Elderly (d) Unusual organism

397. Commonest valve involved in infective endocarditis of IV drug abusers is

(a) Prosthetic valve
(b) Native mitral valve
(c) Native tricuspid valve
(d) Native aortic valve

398. Prosthetic valve endocarditis most commonly occur at

(a) Aortic (b) Mitral
(c) Tricuspid (d) Pulmonary

399. Native valve endocarditis most commonly occurs at which valve

(a) Aortic
(b) Mitral
(c) Tricuspid
(d) Aortic and mitral value

400. Native valve endocarditis less commonly involves

(a) Aortic (b) Mitral
(c) Tricuspid (d) Pulmonary

401. Least common cardiac disease in which endocarditis occurs is

(a) Congenital heart disease
(b) Mitral valve disease
(c) Aortic valve disease
(d) Tricuspid valve disease

402. What is hematocrit in sanguineous pericardial effusion?

(a) £10% (b) 15%
(c) 20% (d) Any of the above

403. What is haematocrit in bloody pericardial effusion?

(a) < 10%
(b) > 10%
(c) 20%
(d) Similar to circulating blood

404. Parasite diseases of pericardium are

(a) Amoebiasis (b) Filariasis
(c) Hydatid disease (d) All of the above

405. Which fungus directly involves pericardium?

(a) Actinomycosis (b) Histoplasmosis
(c) Aspergillosis (d) Candidiasis

406. Most common cause of effusive constrictive pericarditis is

(a) Idiopathic
(b) Rheumatoid arthritis
(c) Renal failure
(d) Neoplastic

407. Physiological cause of pericardial effusion

(a) Elderly
(b) Neonate
(c) During lactation in woman
(d) During pregnancy

408. S4 is heard in chronic AR in all the following situations except

(a) Aortic regurgitation with hypertension
(b) Severe aortic stenosis with mild aortic regurgitation
(c) Mild aortic regurgitation with coronary artery disease
(d) Prosthetic valve malfunction

409. S4 in aortic stenosis indicate the gradient of

(a) 20 mmHg (b) 30 mmHg
(c) 40 mmHg (d) ≥ 50 mmHg

410. All are common causes of acute severe aortic regurgitation except

(a) Infective endocarditis
(b) Trauma
(c) Rheumatic
(d) Dissection of aorta

411. Commonest causes of severe mitral regurgitation (Isolated) is

(a) MVP
(b) Rheumatic
(c) Ischemia
(d) Infective endocarditis

412. Which is the rare symptom in mitral regurgitation?

(a) Dyspnaen (b) Fatigue
(c) Palpitation (d) Hemophysis

413. Giant LA on X-ray in mitral regurgitation suggest which etiology

(a) Rheumatic (b) MVP
(c) Ischemic (d) Dilated CMP

414. Mitral regurgitation in congenital heart disease occurs in all the following except

(a) A-V canal defect
(b) OP ASD
(c) Corrected TGA
(d) VSD

415. Most common cause of acute aortic regurgitation is

(a) Trauma
(b) Dissection of aorta
(c) Infective endocarditis
(d) Rheumatic

416. All are neurological and autonomic dysfunction in MVP except

(a) High adrenergic activity
(b) Abnormal rennin aldosterone regulation
(c) Abnormal calecholamine regulation
(d) Abnormal thyroid function

417. Most frequent consequence of aortic balloon valvouloplasty is

(a) Arrhythmia (b) Embolism
(c) Restenosis (d) Syncope

418. ST elevation in acute pericarditis is seldom present in early stage of pericarditis in which etiological type of acute pericarditis

(a) Trauma (b) Viral
(c) Tuberculosis (d) Idiopathic

419. Common significant murmur in acute rheumatic carditis is

(a) Aortic regurgitation
(b) Carrey coombs
(c) Apical pan systolic
(d) All the above

420. Which statement is correct for normal diastolic pressure is found in aortic regurgitation?

(a) Acute aortic regurgitation
(b) Mild chronic aortic regurgitation
(c) Aortic regurgitation with LVF
(d) All the above

421. In chronic severe aortic regurgitation the usual pulse pressure is

(a) 50 mmHg (b) 60 mmHg
(c) 70 mmHg (d) ≥ 100 mmHg

422. Which skeletal abnormality is not found in MVP?

(a) Straight back
(b) Pectus excavatum
(c) High arched palate
(d) Arachnodactyly

423. All the following connective tissue disorders occur with MVP except

(a) Marfans syndrome
(b) Ehlers-Danls syndrome
(c) Pseudoxanthoma elasticum
(d) Hurlers Syndrome

424. All the following lesions of aortic valve produce dominant stenosis except

(a) Bicuspid valve (b) Unicuspid
(c) Quadricuspid (d) Degenerative

425. All the following AV diseases produces dominant regurgitation except

(a) Rheumatic
(b) Collagen disease
(c) Infective endocarditis
(d) Senile

426. All the following mitral valve disease producespure-mitral regurgitation except

(a) Parachute deformity
(b) Myxomatous
(c) Ischemia
(d) Cleft valve

427. Following are the causes of flail mitral valve leaflet except

(a) Myxomatous chordal rupture
(b) Vegetation with chordal rupture
(c) Ischemic rupture of papillary muscle head
(d) Rheumatic heart disease

428. Lateral movement of earlobe occurs in

(a) Aortic regurgitation
(b) Tricuspid regurgitation
(c) Tricuspid stenosis
(d) None of the above

429. Which is rare physical sign in organic tricuspid stenosis?

(a) Mid diastolic murmur
(b) Presystolic murmur
(c) Loud S1
(d) Opening snap

430. Severe chronic aortic regurgitation usually has all the following features except

(a) Long duration of murmur
(b) S1 decrease
(c) S2 paradoxical split in absence of LBBB
(d) Peripheral signs of aortic regurgitation

431. LV dysfunction in aortic regurgitation is indicated by all the following except

(a) Disappearance of peripheral signs of aortic regurgitation
(b) Sustained apex beat
(c) S3
(d) No change in duration of EDM

432. Commonest cause of constrictive pericarditis

(a) Viral (b) Idiopathic
(c) Pyogenic (d) Neoplastic

433. Commonest cause of constrictive pericarditis in India is

(a) Viral (b) Pyogenic
(c) Tuberculosis (d) Idiopathic

434. Commonest arrhythmia in constrictive pericarditis is

(a) Atrial ectopics
(b) Atrial tachycardia
(c) Atrial fibrillation
(d) Sick sinus syndrome

435. Uremia causes which of the following pericardial disease

(a) Pericarditis

(b) Pericardial effusion
(c) Acute tamponade
(d) Constrictive and effusive constrictive pericarditis
(e) All of the above

436. All are possible associations of pericardial disease except

(a) Atrial septal defect
(b) Aortic regurgitation
(c) Thalassemia
(d) Giant urticaria

437. Which is least quantity of rapid pericardial effusion which produces cardiac tamponade?

(a) 50–100 ml (b) 100–150 ml
(c) 160–190 ml (d) 200 ml

438. All are physiological functions of pericardium except

(a) Lubricator
(b) Protect the heart from contiguous infection
(c) Protect the heart from acute dilatation
(d) Protect the heart from trauma

439. All are causes of hemopericardium except

(a) Acute myocardial infarction
(b) Rupture of pseudo aneurysm
(c) Ascending aortic dissection
(d) Antiplatelet therapy

440. All are hemodynamic features of constrictive pericarditis except

(a) Increase RAP
(b) Increase RV & LV filling pressure
(c) RVP = LVP
(d) No Pulmonary hypertension

441. All are hemodynamic features of cardiac tamponade except

(a) RAP increases
(b) RV/LV filling pressure increased
(c) RVP = LVP
(d) PAP increases

442. Patent ductus arteriosus has all following features except

(a) Communication between proximal descending thoracic aorta 2-10 mm beyond the origin of left subclavian artery to the origin of left pulmonary artery
(b) Usual length 15 mm
(c) Wide pulmonary orifice
(d) Wide aortic orifice

443. Right atrial compression in cardiac tamponade is absent in all the following except

(a) Associated pulmonary hypertension
(b) Associated right heart failure
(c) Associated tricuspid valve disease
(d) Ventricular septal defect

444. Most important echocardiographic sign of cardiac tamponade is

(a) Right atrium collapse
(b) Right ventricle collapse
(c) Exaggerated respiratory variations of in atrioventricular inflow velocity.
(d) Highly exaggerated respiratory variations in the relative size of two ventricles

445. Most rare cause of constrictive pericarditis is

(a) Viral
(b) Tuberculosis
(c) Collagen disease
(d) Rheumatic

446. Intra pericardial pressure of 4–5 mmHg in pericardial effusion has all the following features except

(a) Asymptomatic
(b) No abnormal physical finding
(c) Beginning of cardiac tamponade
(d) Dyspnea on exertion

447. Intra pericardial pressure 8–10 mmHg in pericardial effusion results in all the following except

(a) Asymptomatic
(b) Normal blood pressure
(c) Normal pulse
(d) JVP is normal

448. If intra pericardial pressure is approximately 15 mmHg all following signs of cardiac tamponade appear except

(a) Pulsus paradoxus
(b) Profound fall in blood pressure
(c) Dyspnea
(d) Fatigue

449. If Intra cardiac pressure is ≥ 20 mmHg all following are found except

(a) Pulsus paradoxus
(b) Severe decompensation
(c) Profound fall in blood pressure
(d) Cardiac out put is normal

450. Most frequently encountered intracardiac shunt with coarctation of aorta is

(a) ASD (b) VSD
(c) Single ventricle (d) Single atrium

451. Most frequent shunt lesion in coarctation of aorta is

(a) ASD (b) VSD
(c) PDA (d) All the above

452. Rib notching in coarctation of aorta has all the following except

(a) Occurs on inferior and under surface of ribs
(b) Seldom appears before the age 7 years
(c) Notching is always bilateral
(d) 3rd to 9th ribs are involved

453. Ebstein's anomaly is found in which of teratogenic disorder

(a) Rubella (b) Phenytoin induced
(c) Alcohol induced (d) Lithium induced

454. On ECG presence of RA enlargement left axis deviation and LVH indicates which disorder

(a) Single ventricle (b) Truncus arteriosus
(c) Fallot's tetralogy (d) Tricuspid artesia

455. Left atrial thrombi in mitral stenosis commonly embolize to all except

(a) Brain (b) Kidney
(c) Spleen (d) Liver

456. Ball-valve thrombus in mitral stenosis present with all the following except

(a) Syncope
(b) Angina
(c) Changing auscultatory signs
(d) All of the above

457. PFO may pose all the following problems except

(a) Thrombo embolism
(b) Air embolism
(c) Right-left shunting (desiderated blood)
(d) Vegetable embolism

458. Major clinical problem with PFO is

(a) Thrombo-embolism in young
(b) Air embolism
(c) Vasoactive substance shunted to left side
(d) All of the above

459. In what percentage PFO is present in general population?

(a) 5% (b) 10%
(c) 15% (d) 25%

460. What is minimum size of PFO?

(a) 0.5 mm (b) 1 mm
(c) 5 mm (d) 15 mm

461. What is maximum size of PFO?

(a) 10 mm (b) 15 mm
(c) 18 mm (d) 19 mm

462. What is mean size of PFO?

(a) 2 mm (b) 3 mm
(c) 4 mm (d) 5 mm

463. All are the features of fallot's triology except

(a) Giant 'a' in neck veins
(b) RVH
(c) Dilatation of main pulmonary artery
(d) Right aortic arch

464. All are common associated lesions in fallot's tetralogy except

(a) Left superior vena cava
(b) Right aortic arch

(c) ASD
(d) Subaortic stenosis

465. Rheumatic nodule has all following features except

(a) Firm
(b) Painful
(c) 0.5–2 cm in diameter
(d) Situated over tendon or bony prominences

466. All are causes of central cyanosis with left ventricular hypertrophy except

(a) Tricuspid atresia
(b) Total anomalous systemic venous drainage
(c) IVC to LA shunt
(d) Ebstein's anomaly

467. All are causes of death in eisenmengers complex except

(a) Right heart failure
(b) Haemoptysis
(c) Cerebral abscess
(d) Ventricular arrhythmia

468. All the following signs are usually found in pulmonary valve Stenosis except

(a) Giant 'a' wave
(b) RVH
(c) No click
(d) Loud pulmonary systolic murmur with thrill

469. All are causes of cyanosis central in ASD except

(a) TAPVD
(b) IVC to LA
(c) Eisenmenger syndrome
(d) Mitral regurgitation

470. Most frequent congenital heart disease in elderly persons is

(a) ASD (b) PDA
(c) PS (d) None of the above

471. Most frequent presentation of acute myocardial infarction in elderly is
(a) Acute LVF
(b) CVA
(c) Peripheral embolism
(d) Atypical chest Pain

472. Most common cyanotic congenital heart disease in pregnant women is
(a) Tricuspid atresia (b) Fallot's tetralogy
(c) TGA (d) None of the above

473. Most common L-R shunt resulting in R-L shunt is
(a) VSD
(b) ASD
(c) PDA
(d) Endocardial cushion defect

474. Most common type of supra valvular aortic stenosis is
(a) Hour glass type
(b) Uniform hypoplasia
(c) Fibro muscular
(d) None of these

475. In which of the following Diastolic blood pressure alternans is found with normal pulse?
(a) Acute LVF
(b) Acute myocardial infarction
(c) Acute pulmonary embolism
(d) Congenital absence of pericardium

476. Crochetage sign is found in all the following except
(a) ASD OS (b) SV ASD
(c) PFO (d) OP ASD

477. Crochetage sign is valuable in ASD in predicting all the following except
(a) Location of ASD
(b) Severity of shunt
(c) With rSR pattern the ECG diagnosis is with specificity

(d) Directly correlates with severity of pulmonary hypertension

478. Mechanism of calcification in bicuspid valve are all except

(a) Unequal cusps
(b) Hypercholesterolemia
(c) Mechanical stress
(d) Hypercalcemia

479. All are hemodynamic features in acute severe aortic regurgitation except

(a) Increased peripheral vascular resistance
(b) Ejection fraction not increased
(c) Pulse pressure not significantly increased
(d) Left ventricular end diastolic pressure is normal

480. U shaped tortuous retinal arterioles are found in hypertension associated with

(a) Phaechromocytoma
(b) Hyperthyroidism
(c) Coarctation of aorta
(d) Reno vascular disease

481. Which of the following is rare in congenital mitral stenosis?

(a) Right heart failure
(b) Right axis deviation
(c) Right ventricular hypertrophy
(d) Atrial fibrillation

482. Which test is best for definitive diagnosis of congenital absence of pericardium?

(a) X-ray (b) ECG
(c) Echocardiography (d) MRI Thorax

483. Systolic murmur of tricuspid regurgitation in Ebstein's disease has all the following features except

(a) Heard usually towards apex
(b) Increases with inspiration
(c) Scratchy or rub like
(d) Decrescendo

484. Sail sound in ebstein's anomaly has following feature

(a) Tricuspid component is delayed
(b) Mitral component is loud
(c) Tricuspid component is loud
(d) Heard best between apex and left sternal border

485. S2 has all the following characteristic in ebstein's anomaly except

(a) Wide and fixed splitting
(b) Paradoxical splitting
(c) Single S2
(d) P2 is increased

486. Commonest ECG change in ebstein's anomaly is

(a) WPW-B
(b) Supra ventricular arrhythmia
(c) RBBB
(d) 'P' pulmonale

487. Most consistent feature of ebstein's anomaly on X-ray is

(a) Increase cardiac shadow
(b) Increase right atrium shadow
(c) Decrease pulmonary vascularity
(d) Pulmonary trunk inconspicuous

488. In which cyanotic congenital heart disease both aortic root and pulmonary trunk are likely to be normal or reduced?

(a) Fallot's tetralogy
(b) Truncus arteriosus
(c) Eisenmenger's reaction
(d) Ebstein's anomaly

489. Most common ECG abnormality in acute rheumatic fever is

(a) Conduction defect
(b) T-wave changes
(c) Abnormal rhythm
(d) Abnormal axis deviation

490. ECG is usually abnormal in what percentage of cases of acute Rheumatic fever-

(a) 10 % (b) 20 %
(c) 30 % (d) > 50 %

491. Which is rare valvular defect (Rheumatic) combination?

(a) Mitral stenosis + Aortic stenosis
(b) Mitral stenosis + Aortic regurgitation
(c) Mitral stenosis + TR
(d) Mitral stenosis + TS

492. For pericardiocentasis minimum volume of fluid is required in pericardial cavity

(a) 5 mm Anteriorily
(b) 10 mm Posteraly
(c) 10 mm Anteriorily
(d) A meant of fluid does not matter

493. All following are causes of death in eissen-marg's complex except

(a) Heart failure (b) IE
(c) Brain abscess (d) Hyperviscosity

494. How often aortic regurgitation is present in congenital aortic stenosis?

(a) Not present (b) 10 %
(c) 30 % (d) Approx 50 %

495. Low pressure cardiac tamponade typically occurs in

(a) Purulent pericarditis
(b) Rheumatic pericarditis
(c) Haemopericardium
(d) In CRF during dialysis

496. Which physical sign is rare in cardiac tamponade?

(a) Obliterated Y descent
(b) Increase JV pressure
(c) Pulses paradoxes
(d) Pericardial rub

497. Commonest cause of death in PDA is

(a) Heart failure
(b) Rupture of ductal aneurysm
(c) Hypertensive aneurysm of pulmonary track
(d) Infective endocarditis

498. Pulmonary oligemia develops in PS in which of the following situation?

(a) Mild PS
(b) Mead PS
(c) Severe PS
(d) Severe PS with RVF

499. In which of the following congenital heart disease the berth weight is more than normal?

(a) TGA (b) Fallots tetralogy
(c) Fallots triology (d) Truncus arteriosus

500. In which of the following conditions the pulmonary ejection sound does not decrease with inspiration?

(a) PS (b) PH
(c) Fallots tetralogy (d) TGA

501. Egg shaped heart shadow with narrow pedicle and increase pulmonary vascularly found in

(a) Ebsleceus disease (b) Total APVD
(c) TGA (d) Trumcus arteriesis

502. Trammel values in truncus arteriosus is often

(a) Tricuspid (b) Bicuspid
(c) Qaudricuspid (d) Pentacuspid

503. All following congenital heart disease are associated with congenital animated of coronary arteries except

(a) Congenitally corrected TGA
(b) Bicuspid value
(c) TGA
(d) PDA-Reversed

504. All following ECG founding in anomalous angina of left coronary artery from pulmonary bank except

(a) LVH
(b) LAD
(c) Q in L1 avL
(d) Q in right precedent loads

505. Most common cause of acute aortic regurgitation is

(a) Infective endocarditis
(b) Hypertension

(c) Trauma
(d) Dissection of aorta

506. Auscultation in supine position in mitral stenosis may reveal only which of the following abnormality
(a) OS
(b) Loud S1
(c) Presystolic murmur
(d) Mid diastolic murmur

507. Most common associated cardiac defect with ebstein's anomaly is
(a) WPW syndrome (b) ASD
(c) MVP (d) All of the above

508. Which valvular lesion often presents with systolic hypertension?
(a) Mitral regurgitation
(b) Aortic regurgitation
(c) Mitral stenosis
(d) Aortic stenosis

509. Malignant pericardial effusion commonly occurs from all except
(a) Lung carcinoma (b) Breast carcinoma
(c) Esophagus (d) Lymphoma

510. Beck's triad includes all except
(a) Hypotension
(b) Muffled heart sounds
(c) Juglar neck vein distension
(d) Absent Y descent

511. Poorest prognosis in constrictive pericarditis occurs in which etiological type
(a) Viral (b) Idiopathic
(c) Radiation induced (d) Tuberculosis

512. Most common cause of constrictive pericarditis in west is
(a) Viral
(b) Tuberculosis
(c) Idiopathic
(d) Post cardiac surgery

513. Most common acquired cause of pulmonary stenosis is

(a) Rheumatic (b) Carcinoid
(c) Atherosclerosis (d) None of the above

514. Best results of balloon valvuloplasty are obtained in

(a) Mitral stenosis
(b) Pulmonary stenosis
(c) Aortic stenosis
(d) Tricuspid stenosis

515. Rupture of sinus of valsalva usually occurs in

(a) Right atrium (b) Right ventricle
(c) Left atrium (d) Left ventricle

516. All are pericardial syndromes except

(a) Acute pericarditis
(b) Chronic pericarditis
(c) Pericardial effusion
(d) Constrictive pericarditis

517. Mitral valve narrowing in mitral stenosis progresses at which rate

(a) 0.05 cm/year (b) 0.06 cm/year
(c) 0.08 cm/year (d) 0.09 cm/year

518. The average size of PFO is

(a) < 5 mm (b) 6 – 8 mm
(c) 9 – 12 mm (d) > 12 mm

519. Most likely mechanism of acute rheumatic fever by group a streptococcus

(a) Toxic effect of bacteria
(b) Serum sickness like reaction
(c) Autoimmune phenomena
(d) Molecular mimicry

520. Which manifestation of acute rheumatic fever has potential to cause long-term disability?

(a) Carditis
(b) Rheumatic disease
(c) Dermatic lesions
(d) Neurologic lesion

521. All the following are clinical manifestations of carditis; for diagnosis which is required

(a) New murmur
(b) Cardiomyopathy
(c) Congestive heart failure
(d) Pericarditis
(e) Any of the above

522. Subcutaneous nodules of acute rheumatic fever have all following characteristics except

(a) Comes in crops
(b) Occurs on bony prominences
(c) 0.5 to 2 cm in size
(d) Painful

523. Tricuspid stenosis on X-ray is indicated by all except

(a) Dilated heart
(b) No pulmonary congestion
(c) No pulmonary hypertension
(d) Mild pulmonary hypertension

524. Most common ECG abnormality in myocarditis is

(a) AV block
(b) ST/T changes
(c) Sinus tachycardia
(d) Left bundle branch block

525. Biventricular hypertrophy is usually present in which of the following lesion

(a) VSD (b) AS
(c) MR (d) TR

526. Most common ECG abnormality in MVP is

(a) ST/T changes in inferior lead
(b) QT prolongation
(c) WPW syndrome
(d) Sinus node dysfunction

527. Family history of murmur is commonly found in which of the following?

(a) Congenital valvular aortic stenosis
(b) Congenital subvalvular aortic stenosis
(c) Rheumatic aortic stenosis
(d) HOCM

528. Family history of sudden childhood death is commonly found in

(a) Rheumatic mitral stenosis
(b) HOCM
(c) Congenital valvular aortic stenosis
(d) Congenital subvalvular aortic stenosis

529. All the following biochemical changes causes aortic stenosis to progress more rapidly except

(a) Hypercholesterolemia
(b) Hypocalcemia
(c) Hyperglycemia
(d) Elevated serum creatinine

530. Which is least common cause of mitral stenosis?

(a) Rheumatic
(b) Scarlet fever
(c) Infective endocarditis
(d) Rheumatoid arthritis

531. All the following skeletal abnormalities occur in MVP except

(a) Straight back syndrome
(b) Pectus excavatum
(c) Scoliosis
(d) Kyphosis

532. Which is the commonest combination of valve involvement in RHD?

(a) Mitral + Pulmonary
(b) Mitral + Aortic + Pulmonary
(c) Mitral + Tricuspid + Pulmonary
(d) All four valves

533. Which is characteristic feature of juvenile mitral stenosis?

(a) Retarded growth
(b) Severe pulmonary hypertension
(c) S1 loud
(d) History of frequent soar throat

534. RVH on ECG is consistently found in mitral stenosis at which systolic pressure of RV?

(a) 60 mmHg (b) 70 mmHg

(c) 80 mmHg (d) > 100 mmHg

535. The occurrence of AF in mitral stenosis correlates with all the following except

(a) Degree of atriomegaly
(b) Duration of atriomegaly
(c) Extent of LA fibrosis
(d) Rheumatic carditis

536. The AV block and intraventricular blocks in calcific aortic stenosis are is rolareld all the following except

(a) Septal trauma from high intramyocardial tension
(b) Hypoxic damage
(c) Extension of calcification
(d) LVH

537. ECG indicators for severity of aortic stenosis are all the following except

(a) St. decrease > 3 mm
(b) Total 12 lead voltages
(c) Strain pattern
(d) Loss of R wave in V1-V3

538. Conduction defects in aortic regurgitation are frequently found in all following etiologies of aortic regurgitation except

(a) Rheumatic arthritis
(b) Ankylossing spondylitis
(c) SLE
(d) Congenital

539. Which cyanotic congenital heart disease causes wide pulse pressure?

(a) TGA (b) Single ventricle
(c) Truncus (d) Follots tetralogy

540. Coronary angiography may be required in mitral stenosis in the following situations except

(a) LV dysfunction
(b) Age > 35 years
(c) Clinical history suggestive of coronary artery disease
(d) Male patients

541. Most common cause needing surgery in severe mitral regurgitation in west is

(a) Ischemia mitral regurgitation
(b) MVP
(c) Rheumatic
(d) MAC

542. Molar flush in mitral stenosis is caused by all except

(a) Peripheral cyanosis
(b) Systemic vasdilatation
(c) Severe pulmonary hypertension
(d) Purple-pinkish patches on cheeks

543. Which is the commonest associated condition with MVP?

(a) Tricuspid valve prolapse
(b) Aortic valve prolapse
(c) Pulmonary valve prolapse
(d) ASD (OS)

544. Most common symptom of MVP is

(a) Chest Pain (b) Dyspnea
(c) Palpitation (d) Syncope

545. TR without TS Occurs in all the following except

(a) Functional
(b) Idiopathic hypereosinophilic syndrome
(c) TVP
(d) Post inflammatory

546. Most common cause of TR

(a) Rheumatic (b) Embolism
(c) Functional (d) CHD

547. Most common congenital heart disease apart from MVP and bicuspid aortic valve

(a) ASD
(b) VSD
(c) PDA
(d) Coarctation of aorta

548. Least common cyanotic congenital heart disease is

(a) Truncus arteriosus
(b) Tricuspid atresia
(c) TAPVD
(d) Pulmonary atresia with out VSD

549. The tricuspid valve gradient in severe TS is

(a) 2-3 mmHg (b) 3-5 mmHg
(c) 5 mmHg (d) $\geq$ 6 mmHg

550. Hemoptysis in eissenmengere's occurs because of

(a) Rupture of fragile neovascular channels
(b) Pulmonary infarction
(c) Both of the above
(d) None of the above

551. Immediate cause of death in eissenmenger's include all the following except

(a) Dehydration
(b) CC
(c) Surgery
(d) Infective endocarditis

552. Which is commonest cause of constrictive pericarditis?

(a) Idiopathic (b) Tuberculosis
(c) Uraemia (d) Neoplastic

553. Which is commonest cause of constrictive pericarditis in known etiologies?

(a) Tuberculosis
(b) Neoplastic
(c) Uremia
(d) Acute rheumatic fever

554. What amount of fluid is needed for cardiac sillhoute to enlarge in pericardial effusion?

(a) 50 ml (b) 100 ml
(c) 150 ml (d) > 200 ml

555. New born with cyanotic congenital heart disease which shows LAD on ECG

(a) TGA (b) Truncus arteriosus
(c) AV canal defect (d) Tricuspid atresia

556. Most characteristic X-ray finding in constrictive pericarditis is

(a) Cardiac sithoulte is slighthy enlarged
(b) Pulmonary venous redistribution
(c) Pericardial calcification
(d) Distended azygous vein and superior vena cava

557. Which of the following finding is absent in constrictive pericarditis?

(a) Increase JVP (b) Enlarged vein
(c) Ascites (d) RV not palpable

558. Choice of incision in pericardiectomy in constrictive pericarditis is

(a) Anterolateral thoracotomy
(b) Medial sternotomy
(c) Bilateral anterior thoracotomy
(d) Any of the above

559. Most common manifestation of neoplastic pericardial involvement is

(a) Cardiac tamponade
(b) Constrictive pericarditis
(c) Pericardial effusion chronic
(d) Effusive constrictive pericarditis

560. Functional component in increased pulmonary vascular resistance in eissenmenger's is due to all except

(a) Hypoxia
(b) Acidosis
(c) Increase catecholamines
(d) Decrease PBF

561. Which histological changes pulmonary vascular tree indicates irreversibl pulmonary vascular obstruction?

(a) Medial thickening (b) Intimal thickening
(c) Both of the above (d) Plexi form lesion

562. Ductus patency rate is higher in

(a) Premature birth
(b) Birth at high altitude
(c) Both of the above
(d) None of the above

563. Large PDA (L-R shunt) causes dilation of all the following except

(a) LV (b) LA
(c) Aorta (d) RV

564. All the following are the ECG criteria of complete repair of VSD except

(a) Rapid regression of RV hypertrophy
(b) Rapid regressian left atrial enlargement
(c) Rapid regression of LVH
(d) QRS axis remain abnormally shifted

565. What happens to QRS axis of canal defect is repaired completely?

(a) No change
(b) Regress partially to normal
(c) regress completely to normal
(d) None of the above

566. Most specific indicator of RVP in VSD is

(a) R in V1
(b) Katz watchel's phenomenon
(c) RBBB
(d) RAD

567. Which type of VSD leads to enlargement of all chambers of heart?

(a) Canal defect significant A-V valve Regurgitation
(b) Large gerbodes defect
(c) Both of the above
(d) None of the above

568. Pulmonary artery banding is often restricted to which VSD

(a) VSD with straddling tricuspid valve
(b) Swiss cheese defect
(c) Large VSD with coarctation
(d) All of the above

569. Infective endocarditis is seen in all the following in VSD except

(a) RVOT
(b) Free wall
(c) Tricuspid value apparatus
(d) IVS

570. Which type of VSD produces maximum murmur over the upper sterrium?

(a) Gerbodes defect
(b) Supracristal VSD
(c) Infracrista VSD
(d) None of the above

571. PR internal is prolonged in which types of VSD

(a) Common A-V canal defect
(b) Gerbodes defect
(c) Both of the above
(d) None of the above

572. All 4-chamber enlargement in young patients of ASD suggest

(a) Secondum ASD (b) Primun ASD
(c) SV ASD (d) CS ASD

573. Significant left-right shunting occurs with which type of VSD at birth?

(a) Small defect (b) Muscular defect
(c) Moderate VSD (d) Gerbodes defect

574. Grave prognostic ECG sign of pulmonary valve stenosis is

(a) Height of R wave in V1
(b) T wave inversion V1-V3
(c) RAD
(d) T wave inversion progresses rapidly form V1-V3 to left precordial leads

575. Cyanosis in ASD in absence of pulmonary hypertension is present in

(a) Coronary sinus defect
(b) Sinus venosus defect with straddling SVC
(c) ASD (OS) with large eustachian valve
(d) All of the above

576. Bicuspid valve is most commonly associated with which of the following conditions?

(a) Hypoplastic left heart syndrome
(b) Coarctation of aorta
(c) VSD
(d) Aberrant origin of coronary artery

577. Pulmonary stenosis most commonly occurs at which location?

(a) Valve (b) Infundibulum
(c) PA branch (d) Combination

578. Acquired coarctation of aorta occurs in all the following except

(a) Primary aortitis
(b) Aortic dissection
(c) Extrinsic compression by tumor mass
(d) Syphilis

579. All are radiological signs found in acquired coarctation of aorta except

(a) Dilatation of ascending aorta
(b) Dilatation of left subclavian artery
(c) Rib notching
(d) Cardiac enlargement

580. Which of the following indicates good myocardial function in heart disease?

(a) Sinus bradycardia (b) Sinus tachycardia
(c) Sinus arrhythmia (d) None of the above

581. Which secondary systemic hypertensives usually do not exhibit fundal changes?

(a) Renal
(b) Coarctation of aorta
(c) Hyperaldsteronism
(d) Pregnancy related hypertension

582. Pathognomonic sign of atrioventricular canal defect is

(a) RA + RV enlargement
(b) Increase pulmonary vascular movements
(c) Cleft MV
(d) 'Goose' Neck deformity on selective LV angiocardiography

583. All are common associated lesion with bicuspid aortic valve except

(a) PDA
(b) ASD
(c) VSD
(d) Coarctation of Aorta

584. All following are complication of co-arctation of aorta except

(a) Hypertension
(b) Endarteritis
(c) Aortic aneurysm
(d) Ventricular tachycardia

585. Most common associated anomaly with ebstein's disease is

(a) WPW syndrome
(b) ASD
(c) Tricuspid valve prolapse
(d) Pulmonary stenosis

586. RV out flow tract obstruction in fallots tetralogy is often at

(a) Supravalvular (b) Valvular
(c) Subvalvular (d) Multiple levels

587. What is the usual growth rate of aortic stenosis?

(a) 2 mm/year (b) 5 mm/year
(c) 1 mm/year (d) < 1 mm/year

588. Narrowing at base of heart on X-ray chest is characteristic of

(a) Fallots tetralogy
(b) Truncus arteriosus
(c) Eissenmenger syndrome
(d) Transposition of the great vessels

589. Commonest cause of tricuspid stenosis is

(a) Rheumatic (b) Ebstein's disease
(c) Carcinoid (d) Congenital

590. All following drugs cause valvular heart disease except

(a) Antidepressant (b) Dexfenfluramine
(c) Ergotamine (d) Methysergide

591. Aortic stenosis in elderly exhibits all following except

(a) Wide pulse pressure
(b) Musical murmur often best heard at apex
(c) Hypertension is often found
(d) A2 is loud

592. All following are indication of coronary angiography in aortic stenosis except

(a) Age ≥ 35 years
(b) Age < 35 year with LV dysfunction
(c) Age < 35 year with two or more risk factors for premature CAD excluding gender
(d) In all patients of severe aortic stenosis

593. Hallmark of aortic stenosis on X-ray chest is

(a) LV enlargement
(b) Post stenotic aortic dilation
(c) Calcified aortic valve
(d) Dilatation of left atrium

594. In fallots tetralogy survival normally depends on

(a) Degree of pulmonary stenosis
(b) Degree of overriding
(c) Degree of RVH
(d) Degree of collateral flow

595. Most common congenital heart disease heart hand syndrome is

(a) VSD (b) PDA
(c) OP (ASD) (d) ASD (OS)

596. Which valve is rarely calcified?

(a) Aortic (b) Mitral
(c) Pulmonary (d) Tricuspid

597. Peripheral pulmonary artery stenosis is particularly found with

(a) ASD (b) VSD
(c) PDA (d) AS (Valvular)

598. Pulses paradoxus is best detected in

(a) Carotid artery (b) Femoral artery
(c) Brachial artery (d) Radial artery

599. Which ECG finding is pathognomonic of cardiac tamponade?

(a) ST Segment deviation
(b) T wave inversion
(c) Low voltages
(d) Alternation of P and QRS

600. Enlargement of coronary sinus occurs in following left-right shunt except

(a) Partial anomalous pulmonary venous drainage
(b) Total anomalous pulmonary venous drainage
(c) Coronary arterial-coronary sinus fistula
(d) ASD (OS)

601. Short left veins coronary is found frequently with

(a) Fallots tetralogy (b) TG
(c) DORV (d) Bicuspid AV

602. Which cyanotic congenital heart disease in not associated anomalous coronary arteries?

(a) Tetralogy of fallots
(b) Complete transposition of great arteries
(c) Ebstein's disease
(d) Truncus arteriosus

603. X-ray chest in hypoplastic left heart shows all the following except

(a) RA enlargement
(b) RV dilation
(c) Ascending aorta dilatation
(d) Pulmonary arterial dilatation

604. Which of following congenital heart disease does not cause 1st degree AV block?

(a) ASD (OS) (b) VSD
(c) PDA (d) Ebsteins anomaly

605. Most important clinical finding in MV prolapse

(a) Non ejection systolic click
(b) Ejection systolic click
(c) Multiple ejection systolic click
(d) Mild mitral regurgitation

606. Rheumatic aortic stenosis is always associated with

(a) Mitral valve disease
(b) Aortic fibrillation
(c) (Mild) aortic regurgitation
(d) Heart failure

607. Most common type of truncus arteriosus is

(a) Type I (b) Type II
(c) Type III (d) All the above

608. All are features of dysplastic pulmonary valve stenosis except

(a) Three distinct cusps
(b) No commissural fusion
(c) P2 is soft or absent
(d) Prominent pulmonary ejection sound

609. Truncal valve is usually

(a) Unicuspid (b) Bicuspid
(c) Tricuspid (d) All the above

610. Least common presentation of truncal valve is

(a) Mild atrial regurgitation
(b) Moderate atrial regurgitation
(c) Severe atrial regurgitation
(d) Aortic stenosis

611. Most common congenital heart disease associated with right aortic arch

(a) Fallot's tetralogy
(b) Fallot's triology
(c) Truncus arteriosus
(d) Eisenmenger complex

612. Fetal mortality is highest in mitral stenosis in which of the following

(a) Class III NYHA on medical treatment
(b) NYHA class IV on medical treatment
(c) Mitral valvotomy
(d) Mitral valve replacement

613. Maternal mortality is highest in mitral stenosis with pregnancy in which therapy

(a) Mitral valvotomy
(b) Mitral valve replacement
(c) NYHA class IV on medical treatment
(d) All the above groups

614. All following maternal disease are associated with congenital heart disease in newborn

(a) IDDM (b) Phenylketonuria
(c) Rubella (d) Hypertension

615. All following are ECG indicator's of severe aortic stenosis except

(a) Left atrial enlargement
(b) Left ventricular hypertrophy without ST & T charges
(c) Left ventricular hypertrophy with starts
(d) Left bundle branch block

616. When pulmonary vascular disease is more common in ASD?

(a) ASD (OS) large
(b) In males (ASD OS)
(c) In females (ASD OS)
(d) Sinus venosus ASD

617. All following maternal medication are associated with congenital heart disease in newborn except

(a) Alcohol abuse (b) Lithium
(c) Warfarin (d) Heparin

618. Commonest complication of pregnancy in eisenmenger's syndrome

(a) Spontaneous abortion
(b) IUGR
(c) Premature delivery
(d) Perinatal mortality

619. Which combined valvular lesion has worst hemodynamic state?

(a) Mitral stenosis with aortic stenosis
(b) Mitral regurgitation with aortic stenosis
(c) Mitral regurgitation with atrial regurgitation
(d) Mitral stenosis with atrial regurgitation

620. All following congenital heart disease are associated with supraventricular tachycardia except

(a) ASD (b) Ebsteins disease
(c) TGA (d) PDA

621. Pericarditis does not occurs in all following disorders except

(a) Ankylosng spondylitis
(b) Vasculitis

(c) Polymyositis (d) SLE

622. Left heart is enlarged in all the following congenital heart disease except

(a) Aortic stenosis
(b) Coarctation of aorta
(c) ASD
(d) Tricuspid atresia

623. All following are associated with pericardial disease except

(a) ASD
(b) Thalassemia
(c) Glant urticaria
(d) Aortic regurgitation

624. PR interval is prolonged in all the following ASDs except

(a) Sinus venosus ASD
(b) Ostium primum ASD
(c) Holtoram syndrome
(d) Adult with Large ostium secundum ASD

625. Silent duration has all the feature except

(a) < 1 mm
(b) No continuous murmur
(c) No infective endocarditis
(d) Recognized clinically by abnormal S2

626. Cyanotic spell's are mainly due to

(a) Increased infundibular resistance
(b) Decreased peripheral
(c) Decreased blood pressure
(d) All the above

627. Which ECG criterion in infective endocarditis is indicative of worsening prognosis?

(a) Sinus tachycardia
(b) Bundle branch block
(c) Left ventricular hypertrophy
(d) Prolonged PR interval

628. Which ECG finding in infective endocarditis is probable indication for surgery?

(a) Ventricular extrabeats
(b) RBBB
(c) PR prolongation (d) PR shortening

629. Which is most important complication of infective endocarditis?

(a) Clubbing (b) Splenomegaly
(c) Heart failure (d) Embolism

630. Common organism in late prosthetic valve endocarditis is

(a) Streptococci (b) Staphylococci
(c) Gram –ve bacilli (d) Fungi

631. Pericardial knock in constrictive pericarditis rarely occurs

(a) Children (b) Adults
(c) Middle aged (d) Elderly

632. Aortic enlargement on X-ray is more often seen in

(a) TOF
(b) Hypertension
(c) Coarctation of aorta
(d) None of the above

633. Fetal warfarin syndrome causes which congenital heart disease

(a) Aortic stenosis (b) TOF
(c) PDA (d) ASD

634. Aortic stenosis occurs in which of the following?

(a) Turner's syndrome
(b) Trisomy 21
(c) Trisomy 18
(d) Trisomy 13

635. Highest incidence of congenital heart disease is found in

(a) Trisomy 13 syndrome
(b) Cri-do-cat syndrome
(c) Trisomy 18 syndrome
(d) Turner's syndrome

636. Dextrocardia is found in

(a) Trisomy 13 syndrome
(b) Trisomy 18 syndrome
(c) Trisomy 21 syndrome
(d) Turner syndrome

637. Birth weight is increased in

(a) Corrected TGA (b) TGA
(c) Fallot's tetralogy (d) Truncus arteriosus

638. Most common radiological abnormality MVP is

(a) Pectus excavatum
(b) Straight back syndrome
(c) Scoliosis (d) Kyphosis

639. Which is the rare complication of MVP?

(a) Sudden cardiac death
(b) Stock
(c) Mitral regurgitation
(d) Infective endocarditis

640. Rupture of chordae tendinae is most commonly due to

(a) Rheumatic (b) IE
(c) Idiopathic (d) MVP

641. Most common ECG feature of MVP is

(a) T inversion in inferior leads
(b) T inversion in lateral leads
(c) ST depression in inferior + Lateral leads
(d) Right bundle branch block

642. Which arrhythmia is uncommon in aortic regurgitation?

(a) Bundle branch block
(b) Ventricular arrhythmia
(c) AV blocks
(d) Atrial fibrillation

643. Silent aortic regurgitation develops in all the following except

(a) Paravalvular leak
(b) Aortic regurgitation with heart failure
(c) Aortic regurgitation with marked loss of valve substance
(d) Mild aortic regurgitation

644. Which is the common cardiac abnormality in marfan's syndrome?

(a) Aortic regurgitation
(b) MVP
(c) Mitral annular dilatation
(d) Aortic root dilatation

645. Most reliable tool for assessing severity of aortic regurgitation is

(a) Clinical sign
(b) ECG changes
(c) Doppler echo
(d) Supravalvular aortogram

646. Syncope in aortic stenosis is due to all the following except

(a) Ventricular arrhythmia
(b) Transient electro mechanical dissocation
(c) Peripheral vasodilation
(d) CHB

647. Dyspnea in mitral stenosis indicate MVA of

(a) 2 cm^2
(b) > 2 cm^2
(c) 2 – 1.5 cm^2
(d) < 1.5 cm^2

648. All are clinical manifestation of cardiovascular autonomic neuropathy except

(a) Exercise intolerance
(b) Painless infarction
(c) Orthostatic hypotension
(d) Orthostatic hypertension

649. Ca channel blockers are not

(a) Antihypertensive
(b) Cardiovascular protectives
(c) Antiischaemic
(d) All of the above

650. What is average diameter of PFO?

(a) 2 mm
(b) 3 mm
(c) 4 mm
(d) 4.9 mm

651. Katz wachtel phenomenon in ECG is commonly found in

(a) Advanced ASD (OS)
(b) Advanced VSD
(c) Advanced PDA
(d) None of the above

652. T wave is inverted in only in V1 in which disease?

(a) TOF
(b) Severe PS

(c) Eissenmenger's disease
(d) None of the above

653. Most common congenital heart disease producing LBBB

(a) VSD
(b) Atrial stenosis
(c) Truncus arteriosus
(d) TGA

654. Changes phesiomenon is used for

(a) Atrial aberrant cardioclic
(b) Ventricular aberrant cardioclic
(c) Both above
(d) None of the above

655. Most common ECG finding in single ventricle is

(a) RVH (b) LVH
(c) BVH (d) RAD

656. Murmur of congenital regurgitation has all the following feature except

(a) High pitched
(b) Heard always the left sternal border
(c) Decrescendo
(d) Pulmonary hypertension is absent

657. Which ECG finding is strong indication for aortic stenosis in children?

(a) LA enlargement (b) LVH
(c) LBBB (d) LAD

658. Most specific finding ostium primum ASD in children is

(a) 1 degree AV block
(b) RBBB
(c) LAD
(d) RBBB + LAD

659. Cyanotic child with palpable LV and No RV lift the possibilities are except

(a) Pulmonary atresia eith intact ventricular septum
(b) Tricuspid atresia
(c) Ebsteins disease
(d) Single atrium

660. Moon facies are associated with which cardiac lesion

(a) Severe pulmonary valve stenosis
(b) Aortic stenosis
(c) Mitral stenosis
(d) Tricuspid stenosis

661. All following are common manifestation of infective endocarditis except

(a) Roth spots (b) Oslor nodes
(c) Janeway lesion (d) Renal infarct

662. Reverse coarctation has all following features except

(a) In young adults
(b) More common in females
(c) Pulse less arms
(d) Myocardial infarction more common

663. Which is most common site of coarctation of aorta?

(a) Preductal (b) Juxtaductal
(c) Post ductal (d) Abdominal aorta

664. Acute Aortic regurgitation is characterized by all except

(a) LV compliance not increased
(b) End diastolic pressure markedly increased
(c) Aortic systolic pressure not increased
(d) Ejection fraction is increased

665. Maximum duration of antibiotic therapy is needed in which organism causing infective endocarditis?

(a) Streptococcus viridans
(b) Staphy lococcus epidermides
(c) Culture negative
(d) Penicillin resistant streptococci

666. Which haematologic abnormalities is not found in infective endocarditis?

(a) Leukocytosis
(b) Anaemia
(c) Increase ESR
(d) Thrombocytosis

667. Which immunologic abnormality is not found in infective endocarditis?

(a) Rheumatoid factor
(b) Cryoglobulinemia
(c) Increase complement levels
(d) Increase complexes

668. Normal AV orifice size is

(a) 2–3 cm^2 (b) 3–4 cm^2
(c) 4–4 cm^2 (d) > 4.5 cm^2

669. Symptomatic aortic stenosis develops when AVA is

(a) 1–1.5 cm^2 (b) 2–2.5 cm^2
(c) > 2.5–3 cm^2 (d) < 1 cm^2

670. What is the average decrease in valve area/year in aortic stenosis?

(a) 0.02 cm^2 (b) 0.03 cm^2
(c) 0.04 cm^2 (d) 0.05–0.1 cm^2

671. Average increase in mean pressure gradient/year in aortic stenosis

(a) 2 mm Hg (b) 3 mm Hg
(c) > 15 mm Hg
(d) > 3 to < 11 mm Hg

672. Which aortic stenosis progresses most rapidly?

(a) Degenerative (b) Congenital
(c) Rheumatic (d) All of the above

673. Most common type of VSD is

(a) Perimembranous (b) Muscular
(c) Inlet defect (d) Outlet defect

674. Lithium use in mother causes which heart disease commonly

(a) Ebsteins anomaly (b) ASD
(c) TGA (d) Truncus arteriosus

675. Which complication in ebsteins disease uncommon?

(a) Right ventricular failure
(b) Ventricular tachycardia
(c) Paradoxical embolism
(d) Infective endocarditis

676. What is not found in idiopathic dilatation of pulmonary artery?

(a) Loud P2 (b) Ejection click
(c) Systolic murmur (d) RVH

677. The malformed tricuspid valve in Ebsteins disease in usually

(a) Incompetent
(b) Stenotic
(c) Imperforate
(d) Both incompetent and stenotic

678. Cortriatriatum has all following features except

(a) 1st HS not increase
(b) No murmur
(c) Opening snap rare
(d) Atrial fibrillation common

679. Left atrial pressure is normal in which of following

(a) Rheumatic mitral stenosis
(b) Congenital mitral stenosis
(c) Core triatriatum
(d) Pulmonary vein stenosis

680. All following are found in coarctation of aorta except

(a) Murmur
(b) Hypertensive
(c) LVH
(d) Hypertensive retinopathy

681. Congenital mitral stenosis is most commonly associated with

(a) PDA
(b) Coarctation of aorta
(c) Bicuspid valve
(d) None of the above

682. Maternal ingestion of vitamin D is associated with which congenital heart disease

(a) PS
(b) Supravalvular aortic stenosis
(c) PDA
(d) Pulmonary artery branch stenosis

683. All following are normal in severe Aortic regurgitation except

(a) Effective stroke volume
(b) Effective cardiac output
(c) HR
(d) Ejection fraction

684. All following are increased in acute severe aortic regurgitation except

(a) Peripheral vascular resistance
(b) HR
(c) Left ventricular end-diastolic pressure
(d) Effective stroke volume

685. All following are normal in chronic severe aortic regurgitation

(a) 1st HS
(b) P2
(c) Pulmonary venous vascularity
(d) Aortic root

686. All following conditions are associated with congenital aortic regurgitation except

(a) Bicuspid valve
(b) Tricuspid valve
(c) Discrete sub aortic stenosis
(d) Supravalvular aortic stenosis

687. In chronic severe aortic regurgitation all are increased except

(a) Peripheral vascular resistance
(b) LV compliance
(c) Regurgitant volume
(d) LV ejection velocity

688. Syncope is usually found in

(a) Aortic stenosis
(b) Mitral stenosis
(c) Aortic regurgitation
(d) Mitral regurgitation

689. RVH is found in valvular lesion

(a) Mitral stenosis
(b) Mitral regurgitation
(c) Aortic regurgitation
(d) Aortic stenosis

690. Vasodilators are used in which valvular disease?

(a) Acute mitral regurgitation
(b) Aortic stenosis
(c) Mitral stenosis
(d) None of the above

691. Which antihypertensive causes gingival hyperplasia?

(a) β-blockers (b) Nifedipine
(c) Diuretics (d) Clonidine

692. Marantic endocarditis has all following features except

(a) Paraneoplastic syndrome associated with adenocarcinoma of lung
(b) Embolic phenomena are common
(c) Encephalopathy
(d) Murmurs are often found

693. HDL-C reduced by all the drugs except

(a) Probucal (b) β-blockers
(c) Aspirin (d) Methyldopa

694. Commonest type of truncus arteriosus is

(a) Type I (b) Type II
(c) Type III (d) Type IV

695. Smoking cessation in women is most effective in improving life expectance in which age

(a) 44 – 49 (b) 50 – 54
(c) 55 – 59 (d) 60 – 64

696. All are common congenital defects associated with corrected TGA

(a) PS (b) VSD
(c) MR (d) PDA

697. ECG is acute pericarditis becomes usually normal in what period

(a) 3 Days (b) 7 Days
(c) 10 Days (d) 2 Weeks

698. Pericarditis in ACS occurs in

(a) Transmural myocardial infarction
(b) Subendocardial myocardial infarction
(c) UA (d) All the above

699. Single component of pericarditis has all following features except

(a) Rare
(b) In atrial fibrillation
(c) The early stage
(d) The resolving stage

700. In highest left atrial pressure in mitral stenosis is usually

(a) 10 mmHg (b) 20 mmHg
(c) 25 mmHg (d) 30 mmHg

701. In all following situations presystolic murmur in mitral stenosis may be absent except

(a) Short PR interval (b) Atrial fibrillation
(c) Bradycardia (d) LV dysfunction

702. In all following situations length of murmur of mitral stenosis is unreliable for severity except

(a) Tachycardia
(b) Bradycardia
(c) Low cardiac output
(d) Normal LV function

703. In all following conditions the S2 – OS interval in mitral stenosis is unreliable to predict it severity except

(a) Tachycardia (b) Bradycardia
(c) AR (d) TS

704. Commonest type of commissural pulmonary valve stenosis is

(a) Domed (b) Tricuspid
(c) Bicuspid (d) Dysplastic

705. All following are mechanism of opening snap in mitral stenosis except

(a) Thickening of valve
(b) Doming of valve in LV
(c) High LA pressure (d) Hypotrophy of LV

706. Musical early diastolic murmurs of aortic regurgitation occurs in all the following except

(a) Infective endocarditis
(b) Syphilis
(c) Congenital (d) None of these

707. In all following situation the murmur of significant aortic regurgitation is short or not heard except

(a) Acute aortic regurgitation
(b) Aortic regurgitation with pregnancy
(c) Aortic regurgitation patients receiving vasodilators
(d) Chronic severe aortic regurgitation

708. Which is the commonest cause of secondary hypertension?

(a) Chronic renal disease
(b) Primary aldosteronism
(c) Coarrctation of aorta
(d) Oral contracepturies

709. When pitch of murmur of mitral stenosis becomes high pitched?

(a) Associated mitral regurgitation
(b) Associated aortic regurgitation
(c) Calcified mitral stenosis
(d) None of the above

710. All following cyanotic congenital heart disease causes mid diastolic murmur in MA except

(a) Double outlet RV
(b) Single ventricle
(c) Eissenmenger syndrome
(d) Truncus arteriusus

711. All are causes of AR due to aortic root disease except

(a) Ankylosing spondylitis
(b) Marfan's syndrome
(c) Pseudoxanthoma elasticum
(d) VSD with aortic regurgitation

712. Most common form of pulmonary stenosis is

(a) Endovascular
(b) Supravalvular
(c) Pulmonary artery branch
(d) Valvular

713. All following are poor predictors of surgical outcome in aortic regurgitation except

(a) LVEF < 50%
(b) LV shortening fraction < 25%
(c) LV endsystolic diameter < 55 mm
(d) LV end diastolic diameter > 75 mm

714. Which is least common finding on echo in constrictive pericarditis?
(a) Pericardial calcification
(b) Pericardial – thickening
(c) Abnormal septal diastolic motion
(d) Mildly enlarged atria

715. All are common findings in constrictive pericarditis on echo except
(a) Constrictive doppler pattern of mitral and tricuspid valve inflow increased by inspiration
(b) Left atrial hypertension
(c) Abnormal pulmonary when vein inflow pattern
(d) Pericardial thickening

716. Which of the following has most positive predictive value for diagnosis of cardiac tamponade?
(a) RA collapse
(b) RV collapse
(c) Both RA and RV collapse
(d) Any collapse

717. Most positive predictive valve for detection of cardiac tamponade
(a) Abnormal venous flow
(b) Abnormal venous flow + One Right heart chamber collapse
(c) Abnormal venous flow and two cardiac chamber collapse

718. RA collapse in cardiac tamponade has all following features except
(a) Most common and earliest
(b) Occurs when IPP^3 4 mmHg
(c) Duration valves there 1/3 scardiac cycle
(d) Occurs during early diastole

719. RV collapse in cardiac temponade has all the feature except

(a) More specific
(b) Occurs at IPP ≥ 10 ± 4 mmHg
(c) During late diastole
(d) Best seen RV anterior wall and infundibulum

720. Most common etiology of cardiac tamponade is

(a) Malignancy (b) Uraemia
(c) Idiopathic (d) Infarction

721. Commonest complication of mechanical prosthetic valve

(a) Thrombus (b) Infarction
(c) Stenosis (d) Pannus

722. Which is the rare finding in infective endocarditis?

(a) Fever (b) Anaemia
(c) Polyarthritis (d) Clubbing

723. Commonest complication of biological valve

(a) Thrombus formation
(b) Infarction
(c) Pannus
(d) Degeneration

724. Most common type of extracardiac L-R shunt is

(a) Aorta pulmonary window
(b) PDA
(c) Pulmonary arterio venous fistula
(d) Broncho pulmonary anastomosis

725. Ductus arteriosus usually closes

(a) With in 24 hours of both
(b) With in 48–72 hours of both
(c) Between 5–7th day
(d) After one week of birth

726. Q wave in mitral regurgitation are found in which etiological type

(a) Rheumatic (b) Functional
(c) Ischaemic (d) MVP

727. Most frequent feature of mitral regurgitation (chronic) on ECG is

(a) Atrial fibrillation (b) LA enlargement
(c) LV hypertrophy (d) RV hypertrophy

728. All are the risk factors for thromboembolism in valvular heart disease except

(a) Aortic valve disease
(b) Atrial fibrillation
(c) MV disease
(d) LVEF > 45%

729. Rheumatic aortic stenosis has all following features except

(a) History of rheumatic fever (50%)
(b) No ejection click
(c) Coexisting mitral valve disease common
(d) Post stenotic dilatation of aorta is common

730. Which is commonest arrhythmia found in congenitally corrected TGA?

(a) AV block
(b) BBB
(c) Ventricular preexcitation
(d) Atrial fibrillation

731. Which type of ventricular preexcitation is commonly found in ebsteins disease?

(a) Type A (b) Type B
(c) Type C (d) Unclassified

732. Important causes of papillary muscle dysfunction are

(a) IHD
(b) Cardiomyopathy
(c) LV dilation
(d) Acute rheumatic fever

733. All are causes of rupture of chordiae tendinae except

(a) Infective endocarditis
(b) MVP
(c) Marfan's syndrome
(d) Hypertension

734. Vegetation on echo has all following features except

(a) Usually valvular
(b) Irregular shape
(c) Attached to the proximal side of valve
(d) Motion dependent on valve motion

735. Most sensitive and specific test to defect LA thrombus

(a) Echo TTE (b) Echo TEE
(c) CT (d) Angiography

736. Size of vegetation most likely to embolize

(a) < 5 mm (b) 5 – 7 mm
(c) 7 – 9 mm (d) > 10 mm

737. All are echocardiographic signs of prosthetic valve dysfunction except

(a) Increased antegrade velocity across the valve
(b) Decreased valve area
(c) Increased regurgitant flow
(d) Decreased intensity of regurgitant signal

738. Jugular venous pressure is raised in all the following situations in ASD except

(a) With MV disease (b) RVF
(c) Severe PAH (d) PS

739. Biventricular hypertrophy is found in all the following conditions except

(a) DORV without PS
(b) Truncus arteriosus
(c) Pulmonary atresia with PDA
(d) Tricuspid atresia

740. Which congenital heart disease is with no ventricular enlargement?

(a) TOF
(b) Triology of fallots
(c) Pulmonary arterio-venous fistula
(d) Tricuspid atresia

741. MVP has all following feature except

(a) Chest pain
(b) Abnormal ECG

(c) False positive exercise ECG
(d) Nitrates relieve the pain

742. Po2 is decreased in all the following except
(a) Acute pulmonary edema
(b) Acute pulmonary embolism
(c) Cardiogenic shock
(d) Stable angina

743. Asymptomatic persons with following disease needs surgery except
(a) Cyanotic congenital heart disease
(b) Coarctation of aorta
(c) Large L-R shunt
(d) Moderate mitral stenosis

744. Patient presenting with signs of systemic congestion but deteriorates by diuretic which cardiac diagnosis is likely
(a) CHF
(b) Constrictive pericarditis
(c) Corpulmonule
(d) None of the above

745. Commonest cyanotic congenital heart disease at birth is
(a) D-TGA
(b) Fallots tetralogy
(c) Eissenmenger's syndrome
(d) Truncus arteriosus

746. Commonest location of pulmonary stenosis is
(a) Valvular
(b) Subvalvular
(c) Supravalvular
(d) Combination of (a) & (b)

747. Normsal pulmonary value area is
(a) 1 cm^2/m^2 (b) 1.5 cm^2/m^2
(c) 2 cm^2/m^2 (d) 3 cm^2/m^2

748. Which is last obstruction at pulmonary is required to have prominent 'a' wave in neck wine?
(a) Mild (b) Midrate
(c) Severe (d) All of the above

749. Hall mark of valvular pulmonary stenosis is

(a) ESM
(b) P2 decrease
(c) Ejection click heard in expiration & disappears with inspiration
(d) Narrow split S2

750. Murmur of supravalvular pulmonary stenosis radiates commonly to

(a) Neck
(b) Suprasternal notch
(c) Axilla
(d) Left sternal border

751. In pulmonary valve stenosis at which gradient intervention is cleves not indicated

(a) 40 mmHg (b) 40-50 mmHg
(c) 50-60 mmHg (d) < 25 mmHg

752. Which is most common associated anomaly is

(a) Right aortic arch
(b) Left superior venacava
(c) ASD
(d) Absent ductes arteriosus

753. Most common cyanotic cangenital heart disease is

(a) Eissenmenger's syndrome
(b) Truncus arteriesis
(c) Fallots tetralogy
(d) Total anomalous pulmonary venous drainage

754. Hypoxic spells in fallots commonly occurs

(a) < 1 months of age
(b) < 1.5 month of age
(c) > 2 month of age
(d) > 3 years of age

755. Hypoxic spells most often occurs

(a) In the morning (b) Noon lint
(c) Evening (d) Night

756. Which drug is given for prevention of hypoxic spell?

(a) Sodium bicarbonate

(b) a – Adrenergic agonist
(c) Propranolol
(d) None of the above

757. Wide and fixed splitting of S2 occurs in all the following cyanotic congenital heart disease except

(a) Reversed ASD
(b) Total anomalous pulmonary venous connection
(c) VSD of A-V canal type
(d) Eissenmenger's complex

758. Which tricuspid diastolic murmurs is heard in rupture of sinus of valsalva?

(a) RV (b) RA
(c) LA (d) LV

759. When continuous murmur is not heard in which location of rupture of sinus of valsalva?

(a) RA (b) LA
(c) LV (d) RV

760. Significant aortic regurgitation with short murmur may occurs in all the following except

(a) Acute aortic regurgitation
(b) Aortic regurgitation with hypotension
(c) Aortic regurgitation with patient using vasodilators
(d) Sinus bradycardia

761. All are complication of TAPVD except

(a) Pulmonary vein stenosis after repair
(b) SSS
(c) Heart failure
(d) Infective endocarditis

762. All following complications may occurs in VSD except

(a) Infective endocarditis
(b) Eissenmenger complex
(c) LBBB
(d) Aortic regurgitation

763. Early systolic murmur are found in all following except

(a) Small muscular VSD
(b) TR without PH
(c) Acute mitral regurgitation
(d) Large VSD without significant PAH

764. Commonest conduction abnormality is infective endocarditis is

(a) I Degree AV Block
(b) II Degree AV Block
(c) III Degree AV Block
(d) Bundle Branch Block

765. Which pericardial syndrome is rare in renal disease?

(a) Pericarditis
(b) Cardiac temponade
(c) Lax pericardial effusion
(d) Constrictive pericarditis

766. Most commonly used mechanical aortic valve prosthesis is

(a) Ball and cage (b) Tilting disc
(c) Trileaflet (d) All of the above

767. All following are cardiac complication to elective surgery except

(a) MI < 3 months
(b) Heart failure
(c) Severe aortic stenosis
(d) RBBB with LAHB

768. Depth of inverted T wave is constrictive pericarditis indicate

(a) Non specific
(b) Presence of myocarditis
(c) Degree of pericardial adherence to Myocardium
(d) Drug induced

769. Spontaneous closure of VSD most commonly occurs at which age

(a) By 2 years of age (b) By 5 years of age
(c) By 8 years of age (d) By 10 years of age

770. Loud A2 is found in VSD in all the following except

(a) Associated coarctation of aorta
(b) Bicuspid aortic valve
(c) TGA with VSD
(d) PDA with VSD

771. Commonest microorganism right sided endocarditis is

(a) S. Aureus (b) S. Epidermidis
(c) Pseudomonas (d) Serratia

772. Commonest cause of acute pericarditis is

(a) Viral/idiopathic (b) Bacterial
(c) Fungal (d) Tuberculosis

773. In which valve lesion statin may be given?

(a) Aortic stenosis
(b) Mitral stenosis
(c) Mitral regurgitation
(d) PS

774. Rare presentation of aortic stenosis is

(a) Sudden cardiac death
(b) Angina
(c) Dyspnea (d) Syncope

775. Rib notching may occur in all the following except

(a) Co-arctation of aorta
(b) Pulmonary atresia
(c) Venacaval obstruction
(d) PDA

776. Pericardial thickening is found in which of the following

(a) Constrictive pericarditis
(b) Endomyocardial fibrosis
(c) Amyloid heart disease
(d) Primary restrictive cardiomyopathy

777. PDA murmur is

(a) Crescendo
(b) Decrescendo
(c) Crescendo-decrescendo
(d) Severe intensity

778. All are causes of central cyanosis in ASD except

(a) IVC to LA (b) Bradycardia
(c) TS (d) Mitral stenosis

779. Fallots triology has all following features except

(a) Giant 'a' wave in neck veins
(b) Extreme RVH
(c) RBB
(d) Cyanotic attacks

780. Fallots tetralogy has all following features except

(a) Right aortic arch (b) Cyanotic attack
(c) Giant 'a' wave (d) Squatting

781. Commonest cause of severe aortic regurgitation in young child

(a) Bicuspid valve
(b) VSD with aortic valve prolapse
(c) Infective endocarditis
(d) Acute rheumatic fever

782. Sudden severe aortic regurgitation is due to all following except

(a) Infective endocarditis
(b) Ruptured aneurysm of sinus of valsalva
(c) Acute rheumatic fever
(d) All of the above

783. Commonest cause of mild aortic regurgitation in adult is

(a) Hypertension
(b) Maemia
(c) Anaemia
(d) Acute rheumatic fever

784. All following congenital heart disease are well tolerated during pregnancy except

(a) Uncomplicated ASD
(b) Pulmonary stenosis
(c) Acyanotic ebstein's anomaly
(d) Severe aortic stenosis

785. Which pulmonary vascular change is associated with irreversible pulmonary hypertension?
(a) Medial hypertrophy
(b) Intimal reaction
(c) Fibrotic intimal change
(d) Plexiform lesion

786. In hyperkinetic pulmonary hypertension the pulmonary artery systolic pressure usually does not exceed
(a) 30 mmHg (b) 40 mmHg
(c) 50 mmHg (d) 60 mmHg

787. Which sign suggest primary pulmonary hypertension?
(a) Does not change with respiration
(b) S2 is often single
(c) S1 is split
(d) S1 is vibratory

788. In which cause of eissenmenger syndrome S2 is single?
(a) Single atrium (b) Reversed PDA
(c) Reversed ASD (d) Reversed VSD

789. Commonest presenting symptom in ASD is
(a) Dyspnaea (b) Palpitation
(c) Chest pain (d) Edema

790. Myocardial birdying most commonly occurs in which coronary artery
(a) LAD (b) Cx
(c) PDA (d) RCA

791. Most common symptom in pulmonary hypertension is
(a) Dyspnoea (b) Chest pain
(c) Syncope (d) Pedal edema

792. Most common cause of porto– pulmonary hypertension is
(a) Liver disease
(b) Biliary atresia
(c) Extra hepatic portal veinobstruction
(d) Portal fibrosis

793. Commonest manifestation of acute rheumatic fever

(a) Arthritis
(b) Carditis
(c) Chorea
(d) Sub cutaneous nodules

794. All following congenital heart disease may be associated with atrial fibrillation except

(a) ASD (b) Ebsteins anomaly
(c) TGA (d) Fallots tetralogy

795. Most common cause of junctional escape beat is

(a) Sinus bradycardia (b) AV block
(c) Reserpamia (d) Hyperbalemia

796. Most common infiltrative corp is

(a) Amyloid
(b) Carcinoid
(c) Maetrachromatosis
(d) Sarcoidosis

797. Most common congenital heart associated with VSD

(a) Coarctation of aorta
(b) ASD
(c) PDA
(d) Mitral stenosis

798. Pericardial effusion is found in

(a) Acute myocarditis
(b) Chronic myocarditis
(c) Infiltrative cardiomyopathy
(d) All the above

799. Which is earliest auscutatory finding in mitral stenosis?

(a) Loud S1
(b) Mid diastolic murmur
(c) Presystolic murmur
(d) Opening snap

800. Which finding is found in both acute and chronic severe mitral regurgitation?

(a) LA enlargement
(b) LV enlargement

(c) S3
(d) Apical impulse displacement

801. Commonest cause of constrictive pericarditis

(a) Idiopathic (b) Post CABG
(c) Tuberculosis (d) Radiation

802. Which storage disease of myocardium produces MVP?

(a) Fabrys disease
(b) Glycogen storage disease
(c) Gaucher disease
(d) Sterters syndrome

803. ECG frontal plane axis is normal in all the following except

(a) ASD OS (b) APVD complete
(c) APVD partial (d) Common atrium

804. All are hallmark of significant prosthetic valve haemolysis except

(a) Hemosiderosis
(b) Shistocytosis
(c) Reticulocytosis
(d) Increased heptoglobin

805. Cyanotic Infant in ECG Shows all the following except

(a) 'P' congenital (b) LAD
(c) LVH (d) 'P' mitrate

806. Aortic stenosis as choff nodule consist of all except

(a) Fibrinoid necrosis (b) Lymphocytes
(c) Neutrophills (d) Macrophages

807. Most common cause of rheumatic mitral stenosis is

(a) Commissural fusion
(b) Leaflet fusion
(c) Fusion of chordae (d) Combined

808. Mitral annular calcification is seen in all except

(a) Marfan's syndrome
(b) Hurler's syndrome
(c) Mitral valve prolapse
(d) Rheumatic

809. Symptom of pulmonary venous hypertension occurs at which MVA

(a) 2 cm^2 (b) 1.5 cm^2
(c) 2.5 cm^2 (d) $\leq$ cm^2

810. Which ECG change is not found in acute pericarditis?

(a) ST segment deviation
(b) T wave changes
(c) Voltages changes
(d) Q wave development

811. Major complication of infective endocarditis is

(a) Heart failure (b) Renal failure
(c) Embolism (d) Meningitis

812. Most common pericardial disease is

(a) Pericarditis
(b) Pericardial effusion
(c) Effusive constrictive pericarditis
(d) Constrictive pericarditis

813. Usually Chordal Rupture is due to

(a) Idiopathic degenerative
(b) Rheumatic
(c) Endocarditis (infective)
(d) MVP

814. Bilateral bulging of anterior chest with bulging of upper 2/3 of sternum is commonly found in children with

(a) ASD (b) Large VSD
(c) PDA (d) PS

815. L+ 4th & 5th ICS bulging in adult commonly seen is

(a) ASD (b) VSD
(c) Ebstein's disease (d) None of the above

816. Underdeveloped musculature of lower extremities is commonly found in

(a) PDA
(b) AS
(c) Coarctation of aorta
(d) Aortic aneurysm

817. Which congenital heart is associated as part of syndrome with thromcocytopenia?

(a) OSASD
(b) VSD
(c) PDA
(d) Coarctation of Aorta

818. Stenosis of large arteries occurs with all except

(a) Supravalvular aortic stenosis
(b) Subvalvular aortic stenosis
(c) Neuro fibromatosis
(d) Rubella syndrome

819. Murmur of aortic regurgitation is uncommon in

(a) Congenital valvular aortic stenosis
(b) Acquired valvular aortic stenosis
(c) Congenital subvalvular aortic stenosis
(d) HOCM

820. Which supraventricular tachycardia occurs in L-TGA?

(a) Atrial tachycardia
(b) Sinus node re-entrant tachycardia
(c) AVRT
(d) AVNRT

821. Sudden cardiac death is more common in which congenital heart disease?

(a) Congenital aortic stenosis
(b) Congenital PS
(c) ASD
(d) VSD

822. All following congenital heart disease sudden cardiac death except

(a) Fallot's tetralogy
(b) Aortic stenosis
(c) Ebstein's disease
(d) VSD

823. Commonest complication of MVP

(a) Rupture of chords
(b) Infective endocarditis
(c) Mitral regurgitation
(d) Fibrosideposition

824. Commonest cause of tricuspid valve disease

(a) Rheumatic
(b) Ebstein's
(c) Carcinoid
(d) Infective endocarditis

825. Commonest cause of pulmonary valve disease

(a) Congenital (b) TOF
(c) Carcinoid (d) Rheumatic

826. What is dominant mechanism of rheumatic mitral regurgitation?

(a) Thickening (b) Retraction
(c) Rupture of chord (d) Destrictive lesion

827. Dominant mechanism of mitral regurgitation of marfan's syndrome

(a) Thicking
(b) Prolapse
(c) Rupture chords
(d) Dilatation of anrialop

828. Dominant mechanism of ischemic/hypertensive mitral regurgitation is

(a) Ruptured papillary muscle
(b) Ruptured chord
(c) Prolapse
(d) Destructive lesion

829. Dominant mechanism of mitral regurgitation is dilated cardiomyopathy is

(a) Annular dilatation
(b) Prolapse
(c) Papillary muscle rupture
(d) Thickening

830. Dominant mechanism in restrictive CMP of mitral regurgitation

(a) Thickening (b) Annular dilatation
(c) Leaflet prolapse (d) Chordal rupture

831. Dominant mechanism of mitral regurgitation in infective endocarditis is

(a) Destruction of valve
(b) Thickening of valve
(c) Prolapse of valve (d) Retraction of valve

832. What is mechanism of congenital mitral regurgitation?

(a) Thickening (b) Retraction
(c) Prolapse (d) Cleft

833. Most frequent feature of mitral regurgitation is

(a) Atrial fibrillation (b) Heart failure
(c) LVH (d) LAE

834. Which agent produces pericardial lesions?

(a) Emetine (b) Methysergide
(c) Chloroquine (d) Lithium

835. All following changes occurs in acute pericarditis except

(a) ST Segment elevation
(b) T wave inversion
(c) Reciprocal ST changes don't occurs
(d) PR segment is elevated

836. What hand deformity may occurs in rheumatic heart disease?

(a) Ulnar deviation of 4th finger
(b) Ulnar deviation of 5th finger
(c) Flexion of metacarpophacangeal joints
(d) All the above

837. Which size of VSD closes often spontaneously?

(a) < 0.5 mm
(b) 5 – 10 mm
(c) 10 – 15 mm
(d) < 2 cm > 1.5 cm

838. Dilatation of SVC occurs in which type of ASD?

(a) ASD OS (b) ASD OP
(c) ASD SV (d) All of the above

839. Commonest type of VSD is

(a) Perimembranous (b) Inlet
(c) Trabecular (d) Outlet

840. Infective endocarditis occurs in which type of ASD?

(a) ASD (OS) (b) ASD (OP)
(c) ASD (SV) (d) All the above

841. Which type of ASD is associated with inverted 'P' waves in inferior leads?

(a) ASD (OS) (b) ASD (OP)
(c) ASD (SV) (d) All of the above

842. All are signs of severe pulmonary valve stenosis except

(a) Small volume pulse
(b) Long late peaking murmur
(c) P2 absent
(d) Giant 'a' wave in neck veins

843. All are complications of pulmonary valve stenosis except

(a) RVF
(b) Infective endocarditis
(c) Sudden cardiac death
(d) Pulmonary infarction

844. Intermittent cyanosis is risk in which condition

(a) Fallot's tetralogy (b) Tricuspid atresia
(c) PFO (d) Ebstein's disease

845. Which cyanotic congenital heart disease produces syncope?

(a) Tricuspid atresia (b) TGA
(c) Fallot's tetralogy (d) TAPVD

846. Anabolic steroid can lead to all the following except

(a) Decrease HDL
(b) Hypertension
(c) Clothing abnormalities
(d) Increase LDL

847. All following cyanotic congenital cardiac disease is associated with decreased pulmonary flow except

(a) TOF (b) DORV with PS
(c) ASD with PS (d) TGA

848. Most consistent feature of idiopathic dilatation of pulmonary trunk is

(a) Ejection sound better heard in expiration
(b) Ejection sound better heard in inspiration

(c) Systolic ejection murmur
(d) Variable S2

849. All following are features of heart sound in ebstein anomaly are correct except

(a) Wide split
(b) Second component is more loud
(c) Split S2 wide and fixed
(d) S3 in uncommon

850. What happens to pulmonary artery pressure in pulmonary trunk pulmonary artery branch stenosis?

(a) Only systolic pressure rises
(b) Only diastolic pressure rises
(c) Both pressure rises
(d) Both in are none

851. Which is commonest arrhythmia in constrictive pericarditis?

(a) Premature atrial ectopic
(b) SSS
(c) Atrial fibrillation
(d) AV block

852. All are features of dysplastic pulmonary valve except

(a) Obstructive thickened unmobile cusps
(b) No click
(c) Post stenotic dilatation not prominent
(d) P2 soft

853. Hemoptysis is important feature of

(a) Dome pulmonary stenosis
(b) Dysplastic pulmonary stenosis
(c) Infundibular pulmonary stenosis
(d) Pulmonary artery branch stenosis

854. Commonest cause of chronic pericardial effusion

(a) Viral
(b) Bacterial
(c) Connective tissue disease
(d) Myxaedema

855. Cyanotic congenital heart disease, no ventricular enlargement, no abnormal sound/ murmur/X-ray and ECG are normal, likely diagnosis

(a) Pulmonary arterio venous fistula
(b) Fallots tetralogy
(c) Ebstein's disease
(d) Isolated drainage of vena-cava in to left atrium

856. Acute severe aortic regurgitation on auscultation all the following alternation in heart sounds except

(a) S1 soft absent (b) A2 soft
(c) S4 absent (d) S3 uncommon

857. Which is commonest anatomic type of cortriatriatum?

(a) Diaphragmatic (b) Hour glass
(c) Tubular (d) All of the above

858. Acute severe aortic regurgitation reveals all the following except

(a) Aortic systolic £ 3/6
(b) Aortic regurgitation murmur short medium pitched
(c) Austin flint murmur presystolic
(d) Peripheral signs absent

859. Least common anatomic type of cortriatrium is

(a) Tubular (b) Hour glass
(c) Diaphragmatic (d) All of the above

860. X-ray findings in acute severe aortic regurgitation show all the following except

(a) Left ventricular is round sized
(b) Left ventricle is markedly dilated
(c) Aortic root usually normal
(d) Pulmonary venous vascularity increased

861. Arterial pulse in acute severe aortic regurgitation inhibitors all the following except

(a) Rate rise not increased
(b) Pulse pressure needy none

(c) Single contour of pulse
(d) Pulses alternans uncommon

862. Cortriatriatum reveals all following features except

(a) S1 is not loud
(b) Pulmonary hypertension is present
(c) RVH occurs
(d) Atrial fibrillation common

863. Acute severe aortic regurgitation is characterized by all the following except

(a) Early and sudden heart failure
(b) LV impulse in hyperdynamic
(c) Normal voltage ECG
(d) Major depolarization changes in ECG

864. All following are enlarged on X-ray except

(a) RA (b) RV
(c) Pulmonary trunk (d) LA

865. X-ray in chronic severe aortic regurgitation reveals all the following except

(a) LV massively enlarged
(b) Aortic root prominent
(c) Aortic arch is prominent
(d) Pulmonary vascularity is increased

866. Commonest type of congenital mitral stenosis is

(a) Typical
(b) Parachute MV
(c) Anomalom mitral arched
(d) Accessory mitral valve tissue

867. Pseudcoarctation has all the following features except

(a) Buckling/kinking of aorta at or just beyond ligamentum arteriosus
(b) Elongation/dilatation/tortousity of distal aortic arch and proximal descending aorta
(c) No narrowing of aortic lumen
(d) Always benign condition and not associated with any complication

868. Which of the following does not occur in congenital mitral stenosis?

(a) RVH
(b) Dyspnea
(c) Pulmonary arterial hypertension
(d) Hemoptysis

869. All following signs are infrequent in congenital mitral stenosis except

(a) Loud S1 (b) OS
(c) Diastolic murmur (d) RV enlargement

870. Which shunt lesions is associated with coarctation of aorta?

(a) ASD (b) VSD
(c) .PDA (d) None of these

871. Which is not found in congenital mitral stenosis?

(a) Pulmonary venous congention
(b) Pulmonary arterial hypertension
(c) Left atrial enlargement
(d) MV calcification

872. Collateral arterial pulsations in coarctation of aorta are found in all following locations except

(a) Around and between septal
(b) Around shoulder
(c) Right sternal border
(d) Pulmonary area

873. All statement regarding notching of ribs in coarctation of aorta are correct except

(a) Results from collateral flow through posterior intercostal arteries
(b) Notches originates in costal eroore rather than on the most inferior rib in angina
(c) Occurs on posterior ribs
(d) Occurs on anterior ribs

874. All following are complication of coarctation of aorta except

(a) Hypertension encephalopathy
(b) Heart failure

(c) Infective endocarditis
(d) Rupture/dissection of Aorta

875. Incidences of toxemia of pregnancy is lowest in which type of hypertension?
(a) Essential hypertension
(b) Renal hypertension
(c) Endocranial hypertension
(d) Co-arctation of aorta

876. Arterial pulse in chronic severe aortic regurgitation reveals all the following except
(a) Rate of rise is increased
(b) Pulse pressure is increased
(c) Contour of peak may be bisferiens
(d) Pulsus alternans is common

877. Chronic severe aortic regurgitation shows all the following except
(a) Late and insidious heart failure
(b) LV apex displaced and hyperdynamic
(c) LV voltages are increased
(d) No significant repolarization changes in ECG

878. Chronic severe aortic regurgitation is associated with alterations in heart sounds except
(a) S1 is normal
(b) A2 normal/decreased
(c) P2 is normal
(d) S3 is common

879. Which following is not found in congenital pulmonary vein stenosis?
(a) P2 Loud (b) MDM
(c) RVH (d) PSM of TR

880. Which of statement is incorrect regarding murmurs in chronic severe acute regurgitation?
(a) Aortic systolic murmur ≥ 3/6
(b) EDM high pitched
(c) Peripheral signs are present
(d) Mid diastolic murmur with presystolic accentuation is present

881. ECG in pulmonary vein stenosis slows all the following except

(a) RAD (b) RVH
(c) 'P' pulmonale (d) 'P' mitrale

882. All following are indications of surgery in native valve endocarditis except

(a) Haemodynamic deterioration
(b) Myocardial abscess
(c) Medical treatment failure relapse after adghate treatment
(d) New regurgitant murmur without haemodynamic detonation

883. All are definite indication of surgery in prosthetic valve endocarditis except

(a) Haemodynamic deterioration
(b) Myocardial abscess
(c) Fungal endocarditis
(d) Large vegetation on echo

884. Commonest complication of prosthetic valve endocarditis

(a) Valve ring abscess
(b) Myocardial abscess
(c) Valve obstruction by vegetation
(d) Purulent pericarditis

885. Most uncommon complication of prosthetic valve endocarditis

(a) Ring abscess (b) Myocardial abscess
(c) Valve obstruction by vegetation
(d) Purulent vericarditis

886. All following are the features of marantic thrombotic endocarditis except

(a) Murmurs are found
(b) Embolism occurs
(c) Culture negative
(d) Occurs as complication of chronic disease

887. All are features of fungal endocarditis except

(a) Myocardial abscess
(b) Large systemic embolism
(c) High mortality
(d) Medical therapy usually successful

888. Brucella endocarditis involves which valve

(a) Mitral (b) Aortic
(c) Pulmonary (d) All the above

889. Most common form of renal involvement in infective endocarditis is

(a) Immune complex glomerulonephritis
(b) Focal glomerulonephritis
(c) Renal embolism
(d) Pyelonephritis

890. Which cardiac structure is rarely involved in infective endocarditis?

(a) Myocardium rarely
(b) Conduction tissue
(c) Valves
(d) Pericardium

891. Commonest skin lesion in infective endocarditis is

(a) Petechial rash
(b) Splinter haolmonage
(c) Osler nodes
(d) Janeways lesion

892. All are features of tricuspid stenosis except

(a) Mid diastolic murmur
(b) Split S1
(c) Loud P2
(d) High frequency murmur

893. All following disease have definite association with MVP except

(a) Connective tissue disorders
(b) (OS) ASD
(c) Ebsteins disease
(d) HCM

894. Chick is increased by manouvers in MVP except

(a) Standing and inspiration
(b) Strain phase of valsalva
(c) Amyl nitrite inhalation
(d) Squatting

895. Following skeletomuscular abnormalities occurs in mitral valve prolapse except

(a) High arched palate
(b) Pectus excavatum
(c) Straight back syndrome
(d) Gynecomastia

896. Mitral annular calcification is found in all except

(a) Hypertension (b) DM
(c) HCM (d) Myxedema

897. All are common major risk factor in for VTE except

(a) Malignancy
(b) Major trauma
(c) Paralysis
(d) Heparin induced thrombocytopenia

898. Central cyanosis with pulmonary oligemia is found in all following conditions except

(a) Fallot's tetralogy (b) Pulmonary
(c) Tricuspid atresia (d) TGA

899. Subcutaneous nodule in acute rheumatic fever have all the features except

(a) Firm
(b) Tender
(c) Mobile
(d) On extensor surfaces of body

900. Involvement of MV in non rheumatic heart disease has all the following features except

(a) Mitral stenosis is absent
(b) Sub valvular apparatus involvement is common
(c) Calcification rare
(d) Annular involvement absent

901. Papillary Dysfunction occurs in all the following except

(a) IHD
(b) LV Dilation
(c) Cardiomyopathy
(d) Infective endocarditis

902. All are features of congenital aortic stenosis

(a) No History of RF

(b) Ejection click is present
(c) Aortic regurgitation is absent
(d) MVD is absent

903. Rheumatic aortic stenosis has all the following features except
(a) History of RF in 50%
(b) Ejection click absent
(c) Aortic regurgitation absent
(d) Post stenotic aortic dilation is not prominent

904. Commonest cause of TR
(a) Functional to PH
(b) Carcinoid
(c) Infective endocarditis
(d) Rheumatic

905. Sinequanon for diagnosis of infective endocarditis is
(a) Blood culture (b) Echo
(c) Increase ESR (d) Hematuria

906. The common presentation of right sided endocarditis is
(a) Pneumonia (b) Emphysema
(c) Lung abscess (d) Uremia

907. Coronary arteriovenous fistula exhibits all the following except
(a) Continuous murmur over precordium
(b) 90% of coronary artery fistula drainage in to the right heart
(c) Left coronary artery is more commonly involved
(d) Infection endocarditis may occurs

908. All following congenital heart disease produce RBBB except
(a) PS (b) ASD
(c) VSD (d) PDA

909. Ebsteins occurs in offspring of patient using which drug
(a) Alcohol (b) Thalidomide
(c) Lithium (d) Phenytoin

910. ASD occurs in all the following except

(a) TAR
(b) Down's syndrome
(c) Holtoram
(d) Pseudxanthoma elasticum

911. Compression of Large A-V fistula causes

(a) Sinus tachycardia (b) Premature VE
(c) Atrial fibrillation (d) Sinus bradycardia

912. Hilair dance on fluoroscopy is seen in

(a) ASD (b) VSD
(c) PH (d) PDA

913. Constrictive pericarditis occurs in all the following except

(a) Radiation (b) Neoplastic
(c) Tuberculosis (d) Rheumatic

914. All following cardiac lesion in which IE prophylaxis is not indicated except

(a) Isolated secondary ASD
(b) CABG
(c) Cardiac pacemakers
(d) MVP with mitral regurgitation

915. All following procedures don't need prophylaxis of infective endocarditis except

(a) Endotracheal incubation
(b) Transesophageal echo
(c) Bronchoscopy with flexible bronchoscope
(d) Cystoscopy

916. Shunt reversal in VSD occurs in

(a) 10% (b) 5%
(c) 20% (d) 25%

917. The characteristic ECG findings in tricuspid atresia are all the following except

(a) RA enlargement (b) LA enlargement
(c) LAD (d) LVH

918. Embolic complications maximally occurs when after development atrial fibrillation in mitral stenosis

(a) < 1 years (b) 1–2 years
(c) 2–3 years (d) > 3 years

919. At what levels of systolic pulmonary artery pressure the TR is functional

(a) 30 mmHg (b) 40 mmHg
(c) 50 mmHg (d) > 55 mmHg

920. Most common valvular lesion produces by radiation is

(a) Aortic stenosis
(b) Atrial regurgitation
(c) Aortic stenosis + Aortic regurgitation
(d) Mitral regurgitation

921. Which valvular heart disease is associated with prolonged QT interval?

(a) Mitral stenosis
(b) Mitral regurgitation
(c) TS
(d) MVP

922. What is severe PAH?

(a) > 25 % systemic pressure
(b) 50 % systemic pressure
(c) 70 % systemic pressure
(d) 75 % systemic pressure

923. Frequency of embolic events in mitral stenosis does not relate to all following except

(a) Atrial fibrillation
(b) Cardiac output
(c) Size of LA
(d) Severity of mitral stenosis

924. Mitral in elderly (> 65 years) has all the following features except

(a) Heavy calcification and fibrosis
(b) Success rate of percutaneous vulroformy is similar as that in young
(c) Procedural mortality is high
(d) More frequent complications

925. Which finding is usually not found in mild mitral stenosis on M-mode echo?

(a) Flat EF stope
(b) Decrease excursion
(c) Paradoxical movement of post leaflet
(d) Density of leaflets not markedly increased

926. Following are low frequency signs in IE except

(a) New or changing murmur
(b) Retinal lesion
(c) Renal failure
(d) Splenomegaly

927. Following are the high frequency signs in IE except

(a) Murmur
(b) Skin lesion
(c) Petechiae
(d) Splinter haemorrhage

928. All following are features of acute infective endocarditis except

(a) Shaking chills
(b) Leukocytosis
(c) Increased gamuna globulin
(d) Positive rheumatoid factor

929. All are complication of TAPVD except

(a) Pulmonary vein stenosis after repair
(b) SSS
(c) Heart failure
(d) Infective endocarditis

930. All following complications may occurs in VSD except

(a) Infective endocarditis
(b) Eissenmenger complex
(c) LBBB
(d) Aortic regurgitation

931. Commonest association of atrial septal aneurysm is with

(a) ASD
(b) PFO
(c) Mitral stenosis
(d) Mitral regurgitation

932. Which is rare pericardial syndrome complication renal failure?

(a) Pericarditis
(b) Pericardial effusion
(c) Cardiac tamponade
(d) Constrictive pericarditis

933. Peak flow velocity in tricuspid stenosis (Severe) is

(a) 0.8 m/sec (b) 1.2 m/sec
(c) 1.6 m/sec (d) 1.8 m/sec

934. S2 is single in which of the cause of Eissenmenger's syndrome?

(a) TGA (b) Single ventricle
(c) DORV (d) PDA

935. Infective endocarditis is rare in which of the following disease with age < 60 years?

(a) Rheumatic heart disease
(b) MVP
(c) Degenerative heart disease
(d) Congenital heart disease

936. Commonest heart disease for infective endocarditis in patients > 60 years age

(a) Degenerative heart disease
(b) MVP
(c) Rheumatic heart disease
(d) Congenital heart disease

937. Commonest complication of biologic prothetic valve

(a) Thrombus (b) Infection
(c) Pannus (d) Degomeration

938. Commonest complication of mechanical valve

(a) Infection (b) Stenosis
(c) Pannus (d) Thrombosis

ANSWERS

1. (*e*)	2. (*a*)	3. (*d*)	4. (*b*)	5. (*d*)
6. (*b*)	7. (*c*)	8. (*c*)	9. (*a*)	10. (*d*)
11. (*a*)	12. (*a*)	13. (*c*)	14. (*c*)	15. (*b*)
16. (*c*)	17. (*a*)	18. (*d*)	19. (*a*)	20. (*d*)
21. (*d*)	22. (*d*)	23. (*a*)	24. (*b*)	25. (*c*)
26. (*c*)	27. (*a*)	28. (*a*)	29. (*c*)	30. (*b*)
31. (*c*)	32. (*d*)	33. (*d*)	34. (*a*)	35. (*d*)
36. (*a*)	37. (*b*)	38. (*b*)	39. (*b*)	40. (*d*)
41. (*d*)	42. (*b*)	43. (c)	44. (*d*)	45. (*b*)
46. (*c*)	47. (*a*)	48. (*a*)	49. (*b*)	50. (*a*)
51. (*a*)	52. (*b*)	53. (b)	54. (*b*)	55. (*b*)
56. (*a*)	57. (*d*)	58. (*d*)	59. (*b*)	60. (*d*)
61. (*d*)	62. (*d*)	63. (*c*)	64. (*c*)	65. (*c*)
66. (*d*)	67. (*c*)	68. (*d*)	69. (*d*)	70. (*b*)
71. (*a*)	72. (*d*)	73. (*a*)	74. (*a*)	75. (*d*)
76. (*b*)	77. (*b*)	78. (*d*)	79. (*a*)	80. (*d*)
81. (*a*)	82. (*d*)	83. (*b*)	84. (*a*)	85. (*d*)
86. (*d*)	87. (*a*)	88. (*a*)	89. (*b*)	90. (*d*)
91. (*c*)	92. (*c*)	93. (*d*)	94. (*a*)	95. (*c*)
96. (*a*)	97. (*d*)	98. (*d*)	99. (*a*)	100. (*b*)
101. (*b*)	102. (*d*)	103. (*d*)	104. (*d*)	105. (*a*)
106. (*d*)	107. (*d*)	108. (*c*)	109. (*d*)	110. (*c*)
111. (*d*)	112. (*b*)	113. (*d*)	114. (*a*)	115. (*c*)
116. (*a*)	117. (*a*)	118. (*c*)	119. (*d*)	120. (*g*)
121. (*b*)	122. (*c*)	123. (*b*)	124. (*c*)	125. (*b*)
126. (*b*)	127. (*d*)	128. (*d*)	129. (*b*)	130. (*b*)
131. (*b*)	132. (*d*)	133. (*d*)	134. (*d*)	135. (*b*)
136. (*a*)	137. (*c*)	138. (*a*)	139. (*a*)	140. (*d*)
141. (*c*)	142. (*d*)	143. (*d*)	144. (*a*)	145. (*a*)
146. (*a*)	147. (*d*)	148. (*d*)	149. (*d*)	150. (*d*)
151. (*d*)	152. (*d*)	153. (*a*)	154. (*d*)	155. (*d*)
156. (*d*)	157. (*d*)	158. (*d*)	159. (*d*)	160. (*a*)

161. (*d*)	162. (*b*)	163. (*d*)	164. (*a*)	165. (*a*)
166. (*c*)	167. (*a*)	168. (*d*)	169. (*d*)	170. (*c*)
171. (*d*)	172. (*a*)	173. (*d*)	174. (*d*)	175. (*d*)
176. (*d*)	177. (*b*)	178. (*c*)	179. (*d*)	180. (*d*)
181. (*b*)	182. (*b*)	183. (*b*)	184. (*d*)	185. (*a*)
186. (*c*)	187. (*c*)	188. (*c*)	189. (*d*)	190. (*d*)
191. (*a*)	192. (*a*)	193. (*d*)	194. (*a*)	195. (*d*)
196. (*d*)	197. (*d*)	198. (*d*)	199. (*c*)	200. (*d*)
201. (*d*)	202. (*d*)	203. (*d*)	204. (*d*)	205. (*d*)
206. (*a*)	207. (*b*)	208. (*b*)	209. (*b*)	210. (*b*)
211. (*a*)	212. (*a*)	213. (*a*)	214. (*b*)	215. (*d*)
216. (*a*)	217. (*c*)	218. (*c*)	219. (*c*)	220. (*d*)
221. (*a*)	222. (*a*)	223. (*a*)	224. (*a*)	225. (*d*)
226. (*d*)	227. (*d*)	228. (*a*)	229. (*a*)	230. (*c*)
231. (*d*)	232. (*b*)	233. (*a*)	234. (*b*)	235. (*d*)
236. (*d*)	237. (*d*)	238. (*d*)	239. (*d*)	240. (*d*)
241. (*d*)	242. (*b*)	243. (*d*)	244. (*b*)	245. (*d*)
246. (*d*)	247. (*c*)	248. (*b*)	249. (*a*)	250. (*a*)
251. (*d*)	252. (*c*)	253. (*b*)	254. (*a*)	255. (*c*)
256. (*a*)	257. (*b*)	258. (*a*)	259. (*d*)	260. (*a*)
261. (*d*)	262. (*a*)	263. (*d*)	264. (*d*)	265. (*a*)
266. (*a*)	267. (*d*)	268. (*d*)	269. (*d*)	270. (*d*)
271. (*d*)	272. (*d*)	273. (*c*)	274. (*c*)	275. (*c*)
276. (*d*)	277. (*c*)	278. (*d*)	279. (*b*)	280. (*d*)
281. (*b*)	282. (*b*)	283. (*c*)	284. (*d*)	285. (*a*)
286. (*b*)	287. (*a*)	288. (*a*)	289. (*a*)	290. (*d*)
291. (*a*)	292. (*d*)	293. (*c*)	294. (*b*)	295. (*d*)
296. (*d*)	297. (*a*)	298. (*a*)	299. (*d*)	300. (*b*)
301. (*d*)	302. (*d*)	303. (*d*)	304. (*a*)	305. (*a*)
306. (*c*)	307. (*c*)	308. (*d*)	309. (*d*)	310. (*d*)
311. (*a*)	312. (*a*)	313. (*a*)	314. (*d*)	315. (*d*)
316. (*a*)	317. (*a*)	318. (*d*)	319. (*b*)	320. (*b*)
321. (*a*)	322. (*a*)	323. (*b*)	324. (*d*)	325. (*d*)
326. (*d*)	327. (*d*)	328. (*d*)	329. (*d*)	330. (*b*)
331. (*d*)	332. (*d*)	333. (*d*)	334. (*c*)	335. (*d*)

336. (*c*)	337. (*d*)	338. (*c*)	339. (*b*)	340. (*d*)
341. (*d*)	342. (*d*)	343. (*a*)	344. (*a*)	345. (*b*)
346. (*c*)	347. (*d*)	348. (*d*)	349. (*d*)	350. (*d*)
351. (*d*)	352. (*b*)	353. (*c*)	354. (*c*)	355. (*c*)
356. (*a*)	357. (*b*)	358. (*d*)	359. (*b*)	360. (*d*)
361. (*d*)	362. (*d*)	363. (*c*)	364. (*c*)	365. (*b*)
366. (*d*)	367. (*d*)	368. (*c*)	369. (*c*)	370. (*a*)
371. (*d*)	372. (*a*)	373. (*b*)	374. (*d*)	375. (*d*)
376. (*a*)	377. (*c*)	378. (*c*)	379. (*d*)	380. (*d*)
381. (*d*)	382. (*a*)	383. (*d*)	384. (*c*)	385. (*d*)
386. (*b*)	387. (*d*)	388. (*d*)	389. (*c*)	390. (*d*)
391. (*d*)	392. (*d*)	393. (*b*)	394. (*b*)	395. (*a*)
396. (*d*)	397. (*c*)	398. (*a*)	399. (*b*)	400. (*d*)
401. (*a*)	402. (*a*)	403. (*d*)	404. (*d*)	405. (*b*)
406. (*a*)	407. (*d*)	408. (*d*)	409. (*d*)	410. (*c*)
411. (*a*)	412. (*d*)	413. (*a*)	414. (*d*)	415. (*c*)
416. (*d*)	417. (*c*)	418. (*c*)	419. (*c*)	420. (*d*)
421. (*d*)	422. (*d*)	423. (*d*)	424. (*c*)	425. (*d*)
426. (*a*)	427. (*d*)	428. (*b*)	429. (*d*)	430. (*c*)
431. (*d*)	432. (*b*)	433. (*c*)	434. (*c*)	435. (*e*)
436. (*b*)	437. (*d*)	438. (*d*)	439. (*d*)	440. (*d*)
441. (*d*)	442. (*c*)	443. (*d*)	444. (*d*)	445. (*d*)
446. (*d*)	447. (*d*)	448. (*b*)	449. (*d*)	450. (*b*)
451. (*c*)	452. (*c*)	453. (*d*)	454. (*d*)	455. (*d*)
456. (*d*)	457. (*d*)	458. (*a*)	459. (*d*)	460. (*a*)
461. (*d*)	462. (*d*)	463. (*d*)	464. (*d*)	465. (*b*)
466. (*d*)	467. (*d*)	468. (*c*)	469. (*d*)	470. (*a*)
471. (*a*)	472. (*b*)	473. (*a*)	474. (*a*)	475. (*d*)
476. (*d*)	477. (*d*)	478. (*d*)	479. (*d*)	480. (*c*)
481. (*d*)	482. (*d*)	483. (*b*)	484. (*b*)	485. (*d*)
486. (*c*)	487. (*b*)	488. (*d*)	489. (*a*)	490. (*b*)
491. (*d*)	492. (*c*)	493. (*a*)	494. (*d*)	495. (*d*)
496. (*c*)	497. (*a*)	498. (*d*)	499. (*a*)	500. (*d*)
501. (*c*)	502. (*c*)	503. (*d*)	504. (*d*)	505. (*a*)
506. (*d*)	507. (*b*)	508. (*b*)	509. (*c*)	510. (*d*)

511. (*c*)	512. (*d*)	513. (*b*)	514. (*b*)	515. (*b*)
516. (*b*)	517. (*d*)	518. (*a*)	519. (*d*)	520. (*a*)
521. (*e*)	522. (*d*)	523. (*d*)	524. (*c*)	525. (*a*)
526. (*b*)	527. (*d*)	528. (*b*)	529. (*c*)	530. (*d*)
531. (*d*)	532. (*d*)	533. (*b*)	534. (*d*)	535. (*d*)
536. (*d*)	537. (*d*)	538. (*d*)	539. (*c*)	540. (*d*)
541. (*b*)	542. (*b*)	543. (*a*)	544. (*c*)	545. (*d*)
546. (*a*)	547. (*b*)	548. (*d*)	549. (*d*)	550. (*c*)
551. (*d*)	552. (*a*)	553. (*a*)	554. (*d*)	555. (*d*)
556. (*c*)	557. (*d*)	558. (*b*)	559. (*a*)	560. (*d*)
561. (*d*)	562. (*c*)	563. (*d*)	564. (*d*)	565. (*a*)
566. (*d*)	567. (*c*)	568. (*d*)	569. (*b*)	570. (*a*)
571. (*c*)	572. (*b*)	573. (*d*)	574. (*d*)	575. (*d*)
576. (*b*)	577. (*a*)	578. (*d*)	579. (*d*)	580. (*c*)
581. (*b*)	582. (*d*)	583. (*b*)	584. (*d*)	585. (*b*)
586. (*d*)	587. (*c*)	588. (*d*)	589. (*a*)	590. (*a*)
591. (*d*)	592. (*d*)	593. (*c*)	594. (*d*)	595. (*d*)
596. (*c*)	597. (*c*)	598. (*b*)	599. (*d*)	600. (*d*)
601. (*d*)	602. (*c*)	603. (*c*)	604. (*b*)	605. (*a*)
606. (*a*)	607. (*a*)	608. (*d*)	609. (*c*)	610. (*d*)
611. (*c*)	612. (*b*)	613. (*c*)	614. (*d*)	615. (*b*)
616. (*c*)	617. (*d*)	618. (*c*)	619. (*b*)	620. (*d*)
621. (*d*)	622. (*c*)	623. (*d*)	624. (*a*)	625. (*d*)
626. (*a*)	627. (*d*)	628. (*c*)	629. (*c*)	630. (*b*)
631. (*a*)	632. (*a*)	633. (*b*)	634. (*a*)	635. (*c*)
636. (*a*)	637. (*b*)	638. (*a*)	639. (*a*)	640. (*c*)
641. (*c*)	642. (*d*)	643. (*d*)	644. (*b*)	645. (*d*)
646. (*d*)	647. (*d*)	648. (*d*)	649. (*b*)	650. (*d*)
651. (*b*)	652. (*a*)	653. (*b*)	654. (*a*)	655. (*d*)
656. (*a*)	657. (*c*)	658. (*d*)	659. (*d*)	660. (*a*)
661. (*d*)	662. (*d*)	663. (*c*)	664. (*d*)	665. (*c*)
666. (*d*)	667. (*c*)	668. (*b*)	669. (*d*)	670. (*d*)
671. (*d*)	672. (*a*)	673. (*a*)	674. (*a*)	675. (*a*)
676. (*d*)	677. (*a*)	678. (*d*)	679. (*d*)	680. (*d*)
681. (*b*)	682. (*b*)	683. (*d*)	684. (*d*)	685. (*d*)

686. (*b*)	687. (*a*)	688. (*a*)	689. (*a*)	690. (*a*)
691. (*b*)	692. (*d*)	693. (*c*)	694. (*a*)	695. (*b*)
696. (*a*)	697. (*d*)	698. (*a*)	699. (*c*)	700. (*d*)
701. (*a*)	702. (*c*)	703. (*d*)	704. (*a*)	705. (*d*)
706. (*c*)	707. (*d*)	708. (*a*)	709. (*c*)	710. (*c*)
711. (*d*)	712. (*d*)	713. (*c*)	714. (*a*)	715. (*d*)
716. (*b*)	717. (*c*)	718. (*d*)	719. (*c*)	720. (*a*)
721. (*a*)	722. (*c*)	723. (*d*)	724. (*b*)	725. (*b*)
726. (*c*)	727. (*b*)	728. (*d*)	729. (*d*)	730. (*a*)
731. (*b*)	732. (*d*)	733. (*d*)	734. (*d*)	735. (*b*)
736. (*d*)	737. (*d*)	738. (*d*)	739. (*a*)	740. (*c*)
741. (*d*)	742. (*d*)	743. (*d*)	744. (*b*)	745. (*a*)
746. (*a*)	747. (*c*)	748. (*b*)	749. (*c*)	750. (*c*)
751. (*d*)	752. (*a*)	753. (*c*)	754. (*c*)	755. (*a*)
756. (*c*)	757. (*d*)	758. (*b*)	759. (*c*)	760. (*d*)
761. (*d*)	762. (*c*)	763. (*d*)	764. (*a*)	765. (*d*)
766. (*c*)	767. (*d*)	768. (*c*)	769. (*a*)	770. (*d*)
771. (*a*)	772. (*a*)	773. (*a*)	774. (*a*)	775. (*d*)
776. (*a*)	777. (*c*)	778. (*d*)	779. (*d*)	780. (*c*)
781. (*b*)	782. (*c*)	783. (*a*)	784. (*d*)	785. (*d*)
786. (*d*)	787. (*d*)	788. (*d*)	789. (*a*)	790. (*a*)
791. (*a*)	792. (*a*)	793. (*b*)	794. (*d*)	795. (*a*)
796. (*a*)	797. (*a*)	798. (*a*)	799. (*a*)	800. (*c*)
801. (*a*)	802. (*a*)	803. (*d*)	804. (*d*)	805. (*d*)
806. (*c*)	807. (*d*)	808. (*d*)	809. (*d*)	810. (*d*)
811. (*a*)	812. (*a*)	813. (*a*)	814. (*b*)	815. (*b*)
816. (*c*)	817. (*a*)	818. (*b*)	819. (*d*)	820. (*c*)
821. (*a*)	822. (*d*)	823. (*c*)	824. (*a*)	825. (*b*)
826. (*a*)	827. (*c*)	828. (*a*)	829. (*a*)	830. (*a*)
831. (*a*)	832. (*d*)	833. (*a*)	834. (*b*)	835. (*d*)
836. (*d*)	837. (*a*)	838. (*c*)	839. (*a*)	840. (*b*)
841. (*c*)	842. (*d*)	843. (*d*)	844. (*d*)	845. (*c*)
846. (*d*)	847. (*d*)	848. (*a*)	849. (*d*)	850. (*d*)
851. (*c*)	852. (*d*)	853. (*d*)	854. (*d*)	855. (*d*)
856. (*d*)	857. (*a*)	858. (*c*)	859. (*a*)	860. (*b*)

861. (*d*)	862. (*d*)	863. (*d*)	864. (*d*)	865. (*d*)
866. (*a*)	867. (*d*)	868. (*d*)	869. (*d*)	870. (*a*)
871. (*d*)	872. (*d*)	873. (*d*)	874. (*a*)	875. (*d*)
876. (*d*)	877. (*d*)	878. (*d*)	879. (*b*)	880. (*d*)
881. (*d*)	882. (*d*)	883. (*d*)	884. (*a*)	885. (*d*)
886. (*c*)	887. (*d*)	888. (*b*)	889. (*a*)	890. (*d*)
891. (*a*)	892. (*c*)	893. (*c*)	894. (*d*)	895. (*d*)
896. (*d*)	897. (*d*)	898. (*d*)	899. (*b*)	900. (*d*)
901. (*d*)	902. (*c*)	903. (*d*)	904. (*a*)	905. (*a*)
906. (*d*)	907. (*c*)	908. (*d*)	909. (*c*)	910. (*d*)
911. (*d*)	912. (*a*)	913. (*d*)	914. (*d*)	915. (*d*)
916. (*d*)	917. (*b*)	918. (*a*)	919. (*d*)	920. (*c*)
921. (*d*)	922. (*d*)	923. (*a*)	924. (*b*)	925. (*c*)
926. (*d*)	927. (*d*)	928. (*c*)	929. (*d*)	930. (*c*)
931. (*b*)	932. (*d*)	933. (*d*)	934. (*d*)	935. (*c*)
936. (*a*)	937. (*d*)	938. (*d*)		

SECTION–6

MISCELLANUEOUS

1. **Renal artery embolism is characterized by**
   (a) Flank pain (b) Haematuria
   (c) Hypertension (d) All the above

2. **Potassium rich food include all except**
   (a) Watermelon (b) Guawa
   (c) Banana (d) Tomato

3. **Which is the best drug for patients of seizures in ecclampsia?**
   (a) Phenytoin (b) Barbiturates
   (c) Magnesium (d) Diazepam

4. **Highest fetal and maternal mortality occurs during pregnancy in which of the following cardiac condition?**
   (a) HCM
   (b) Acyanotic ebsteins anomaly
   (c) Severe aortic stenosis
   (d) Pulmonary stenosis

5. **All the following occurs physiological during pregnancy except**
   (a) Increased blood volume
   (b) Heart rate is increased
   (c) Pulse pressure is decreased
   (d) Cardiac output increases

6. **All of the following cardiac complications are associated with sleep apnea except**
   (a) Pulmonary hypertension
   (b) Right ventricular failure
   (c) Systemic hypertension
   (d) Hypertrophic cardiomyopathy

7. Left atrial myxomia is characterized by all except

(a) Marked constitutional symptoms
(b) History of syncope
(c) Large left atrium
(d) Tumour plop

8. Which is the least common manifestation of left atrial myxoma?

(a) Embolism (b) Anorexia
(c) Weight loss (d) Hemoptysis

9. All following hematological disorders are associated with myocardial Infarction except

(a) Polycythemia rubra vera
(b) Thrombocytopenia
(c) DIC
(d) Aplastic anemia

10. Most common cause of cardiac death in chronic renal failure is

(a) Heart failure
(b) Myocardial infarction
(c) Pericardial effusion
(d) Constrictive pericarditis

11. Smaller than average heart is found in all the following except

(a) COPD
(b) Addison disease
(c) Anorexia nervosa
(d) Acute mitral regurgitation

12. Hamman's sign has all the following features except

(a) Indicates air in mediastinum
(b) Commonly occurs following cardiac surgery
(c) Related to both heart beat and respiration
(d) It is short ejection murmur

13. Which cardiac chamber hypertrophy occurs in freidrichs ataxia?

(a) RA hypertrophy (b) LA hypertrophy
(c) RV hypertrophy (d) LV hypertrophy

14. Most Common ECG finding in myotonic dystrophy is

(a) 1 degree AV block
(b) RBBB
(c) LBBB
(d) Sinus bradycardia

15. Most distinctive cardiac abnormality in facioscapulohumeral myopathy is

(a) Valve regurgitation
(b) Coronary artery disease
(c) Myocardial infarction
(d) Atrial paralysis

16. Which cardiac manifestation is rare in myxodema?

(a) Bradycardia (b) Pericardial effusion
(c) Hypertension (d) Heart failure

17. Most common arrhythmia in hyperthyroidism is

(a) Resting sinus tachycardia
(b) Atrial fibrillation
(c) Atrial ectopics
(d) PVCS

18. All following cardiovascular diseases are related to pregnancy except

(a) Dilated cardiomyopathy
(b) Pulmonary embolism
(c) Systemic hypertension
(d) Pulmonary hypertension

19. Physiological hemodynamic changes during pregnancy in 1st trimester includes all except

(a) Increase systolic blood pressure
(b) Increase diastolic blood pressure
(c) Increase cardiac output
(d) Increase stroke volume

20. Diastolic blood pressure is decreased most in which trimester of pregnancy?

(a) Ist (b) IInd
(c) IIIrd (d) In all similar fall

21. All cardiac complication occur in sleep apnea except

(a) Nocturnal arrhythmia
(b) Pulmonary hypertension
(c) Right ventricular failure
(d) Valvular heart disease

22. Cardiac encephalopathy with normal renal hepatic pulmonary and furation electrolyte is due to

(a) Decrease brain perfusion due to decrease cardiac output
(b) High central venous pressure
(c) Intravanial fluid retention
(d) All the above

23. Which of the following is not found in left atrial myxoma?

(a) Anemia (b) Thrombocytosis
(c) Increased ESR (d) Leucocytosis

24. All the following features are present in left atrial myxoma except

(a) Mid diastolic murmur
(b) Mitral regurgitation murmur
(c) Opening snap (d) Positional syncope

25. Definitive diagnosis of left atrial myxoma is made by

(a) X-ray
(b) Clinical
(c) Echocardiography
(d) Ventricular angiography

26. Which is the commonest type of left ventricular tumor?

(a) Myxoma (b) Fibroma
(c) Rhabdomyoma (d) None of the above

27. Thyrotoxicosis may cause all the following cardiac features except

(a) Ejection systolic murmur in pulmonary area
(b) S_3
(c) Mid diastolic murmur in mitral area
(d) Mitral regurgitation

28. Best position to treat air embolism is

(a) Supine position
(b) Right lateral position
(c) Head up position
(d) Left lateral and head down position

29. Which of the following is characteristic of fat embolism?

(a) Hemoptysis (b) Cyanosis
(c) Convection (d) Stem patchiest

30. In elderly persons which is a true statement?

(a) LV stiffness increases due to increased thickness and fibrous tissue
(b) LV wall thickness preserves ventricular performance in early stages
(c) Bar reflex arch has heightened sensitivity
(d) B receptor sensitivity is increased

31. In normal age related changes all are true except

(a) Diastolic dysfunction is frequent as seen in doppler studies
(b) Endocardium appears highly refractile in echocardiographic studies
(c) With exercise heart rate rises markedly compared to younger subjects
(d) Maximum O_2 consumption is decreased

32. All are contra indicated in goitrous hypothyroidism except

(a) Cauliflower (b) Rapeseed
(c) Drum stick (d) Cabbage

33. Levothyroxine is used as single daily dose because

(a) It is very toxic drug
(b) Its half-life is long
(c) Repeated use may disturb sleep
(d) More than one use per may be associated with hyper defaecation

34. While treating hypothyroid with angina pectoris, one should start with Eltroxin

(a) 25 μg (b) 50 μg
(c) 75 μg (d) 100 μg

35. Decreased peripheral conversion of T_4 to T_3 is associated with all except

(a) Dexamethasone (b) Amiodarone
(c) Enalapril (d) Propranolol

36. Decreased thyroxine binding globulin is seen in all except

(a) Pregnancy (b) Nephrosis
(c) Acromegaly (d) Chronic hepatitis

37. A subnormal response of the serum TSH to administration of TRH confirms presence of

(a) Hypothalamic hypothyroidism
(b) Pituitary hypothyroidism
(c) Postradiation hypothyroidism
(d) Iodine deficiency

38. All are useful in investigating hypothyroidism except

(a) Serum TSH level
(b) Thyroid antimicrosomal antibodies
(c) Radio iodine uptake
(d) Serum cholesterol

39. The concentration of free T_4 and T_3 in serum is

(a) 1% (b) 2%
(c) 3% (d) 4%

40. The half-life of L-thyroxine is

(a) 24 hours (b) 8 hours
(c) 7 days (d) 28 days

41. All decreases thyroid hormone secretion except

(a) Dopamine (b) Lithium
(c) Amiodarone (d) Iodine

42. Hormone replacement therapy adversely affects all cancers except

(a) Ovarian cancer
(b) Breast cancer
(c) Colorectal cancer
(d) Endometrial cancer
(e) Both (a) + (c)

43. Oestrogen receptors are present in all of the following tissues except

(a) Skin (b) Vagina
(c) Urethra (d) None of the above
(e) All of the above

44. Which of the following oestrogenic preparations has the highest receptor binding affinity?

(a) Estrone (b) Estriol
(c) Estradiol 17 β (d) Oestrogen sulphate
(e) 17 alpha dihydroquilin

45. Hot flushes are associated with all of the following except

(a) Gradual fall in estradiol level
(b) Sudden fall in estradiol level
(c) Leuteinizing hormone peak
(d) Catecholamine surge
(e) None of these

46. Contraindications for hormonal replacement therapy includes all of the following except

(a) Thrombo embolic disease
(b) Undiagnosed vaginal bleeding
(c) Breast and endometrial cancer
(d) Chronic liver disease
(e) None of these

47. Progesterone is added in hormonal replacement therapy for all the following reasons except

(a) Protection against breast cancer
(b) Protection against endometrial cancer
(c) As a CNS sedative
(d) For down regulation of E_2 receptors

48. All of the following modalities of treatment are effective in the treatment of postmenopausal osteoporosis except

(a) HRT
(b) Alendronate
(c) Alfacalcidol
(d) Parathyroid hormone
(e) None of the above

49. Which of the following is not a biochemical marker of bone formation?

(a) Serum alkaline phosphates
(b) Serum osteocalcin
(c) Serum C- and N-propeptides of type I collagen
(d) Serum tartrate-resistant acid phosphatase
(e) All of the above

50. Cardio protective effects of oestrogen are related to the following mechanisms except

(a) Raised HDL (High density lipoprotein)
(b) Lower LDL (Low density lipoprotein)
(c) Lowered homocysteine
(d) Raised PAI-1 (Plasminogen activator inhibitor-1)
(e) Altered vascular reactivity

51. Which of the following is not a natural oestrogen?

(a) Diethyl stilboestrol
(b) Estrone sulphate
(c) Estrone E_1
(d) Estradiol E_2
(e) Estrial E_3

52. Elevated central venous pressure is seen in

(a) Application of PEEP
(b) CPAP mode of ventilation
(c) All of the above (d) None of the above

53. An average smoker has a shorter lifespan compared to a non smoker by

(a) 3 years (b) 4 years
(c) 5 years (d) 6 years

54. The following are observational studies except

(a) The Framingham study
(b) The PROCAM study
(c) The seven countries study
(d) Physician's health study

55. The prescribed limit of total energy through dietary fats for Asians is

(a) 20% (b) 21%
(c) 22% (d) 23%

56. Which procedure is avoided during pregnancy?

(a) Echocardiography
(b) Radionucleotide studies
(c) MRI
(d) ECG

57. During sleep the normal lowest heart rate is

(a) 70/min (b) 60/min
(c) 50/min (d) 35–40/min

58. Osteoporosis may occur by which drug?

(a) β-blockers
(b) Ca-blockers
(c) Aspirin
(d) Prolonged heparin use

59. Hyperkalemia occur with all the following except

(a) K sparing diuretics
(b) β-blockers
(c) ACE inhibitors
(d) Nitrates

60. Pigmented skin is found in which type of ulcer

(a) Arterial (b) Venous
(c) Neuropathic (d) Small vessel

61. Which type of ulcer is located above malleoli?

(a) Arterial (b) Venous
(c) Neuropathic (d) Small vessel

62. Severe pain occur in which type of ulcer?

(a) Venous (b) Small vessel
(c) Arterial (d) Neuropathic

63. Wet base is found in which type of ulcer?

(a) Venous (b) Neuropathic
(c) Arterial (d) Small vessel

64. Cellulitis is not found in which type of ulcer?

(a) Venous (b) Arterial
(c) Neuropathic (d) Small vessel

65. Fluid retention occur with all the following except

(a) Estrogen (b) Indomethacin
(c) Steroids (d) ACE inhibitors

66. All are features of osteogenesis imperfecta except
(a) Blue sclera (b) Aortic dissection
(c) VSD (d) Atrial regurgitation

67. Commonest clinical manifestation of penetrating injury to heart is
(a) A-V fistula
(b) Heart failure
(c) Cardiac tamponade
(d) Intracardiac shunts

68. Which of the following cardiac findings extremely uncommon in myxoedema?
(a) Pericardial effusion
(b) T wave inversion on ECG
(c) Heart failure (d) Low voltage QRS

69. All are uncommon cardiac findings in myxoedema except
(a) Constrictive pericarditis
(b) Arrhythmia
(c) Heart failure
(d) Pericardial effusion

70. Anabolic steroids may cause all the following except
(a) Left ventricular hypertrophy and hypertension
(b) Increased lipids
(c) Diabetes mellitus
(d) Increased atherosclerosis

71. Myxoedema produces all the following ECG changes except
(a) Low voltage of QRS
(b) Normal voltage P & T wave
(c) High incidence of digitalis toxicity
(d) Left bundle branch block

72. Regarding estrogen replacement therapy all are true except
(a) Might lower CVS risk
(b) Decreases incidence of stroke
(c) Increases thrombo embolisms
(d) Increases risk of breast cancer

73. Optimal approach to diabetic nephropathy includes all except

(a) Na-restriction
(b) Glycemic control
(c) Treatment of hypertension with ACE inhibitors
(d) Treatment of hypertension with beta-blockers

74. All are risk factors of diabetic nephropathy except

(a) Poor glycemic control
(b) Hypertension
(c) Occurs only in type II DM
(d) Common in blacks

75. Earliest finding in diabetic nephropathy

(a) Micro albuminuria
(b) Macro albuminuria
(c) Abnormal renal histology
(d) Abnormal renal ultrasound

76. Low molecule weight heparin is better than standard heparin except for

(a) More predictable anticoagulation response
(b) Less expensive
(c) More safe
(d) Easily administered

77. Most frequent cardiac disease in infant born to mother with SLE is

(a) ASD (b) VSD
(c) AS (d) CHB

78. Pagets disease of bone may be associated with all the following except

(a) High output state
(b) Conduction defects
(c) Calcific AV disease
(d) Cardiomyopathy

79. Usual cardiac finding in hemochromatosis are all the following except

(a) Heart failure (b) Atrial fibrillation
(c) AV block (d) Pericarditis

80. Anemia is found in all the following cardiac disease except
- (a) Infective endocarditis
- (b) Left atrial myxoma
- (c) Prosthetic valves
- (d) Aortic stenosis

81. Highest prevalence of heart disease in elderly male is
- (a) Coronary artery disease
- (b) HTN
- (c) Valvular
- (d) Cor pulmonale

82. Highest prevalence of heart disease in elderly female is
- (a) Hypertension
- (b) Coronary artery disease
- (c) Valvular
- (d) Cor pulmonale

83. Lithium results in following congenital cardiac defects commonly except
- (a) Ebstein's anomaly
- (b) ASD
- (c) Tricuspid atresia
- (d) A-V canal defect

84. All are important cardiovascular teratogens except
- (a) Rubella (b) Lithium
- (c) Thalidomide (d) Ca-blockers

85. All are common defects encountered in rubella infection except
- (a) Patient ductus arteriosus
- (b) Pulmonary stenosis (valvular)
- (c) Peripheral pulmonary artery stenosis
- (d) Septal defects

86. All are cocaine induced cardiovascular diseases except
- (a) Ventricular arrhythmia
- (b) Myocardial infarction
- (c) Pericarditis
- (d) Hypertension

87. Hypotension during dialysis is cause by all except

(a) Pericardial effusion
(b) LV failure
(c) Arrhythmia
(d) Dilated CMP

88. Commonest ECG change in freidrich's ataxia

(a) ST/T changes
(b) RAD
(c) LAD
(d) Infero lateral Q waves

89. Lithium can cause all the following except

(a) T wave inversion
(b) Prominent U wave
(c) QT prolongation
(d) Sinus tachycardia

90. Oral contraceptives may cause all the following except

(a) Pulmonary hypertension
(b) Myocardial infarction
(c) Systemic hypertension
(d) Deep vein thrombosis

91. Anabolic steroids may cause all the following except

(a) Dyslipidemia
(b) Left ventricular hypertrophy
(c) Hypertension
(d) Cardiomyopathy

92. Cocaine can cause all the following except

(a) Acute myocardial infarction
(b) Acute severe hypertension
(c) Acute aortic dissection
(d) Acute pericarditis

93. All statements regarding cyclophosphamide cardiotoxicity are correct except

(a) Causes pericarditis
(b) Systolic dysfunction
(c) Arrhythmias
(d) Related to dose of the drug

94. **Angioedema is rare with which ACE inhibitor?**
(a) Ramipril (b) Captopril
(c) Lisinopril (d) Enalapril

95. **Which of the following drug needs loading dose?**
(a) Propranolol (b) Digoxin
(c) Captopril (d) Nifedipine

96. **Smoking decreases the effect of which of the following drugs?**
(a) Propranolol (b) Verapamil
(c) Enalapril (d) Digoxin

97. **Which of the following drug is not used by transdermal route?**
(a) Nitroglycerine (b) Methyldopa
(c) Clonidine (d) All of the above

98. **All are causes of electromechanical dissociation except**
(a) Hypovolemia
(b) Pulmonary embolism
(c) Cardiac tamponade
(d) Uncomplicated acute myocardial infarction

99. **Which chamber is most commonly hypertrophied in athletes?**
(a) Left ventricular (LV)
(b) Right ventricular (RV)
(c) Right atrium (RA)
(d) Left atrium (LA)

100. **Which cardiovascular disease dose not produces epistaxis?**
(a) Severe hypertension
(b) Acute rheumatic fever
(c) Congenital aortic stenosis
(d) All of the above

101. **Hoarseness of voice occurs in all the following except**
(a) Mitral stenosis
(b) Aortic aneurysm
(c) Idiopathic dilation of PA
(d) Aortic stenosis

102. Most common cardiovascular abnormality in marfans syndrome is

(a) Mitral valve prolapse
(b) Aortic root dilation
(c) Mitral regurgitation
(d) ASD

103. Pulse less electrical activity of heart is found in all the following except

(a) Cardiac tamponade
(b) Acute massive pulmonary embolism
(c) Tension pneumothorax
(d) Acute severe mitral regurgitation

104. Commonest cardiac lesion in rheumatoid arthritis is

(a) Conduction defect
(b) Aortic regurgitation
(c) Pericarditis
(d) Cardiomyopathy

105. Excessive sweating occur in all except

(a) During acute myocardial infarction
(b) Thyrotoxicoses
(c) Heart failure
(d) Aortic stenosis

106. Hoarseness of voice may suggest all the following cardiac disease except

(a) Primary pulmonary hypertension
(b) Large PDA
(c) Mitral stenosis
(d) Aortic stenosis

107. Drug induced pedal edema occurs in all except

(a) Nifodipine (b) NSAIDS
(c) Hydralazine (d) β-blockers

108. Commonest cardiac lesion with rheumatoid arthritis is

(a) Pericarditis
(b) Myocarditis
(c) Aortic regurgitation
(d) Conduction defects

109. Malar flush is severe in all the following except

(a) Mitral stenosis
(b) Increase venous pressure
(c) Cardiac cachexia
(d) Aortic stenosis

110. Which is commonest tumor (Benign) in heart?

(a) Lipoma (b) Teratoma
(c) Fibroma (d) Myxoma

111. Myocardium is most commonly involved in

(a) SLE
(b) Scleroderma
(c) Rheumatoid arthritis
(d) Ankylosing spondylitis

112. All following disorders may arise during pregnancy except

(a) Hypertension systemic
(b) Pulmonary embolism
(c) Peripartum cardiac myopathy
(d) Pericardial disease

113. All are high risk cardiac lesion for pregnancy except

(a) Primary pulmonary hypertension
(b) Eissermemgers syndrome
(c) Aortic stenosis
(d) ASD

114. All are low risk cardiac patients for pregnancy except

(a) Mitral regurgitation
(b) Aortic regurgitation
(c) VSD without PAH
(d) Marfances syndrome

115. Circulatory changes in pregnancy are all except

(a) Vascular resistance increase
(b) Cardiac resistance increase
(c) Venous resistance increase
(d) Blood volume increase

116. Commonest cardiac feature of sarcoidosis

(a) BBB
(b) CHB

(c) Pericarditis
(d) Supraventricular arrhythmia

117. All feature are found in amyloid heart disease except

(a) PAP > 50 mmHg
(b) LVEDP > 20 mmHg
(c) LVEDP – RVEP = > 5
(d) No kussmull's sign

118. Cardiovascular protective effect of alcohol is mediated by all the following mechanisms except

(a) Improves insulin sensitivity
(b) Increase Lp (a)
(c) Decrease HDL-C
(d) Increase sympathetic activity

119. The most common cardiac finding in addison's disease is

(a) Heart failure
(b) Prolonged QT interval
(c) Sinus bradycardia
(d) Hypertension

120. All the following lipid lowering drugs require dose modification with renal insufficiency except

(a) Statins (b) Beno fibrate
(c) Feno fibrate (d) Resins

121. Characteristic lesion in coronaries following radiotherapy is located at

(a) Proximal (b) Distal
(c) Mid (d) Any where

122. All the following statements regarding arrhythmia in pregnancy are correct except

(a) SVT in absence of heart often occur
(b) SVT dine city related to projectance
(c) SVT dine city related to stinger
(d) ICD patients have no contrandication to pregnancy

123. Most common site of cardiovascular involvement in HIV infection is

(a) Myocardium (b) Endocardium
(c) Pericardium (d) Conducting tissue

124. In left atrial myxoma tumor plop has all the following features except

(a) Early diastolic sound
(b) Usually after 3rd heart sound
(c) Low pitched
(d) Transient sound

125. Which is usually not the feature of left atrial myxomia?

(a) Syncope
(b) Tumous plop
(c) Atrial fibrillation
(d) Murmur vary with position

126. Most common clinical manifestation of left atrial myxoma is

(a) Embolism (b) Arthalgia
(c) Syncope (d) Haemoptysis

127. All are common sites of embolism from left atrial myxomia except

(a) Coronary (b) Kidney
(c) Brain (d) Lower extremity

128. Antidepressant overdose is suggested by all except

(a) Sinus tachycardia
(b) QRS prolongation
(c) QT prolongation
(d) Generalized T wave inversion

129. Most common cause of death in chronic renal failure is

(a) Heart failure
(b) Myocardial infarction
(c) Stroke
(d) Sepsis

130. Which of the fallowing physiological change remains unchanged during pregnancy?

(a) O_2 consumption
(b) Cardiac output
(c) Peripheral vascular resistance
(d) Pulmonary artery pressure

131. Myxoedema causes all the following cardiac abnormalities except

(a) Bradycardia (b) Pericardial effusion
(c) Hyperlipidemia (d) Valvular defects

132. Hyperthyroidism may cause all the following except

(a) Atrial fibrillation
(b) Systolic hypertension
(c) Sinus tachycardia
(d) Pericarditis

133. Which is least common manifestation of RA?

(a) Venous thrombosis
(b) Myocarditis
(c) Conduction defect
(d) CAD

134. In cardiac contusion the ECG usually shows following change except

(a) ST-T changes
(b) Q wave
(c) Supra ventricular and ventricular arrhythmia
(d) AV block

135. Only known cardiac effect of SSRIS is

(a) Myocarditis
(b) VES
(c) Sinus tarchycardia
(d) Sinus bradycardia

136. All the following psychotropic drugs have no know CV effects except

(a) Citalopram (b) Escitalopram
(c) Mitrazapine (d) Benzodiazepine

137. Which of the following psychotropic agent cause orthostatic hypotension?

(a) Venflexine (b) Bupropion
(c) Nefazodone (d) Trazodone

138. All the following cause orthastatic hypotension except

(a) Tricyclic antidepressant
(b) Monoamine oxidase inhibitor
(c) Trazodone
(d) Floxnoxetinal

139. All are common cardiac signs in normal pregnancy except

(a) Pedal edema (b) PND
(c) DOE (d) Hemophysis

140. Obstruction of cardiac lymphatics may cause following except

(a) Myocardial edema
(b) Pericardial effusion
(c) Pleural effusion
(d) None of the above

141. Which drug is removed by peritoneal dialysis?

(a) Quinidine
(b) Sotalol
(c) Amiodasone
(d) None of the above

142. Most common lesion in marfan's syndrome is

(a) MVP
(b) Aortic root dilation
(c) Aortic regurgitation
(d) All the above

143. All are cardiovascular manifestation of hurler's in MPS except

(a) HT
(b) Valvular dysfunction
(c) Arterial disease
(d) Pericardial disease

144. In marquio syndrome commonly seen cardiac lesion is

(a) HT (b) Pericarditis
(c) Valvular defect (d) Septal defect

145. MPS (VI) presents with which cardiac lesion?

(a) Calcific stenolic AV
(b) MAC
(c) Septal defect
(d) Coronary calcification

146. Pseudohurler polydystrophy presents with which cardiac lesion?

(a) Valvular lesion (b) Pericarditis
(c) CHB (d) CMP

147. LCAD deficiency causes which cardiac lesion?

(a) Valvular defect (b) Pericardial disease
(c) HCM (d) Septal defects

148. Primary hyperoxaluria causes which cardiac defect?

(a) Valvular (b) Pericardial
(c) Myocarditis (d) CHB

149. Cerebro tendinous xanthomahosi's causes which cardio vascular disease?

(a) Valvular
(b) CMP
(c) CHB
(d) Premature atherosclerosis

150. Wilsar's disease causes commonly which cardiac disorder?

(a) Pericarditis (b) Valvular lesion
(c) CHB (d) Cardiomyopathy

151. Homocysteinuria causes commonly which cardiovascular disorder

(a) Pericarditis
(b) Thrombosis of large and small arteries and veins
(c) Valvular lesion
(d) Conduction defects

152. Antiphospholipid antibodies cause all the following cardiac disorder except

(a) Coronary thrombosis
(b) Endocarditis
(c) Aortic/Mitral valvular stenosis regurgitation
(d) Pericarditis

153. SLE produces all the following cardiac disorders except

(a) Pulmonary hypertension
(b) Systemic hypertension
(c) Endocarditis
(d) Premature atherosclerosis

154. Which is commonest pericardial involvement in rheumatoid arthritis?

(a) Pericardial thickening
(b) Acute pericarditis
(c) Constrictive pericarditis
(d) Pericardial tamponade

155. The characteristic cardiac finding in Becker's muscular dystrophy is

(a) Dilated CMD (b) CHB
(c) Q waves (d) Tall R in V1

156. The most common cardiac finding in farcioscopulohumeral muscular dystrophy is

(a) Atrial enlargement
(b) PR increase
(c) Atrial flutter
(d) VES

157. Most common arrhythmia in severe form of myotonic dystrophy is

(a) Atrial flutter
(b) AV block
(c) Intraventricular conduction defect
(d) Ventricular arrhythmia

158. Most common echo finding in fredrichis ataxia is

(a) RWMA
(b) LVH
(c) Normal LV function
(d) Dilated CMP

159. Alcohol can cause all is of the following cardiac disorders except

(a) Dilated CMP (b) Arrhythmias
(c) Hypertension (d) CAD

160. Commonest ECG finding in duchenne muscular dystrophy is

(a) Tall R with high R/S ratio in V1
(b) RAD
(c) Short PR interval
(d) Deep narrow q in Ant Lat leads

161. All of the following changes occur in ECG is myotomic dystrophy except

(a) AV block
(b) Fascicular block
(c) Prolongation of QRS interval
(d) Sinus techycardia

162. All are hemodynamic charges normal pregnancy in 1st trimester except

(a) Cardiac output
(b) Systolic blood pressure unchanged
(c) Diastolic blood pressure
(d) LVEF unchanged

163. All of the following hemodynamic changes occur during 2nd trimester in normal pregnancy except

(a) Cardiac output increase
(b) Systolic blood pressure decrease
(c) Diastolic blood pressure
(d) LVEF increased

164. All of the following changes occur in 3rd trimester during normal pregnancy except

(a) Cardiac out put increases
(b) Both systolic/diastolic blood pressure remain unchanged
(c) Left ventricular volume increases
(d) LVEF is decreased

165. Rarest benign tumor of heart is

(a) Teratoma
(b) Hemongioma
(c) Mesothelioma of AV node
(d) Fibroma

166. Commonest malignant tumour of heart is

(a) Angiosarcoma
(b) Fibrosarcoma
(c) Malignant lymphoma
(d) Neurogenic sarcoma

167. All are homodynamic effects of ureteric contraction except

(a) Increase blood volume
(b) Increase cardiac output
(c) Increase blood pressure
(d) Increase PVR

168. CHB developing during pregnancy is related to all the following except

(a) Acute myocarditis
(b) Calcific aortic stenosis
(c) After surgical correction of VSD
(d) Severe calcific mitral stenosis

169. Which is the commonest lipid disorder seen in chronic renal failure (non-nephrotic)?

(a) Increase TG
(b) Increase TC
(c) Increase TG + TC
(d) None of the above

170. Commonest cardiovascular cause of death in ESRD is

(a) Myocardial infarction
(b) Hemorrhagic pericarditis
(c) Heart failure
(d) CVA

171. Rheumatoid arthritis may cause all the following except

(a) Pericarditis
(b) Valvulitis
(c) Coronary vasculitis
(d) Aortitis

172. SLE produces all the following except

(a) Myocarditis
(b) Pericarditis
(c) Valvulitis
(d) Aortitis

173. Scleroderma causes which of the following?

(a) Myocarditis
(b) Valvulitis
(c) Coronary vasculitis
(d) Aortitis

174. Ankylosing spondylitis produces which of the following?

(a) Aortitis
(b) Myocarditis
(c) Pericarditis
(d) Coronary vasculitis

175. Polymyositis produces which of the following?

(a) Myocarditis
(b) Pericarditis
(c) Valvulitis
(d) Aortitis

176. All are nutritional causes of heart muscle disease except

(a) Kwashiorkor
(b) Magnesium deficiency
(c) Beri beri
(d) Pertubations of Na metabolism

177. Usual cardiac causes of hoarseness of voice

(a) Idiopathic dilation of PA
(b) Pulmonary hypertension
(c) Aortic syndrome
(d) Aortic regurgitation

178. Which cardiac disease produces anemia?

(a) Infective endocarditis
(b) Prosthetic valve
(c) Aortic stenosis
(d) All of the above

179. Which vasodilator has similar arterial and venous dilation capacity?

(a) Hydralazine (b) Minoxidil
(c) β-blocker (d) ACE inhibitors

180. Which Ca-blocker always increases heart rate?

(a) Amlodipine (b) Nifedipine
(c) Diltiazem (d) Verapamil

181. All of the following are aldosterone antagonists except

(a) Aldactone (b) Trimethaphan
(c) Eprinilone (d) β-blockers

182. AT1 receptors are located in all the following sites except

(a) Vessels (b) Brain
(c) Heart (d) Adrenal gland

183. AT2 receptors are located at all following sites except

(a) Heart
(b) Brain
(c) Uterus (Myometrium)
(d) Nerves

184. AT3 receptors are located in which of the following?

(a) Vessels
(b) Adrenal gland
(c) Neuroblastoma cells in amphibian
(d) Heart

185. Which receptor has anti proliferative effect?

(a) AT1 (b) AT2
(c) AT3 (d) AT4

186. Upper respiratory tract infection occurs maximally with which of the following

(a) Irbisartan (b) Losartan
(c) Candisartan (d) Valsartan

187. AT4 are located in all the following except

(a) Brain (b) Lungs
(c) Prostate (d) Nerves

188. Which of the following receptors is involved in increasing vasopressin release?

(a) AT1 (b) AT2
(c) AT3 (d) AT4

189. Which receptors are increased in stimulation of PAI-1?

(a) AT1
(b) AT4
(c) Both of the above
(d) None of the above

190. Proneness to viral infection occurs with which ARB

(a) Valsartan (b) Tirbisartan
(c) Losartan (d) Candisartan

191. Arthralgia occurs with which of the following?

(a) Losartan (b) Olmesartan
(c) Irbisartan (d) Iprosartan

192. Insulin sensitizers in type 2 Diabetes mellitus cause all the following effects except

(a) Intima-medial thickness
(b) Induces coronary artery relaxation
(c) Increases cardiac output
(d) Increases blood pressure

193. ARB's cause all of the following except

(a) No change in bradykinin
(b) Cough occurs with equal frequency as with ACE inhibitors
(c) Less angioedema than ACE inhibitors
(d) Hyperkalemia less common than ACE inhibitor

194. For persistent hyperkalemia the choice of treatment is

(a) Calcium gluconate
(b) Glucose with insulin
(c) B2 adrengic agonist
(d) Dialysis

195. All of following are the causes of electro-mechanical dissociation except

(a) Cardiac tamponade
(b) Hyperkalemia
(c) Alkalosis
(d) Hypovolemia

196. All are non cardiac uses of beta-blockers except

(a) Hypothyroidism (b) Migraine
(c) Glaucoma (d) Essential tremors

197. All are compelling contraindication to ACE inhibitors except

(a) Pregnancy
(b) Bilateral renal artery stenosis
(c) Hyperkalemia
(d) ESRD

198. Thiazide diuretics are not effective at which level of serum creatinine

(a) 1 mg % (b) 1.5 mg %
(c) 2.0 mg % (d) ≥ 2.5 mg %

199. In all the following situations risk of diabetes mellitus may not beard except

(a) AF with for VR
(b) PH severe
(c) Very disorganized and immobile valve
(d) Mod mitral stenosis in NSR and normal rate

200. All of the following cardiac lesions occur in AIDS except

(a) Cardiomyopathy
(b) Pericardial effusion
(c) Infective endocarditis
(d) Left atrial myxoma

201. Which is the commonest manifestation of rheumatic pericarditis?

(a) Valvulitis (b) Myocarditis
(c) Pericarditis (d) All of the above

202. Anabolic steroid may cause all the following except

(a) Decrease HDL-C
(b) Precipitate heart failure
(c) Causes hypertension
(d) Valvular defects

203. All are clinical features of left atrial myxomia except

(a) Changing murmur with position
(b) Enlarged LA
(c) Tumor plop
(d) Sinus rhythm

204. Which is the most common finding in left atrial myxoma?

(a) Embolism (b) Syncope
(c) Arthralgia (d) Hemoptysis

205. Osteogenesis imperfecta is not associated with

(a) VSD (b) AR
(c) MVP (d) Dissection of aorta

206. Which lipid fraction is not decreased in diabetic dyslipidemia?

(a) HDL-C (b) Apo A1
(c) Both (a) and (b) (d) Apo B

207. Endothelial dysfunction in diabetes mellitus causes all the following except

(a) Increase in angiotensin II
(b) Increase in PAI-1 production
(c) Increase NO production
(d) Increase in DAG synthesis

208. Primary cause of death in woman is

(a) Cardiovascular disease
(b) Cancer
(c) Inflectional
(d) Anaemia

209. Which is most sensitive test in cardiac amydoidosis?

(a) Skin biopsy
(b) Rectal biopsy
(c) Endomyocardial biopsy
(d) Bone marrow biopsy

210. Cardiac amyloid patients are usually sensitive to which of the following drug?

(a) Dimeters
(b) Ca-blockers
(c) Beta-blockers
(d) ACE inhibitors

211. Following are echocardiographic predicting poor prognosis in aneroid heart except

(a) LA enlargement
(b) RV dilatation
(c) Increased LV thickness
(d) Decrease EF

212. All are left atrial causes of cardiogenic embolism to brain except

(a) Atrial flutter/fibrillation
(b) Left atrial myxomia
(c) Atrial septal aneurysm
(d) Atrial tachycardia

213. Embolism presents in all the following MV lesions except

(a) Infective endocarditis
(b) MVP
(c) Prosthetic value
(d) All the above

214. All the following cardiac drugs decrease blood viscosity except

(a) Prazocin
(b) Nitrates
(c) Nicardipine
(d) Hydrochlore thiazide

215. All the following drugs increase erythrocytes deformability except

(a) Verapanil
(b) Clazapil
(c) Carvedilal
(d) Hydrochloric thiazide

216. Antibiotic therapy should be targeted to bring the HbAIC level to for reducing cardio vascular events

(a) 7.5% (b) 7%
(c) 65% (d) < 6%

217. Neutropemia with ACE inhibitor is maximum when

(a) Given alone
(b) Given with renal insufficiency
(c) Given with collagen disease
(d) Given with collagen disease and renal insufficiency

218. First dose hypotension with ACE inhibitor is more likely in all of the following saturation except

(a) Renal artery stenosis
(b) Malignant hypertension with low age + K
(c) Severs HF treated with diameter
(d) Increase sensitivity to drug

219. Smoking causes highest risk ratio of which of the following

(a) Sudden cardiac death
(b) Myocardial infection
(c) All coronary related deaths
(d) UA

220. Following dimities produce neutropemis except

(a) Ethaerynic acid
(b) Hydrochlor thiazide
(c) Mereuratt (d) Splronalectone

221. All of the following drugs produce thrombocytopenia except

(a) Acetazalamide (b) Chlorthiazide
(c) Chlorthalidone (d) Ethererynic acid

222. Thrombocytopenia occurs with

(a) Hydralazemil (b) Methyldopa
(c) Reserpine (d) All of the above

223. All of the following drugs may produce agramulocytosis except

(a) Procainamide (b) Tocuenide
(c) Propaphenone (d) Digoxin

224. Pure red cell aphasia may occurs with which of the following drug?

(a) Captopril (b) Heparin
(c) Acetazalamide (d) Tocaenide

225. Which of the following drug produces Megaloblastic anemia?

(a) Triamterine (b) Procairamide
(c) Quinidine (d) Reserpime

226. Autopsy incidence which cardiac disease in india is highest?

(a) Rheumatic (b) Hypertensive
(c) IHD (d) Cor pulmonale

227. Radiation does not cause which cardiovascular disease?

(a) Pericardial (b) Myocardial
(c) Valvular (d) Hypertension

228. Common neonatal cardiac abnormality when mother is taking ACE inhibitors

(a) Coarctation of aorta
(b) PDA
(c) Fallots tetralogy
(d) ASD

229. All following drugs used in pregnancy can cause neonatal bradycardia except

(a) β-Blockers (b) Nitrates
(c) Mexiletin (d) Procainamide

230. All following drugs may cause raynauds phenomenon except

(a) β-blockers (b) Ergolamine
(c) Methysergide (d) Clonidine

231. Most common cardiac manifestation of HIV disease is

(a) Pericardial effusion
(b) Dilated cardiomyopathy
(c) Pulmonary hypertension
(d) Cardiac tumors

232. In acromegaly all of the following may be found except

(a) Hypertension
(b) Heart failure
(c) Premature coronary artery disease
(d) Heart blocks

233. Least common cause of hypotension is

(a) Right ventricular infarction
(b) Cardiogenic shock
(c) Cardiac tamponade
(d) Hypothyroid heart disease

234. TG is increased by all the following except

(a) Diabetes mellitus
(b) Atenolol
(c) Oral contraceptives
(d) Primary biliary cirrhosis

235. When are anticoagulants used in superficial thrombophlebitis?

(a) Every case
(b) When anti inflammatory drugs fail
(c) Extension to deep venous thrombosis
(d) All of the above

236. Which heart disease has highest prevalence in elderly female?

(a) Coronary artery disease
(b) Hypertension
(c) Valvular
(d) Pulmonary

237. Hoarseness of voice occurs in all of the following except

(a) Enlarged left atrium
(b) Enlarged (dilated) pulmonary artery
(c) Aortic aneurysm
(d) Enlarged left ventricle

238. Which heart disease has highest prevalence in elderly male?

(a) Coronary artery disease
(b) Hypertension
(c) Valvular
(d) Pulmonary

239. All of the following are the hemodynamic alteration in amyloid heart disease except

(a) PAP > 50 mmHg
(b) LVEDP > 20 mmHg
(c) LVEDP – RVEDP > 5
(d) Equalization of end diastolic pressure in all 4 chambers

240. Cardiovascular changes in anemia usually occur when Hb concentration is reduced by

(a) 10% (b) 20%
(c) 30% (d) 40%

241. Which is characteristic finding of cardiovascular system due to anemia?

(a) Systemic congestion
(b) Pulmonary congestion
(c) Dilatation of heart
(d) Presence of murmurs

242. Which is rare finding in myxoedema?

(a) Increase incidence of coronary atherosclerosis
(b) Cardiac out put is reduced
(c) Pericardial effusion
(d) Cardiac tamponade

243. Commonest cause of coronary artery embolism is

(a) Infective endocarditis
(b) Prosthetic valve thrombosis
(c) Mural thrombi in left heart
(d) Valve fragments emboli during surgery

244. The exchange function is carried by which part of arterial tree?

(a) Medium sized arteries
(b) Small arteries
(c) Arterioles (d) Capillaries

245. Which part of arterial tree is responsible for vascular resistance?

(a) Small arteries (b) Arterioles
(c) Capillaries (d) All of the above

246. Redistribution of blood is carried by which part of arterial tree?

(a) Large arteries (b) Arterioles
(c) Capillaries (d) All of the above

247. Which part of arterial tree has maximum wall thickness?

(a) Aortic (b) Large arteries
(c) Arterioles (d) Capillaries

248. Endothelium is the predominant structure in which part of arterial tree?

(a) Small artery (b) Arterioles
(c) Capillaries (d) Large arteries

249. Elastin is predominantly found in which part of arterial tree?

(a) Aorta
(b) Large arteries
(c) Medium sized artery
(d) Small sized artery

250. Neutropenia is most frequently linked tos

(a) Captopril (b) Enalapril
(c) Lisinopril (d) Terindopril

251. Cough induced by ACE inhibitors has all the following features except

(a) Increase sensitivity of cough reflex
(b) Start with tickling sensation in throat
(c) More in men than women
(d) Related to prostaglandin formation

252. Visceral obesity is associated with all except

(a) Hypertension
(b) Type 2 diabetes mellitus
(c) Coronary artery disease
(d) ASD

253. Perioperative cardiac events peak at which time?

(a) During surgery
(b) On Ist operative day

(c) Between 2nd and 5th post operative day
(d) After one week of surgery

254. Which is the most common cardiovascular abnormality in arteriohepatic dysplasia?

(a) Diffuse pulmonary artery stenosis
(b) Pulmonary atresia
(c) TOF
(d) Coarctation of aorta

255. Most common cardiovascular abnormality in turner's syndrome

(a) Aortic stenosis
(b) TAPVD
(c) Bicuspid aortic valve
(d) Ventricular septal defect

256. Most common cardiac abnormality is down's syndrome

(a) A-V canal defect (b) VSD
(c) ASD (d) Fallot's tetralogy

257. Which is the most common neoplastic disorder involving pericardium by direct extension?

(a) Breast (b) Lung
(c) Lymphoma (d) Leukemia

258. Sinns tachycardia is not found with fever in all following conditions except

(a) Typhoid fever
(b) Viral hemorrhagic fever
(c) Lessa fever
(d) Pulmonary turberculosis

259. Most common cause of ESRD is

(a) Diabetic nephropathy
(b) Hypertensive nephrosclerosis
(c) Primary glomerular disease
(d) Tubulo interstitial disease

260. Anabolic steroids may causes following cardiovascular disorders except

(a) Increase atherocosclerosis
(b) Hypertension
(c) LVH
(d) Cardiomyopathy

261. Most common symptom of cocaine is

(a) Sudden cardiac death
(b) Chest pain
(c) Dyspnaea
(d) Edema

262. In which CNS lesion cardiac arrhythmias are most common

(a) Meningitis
(b) Encephalitis
(c) Brain sten lesion
(d) Internal capsule lesion

263. Horse chest nut tree extract is useful in edema (Leg) of which origin

(a) Renal failure
(b) Heart failure
(c) Myxoedema
(d) Edema venous in sufficiency

264. Which of the following May be the only manifestation of apathetic hyperthyraidison in elderly

(a) AE (b) AT
(c) Atrial fibrillation (d) Atrial flutter

265. Gibson's murmur is found in

(a) Fallot's tetralogy
(b) Pulmonary arterio venous fistula
(c) VSD with atrial regurgitation
(d) PDA

266. All the following are common cardiac complications of acromegaly except

(a) Heart failure
(b) Acute coronary syndromes
(c) Tachyarrhythmias
(d) Heart block complete

267. Adrenal insufficiency produces all the following except

(a) Hypotension
(b) Sinus bradycardia
(c) Nonspecific ST/T changes
(d) Long QT interval

268. Which is most common cardiac pathology in AIDS?

(a) Myocarditis
(b) Pericardial effusion
(c) Pulmonary hypertension
(d) Long QT interval

269. Which of the following is rare in cardiac allograft vasculopathy?

(a) Dyspnoea
(b) Ventricular arrhythmia
(c) Sudden death
(d) Angina

270. All following are used to prevent development of anthracycline induced cardiomyopathy except

(a) Limit the dose
(b) Liposomal encapsulated formulation
(c) Modified dosing schedule
(d) ACE inhibitors

271. Myoxomas occur most commonly in which cardiac chamber?

(a) Left ventricular (b) Right ventricular
(c) Right atrium (d) Left atrium

272. Sildenafil is useful in which cardiac condition?

(a) Angina
(b) Systemic hypertension
(c) Pulmonary hypertension
(d) All the above

273. Endocardial metastasis most often occurs with

(a) Adencarcinoma
(b) Bronchogenic carcinoma
(c) Breast cancers
(d) Lymphoma

274. Which is primary malignant tumour of heart?

(a) Papillary fibroelastoma
(b) Lymphoma
(c) Fibroma
(d) Lipoma

275. Which systemic manifestation is not found in left atrial myxomia as against infective endocardia?

(a) Fever (b) Anemia
(c) Spleenomegaly (d) Clubbing

276. All of the following drugs increase cyclosporine levels except

(a) Diltiazem (b) Erythromycin
(c) Metoclopramide (d) Hydantoins

277. Which of the following cardiac vascular disorders has highest risk for pregnancy?

(a) Coarctation of aorta
(b) Eisenmenger syndrome
(c) Peripartum cardiomyopathy
(d) TOF

278. Which chromosome abnormalities causes highest % of CV abnormalities?

(a) + 21, down syndrome
(b) × 0, turner syndrome
(c) + 18, edward syndrome
(d) + 13, patau's syndrome

279. All following endocardial lesion are produce in systemic lupus erythematosis except

(a) Libman sacks endocarditis
(b) Valvular thickening
(c) Intracardiac thrombi
(d) Endocardial fibroelastosis

280. All following coronary arterial lesion can occur SLE except

(a) Premature atherosclerosis
(b) Arteritis
(c) Thrombosis
(d) Coronary artery dissection

281. Which is the commonest ECG funding the systemic sclerosis?

(a) Normal ECG (b) RBBB
(c) Atrial ectopic (d) LVH

282. Which cardiac drugs doesn't cause lupus like syndrome?

(a) Procainamide (b) Quinidine
(c) Methyldopa (d) Reserpine

283. Which of the following anaesthetic is marked myocardial depressant?

(a) Morphine (b) Fentanyl
(c) Isoflurane (d) Halothane

284. All of the following anaesthetic agents produce no change in heart rate except

(a) Halothane (b) Sevoflurane
(c) Nitrous oxide (d) Fentanyl

285. Narcotic based anaesthetic agents are choice in all the following except

(a) MV disease
(b) Aortic stenosis
(c) Cardiomyopathy
(d) Constrictive pericarditis

286. Halogen based anaesthetic agents are choice in

(a) Aortic stenosis
(b) Aortic aneurysm
(c) Coronary artery disease
(d) Aortic regurgitation

287. Which is the commonest benign tumor of heart?

(a) Lipoma (b) Myxoma
(c) Fibroma (d) Haemangioma

288. Which is commonest malignant cardiac tumor?

(a) Angiosarcoma (b) Mesothliomia
(c) Fibro sarcoma (d) Thynoma

289. Maximum distribution of cardiac output during rest occurs in which organ?

(a) Kidneys (b) Liver
(c) Heart (d) Brain

290. Maximum distribution of cardiac out during exercise occurs in which organ?

(a) Muscles (b) Heart
(c) Liver (d) Brain

291. Which nutritional deficiency in mother is associated with congenital heart disease in newborn?

(a) Fat (b) Protein
(c) Vitamin A (d) Folate

292. Which physiological change occurs maximally in pregnancy?

(a) Cardiac output
(b) HR
(c) Stroke volume
(d) Pulmonary artery pressure

293. Commonest cardiovascular manifestation of kawasaki disease

(a) Pericardial effusion
(b) Coronary artery aneurysm
(c) Mitral regurgitation
(d) Myocarditis

294. Lymphocytic myocarditis is found in all except

(a) Viral
(b) Polymyositis
(c) Mycoplasma pneumonia
(d) Parasitic infestation

295. Granulomatons myocarditis is found in all except?

(a) Rheumatoid (b) Rheumatic
(c) Sarcoid (d) Kawasaki disease

296. All of the following drugs have hepatic route of elimination except

(a) Propranolol (b) Diltiazem
(c) Verapamil (d) Bretyllium

297. All of the following endocrine disorders may cause heart musle disease except

(a) Thyrotoxicosis
(b) Myxoedema
(c) Phaeochromocytoma
(d) Hypoparathyroidism

298. All are radiation induced cardiovascular disease except

(a) Pericardial disease

(b) Hypertension
(c) Valvular dysfunction
(d) Myocardial disease

299. Rheumatoid arthritis does not involve

(a) Coronaries (b) Valves
(c) Myocardium (d) Pericardium

300. Ankylosing spondylitis particularly involve

(a) Valves (b) Coronaries
(c) Pericardium (d) Myocardium

301. Systemic sclerosis does not involve

(a) Valves (b) Coronaries
(c) Myocardium (d) Pericardium

302. Myocardial biochemical alterations in heart failure include all except

(a) Increased collagen
(b) Decreased myocardial nor epinephrine
(c) Decreased synthesis of alerepibephone
(d) Increased function of sarcoplasmic reticulum

303. All of the drugs cause autonomic failure except

(a) Phenothiazines
(b) Tricyclic antidepressants
(c) Diuretics
(d) ACE inhibitors

304. Drug used in prevention of post prandial hypotension

(a) Clonidine (b) Dihydroegotamine
(c) Propanolol (d) Caffeine

305. Which drug inhibits negative inotropic and chronotropic effect of β-blockers?

(a) Adrenaline
(b) Methyldopa
(c) Glycogen
(d) Tricyclic antidepressants

306. Fetal alcohol syndrome does not cause which congenital heart disease?

(a) ASD (b) VSD
(c) PDA (d) Aortic stenosis

307. Which congenital heart disease is common in congenital hypothyroidism?

(a) PDA (b) ASD
(c) VSD (d) Aortic stenosis

308. High incidence of congenital heart block in offspring occurs when mother suffers from

(a) DM
(b) Rheumatoid arthritis
(c) SLE
(d) All the above

309. Offsprings of diabetic mother are usually

(a) Over weight (b) Under weight
(c) Both (a) and (b) (d) Average weight

310. Phenytoin by mother is associated with all following congenital heart disease except

(a) PS (b) AS
(c) Coarctation of AV (d) VSD

311. All following are effects of insulin sensitisers or lipids except

(a) Decrease TG Levels
(b) Increase HDL levels
(c) Decrease LDL-C oxidation
(d) Decrease LDL-C

312. Insulin sensitizers have the following vascular effects except

(a) Decrease intima-media thickness
(b) Lower blood pressure
(c) Induce coronary artery relaxation
(d) Increase vascular smooth muscle cell migration

313. All are advantages of metformin therapy except

(a) Weak insulin sensitizer
(b) Improve insulin resistance
(c) Improve endothelial resistance
(d) Indicated in CHF

314. Thiazaliadinediones have all the following advantages except

(a) Potent insulin sensitizer

(b) Improves endothelial function
(c) Benefit cardiovascular system
(d) Contraindicated in NYHA III IV

315. Most common cardiac manifestation of cardiac sarcoidosis is

(a) Ventricular arrhythmia
(b) CHB
(c) RBBB
(d) LBBB

316. Which is most sensitive parameter for detection of HIV associated myocarditis?

(a) Increase of troponin I
(b) Increase of Ck–MB
(c) ST elevation
(d) Ventricular ectopics

317. Which is most specific parameter for detection of HIV associated myocarditis?

(a) ST elevation
(b) Increase in Troponin I
(c) Increase in CKMB
(d) Ventricular ectopics

318. Most important side effect reported during 1st month of interferon â treatment

(a) Injection site reaction
(b) Arthralgia
(c) Dyspnaea
(d) Angina

319. All of the following drugs may cause post operative encephalopathy except

(a) Haloparidol (b) Narcotics
(c) Sedatives (d) Nitrous oxide

320. All are endoscopic manifestation of cardiac disease except

(a) Villous hypertrophy
(b) Ulcers
(c) Strictures
(d) Adenocarcinoma

321. All of the following are protective effects on cardiovascular system of metformin therapy except

(a) Improved diastolic function
(b) Decreased total cholesterol
(c) Increased HDL cholesterol
(d) Increased platelet aggregation

322. All of the following drugs are safe in curing torch infection during pregnancy except

(a) Penicillins (b) Cephalosporins
(c) Nitrofurantoin (d) Amioglycosides

323. Colostrum contains all the following except

(a) Cytokines
(b) Interleukin 1α
(c) Tumour necrosis factor
(d) Interleukin II

324. All of following are laboratory findings in acute mesenteric ischemia except

(a) Leucopoenia
(b) Metabolic acidosis
(c) Increased serum lipase
(d) Increase amylase

325. All of the following cardiac conditions are associated with blue sclera except

(a) Osteogenesis imperfecta – aortic regurgitation
(b) Marfan's syndrome – great vessel aneurysm
(c) Ehler's danlos syndrome – aorta
(d) Down syndrome

326. All of the following viruses are commonly in involved is myocarditis except

(a) Adenoviruses (b) Coxsackie virus B
(c) Echo viruses (d) Mumps

327. Which is most common ECG abnormality in chagas disease is?

(a) PR prolongation (b) RBBB
(c) LBBB (d) CHB

328. Which valvular dysfunction is common in ankylosing spondylitis?

(a) Aortic regurgitation
(b) Mitral regurgitation
(c) Mitral stenosis
(d) Aortic stenosis

329. How common are cardiac manifestation of ankylosing spondylitis?

(a) < 1% (b) 1%
(c) 1–2% (d) 3–10%

330. All are cardiac features of GERD except

(a) Atypical chest pain
(b) Arrhythmias
(c) Ischemia
(d) Hypertension

331. Smoking cessation is most effective in men in which age group in improving life expectation?

(a) 35–30 years (b) 40–44 years
(c) 45–49 years (d) 65–69 years

332. Which of the following doesn't cross placenta during pregnancy?

(a) Heparin
(b) Aspirin
(c) Oral anticoagulants
(d) None of the above

333. All are metabolic causes of myocarditis except

(a) Hypocalcaemia
(b) Hypophosphatemia
(c) Carnitine
(d) Hypercalcemia

334. Hypoxia causes all the following except

(a) Cyanosis (b) Polycythemia
(c) Heart failure (d) CVA

335. Standard heparin has all following features except

(a) Don't in activate clot bound thrombin
(b) Increases vascular permeability
(c) Thrombocytopenia occurs
(d) Liver toxicity uncommon

336. Low molecular weight heparin has all the following features except

(a) Don't inactivate clot bound thrombin
(b) Vascular permeability is increased
(c) Thrombocytopenia is rare
(d) Liver toxicity is uncommon

337. Low molecular weight heparin has all the following features except

(a) Increase molecular weight 4000–6500 Dalton
(b) Platelet inhibition is more
(c) Renal clearances is more
(d) Given subcutaneosly

338. Standard heparin has all the following features except

(a) Molecular weight is 12000–15000
(b) Platelet inhibition is more
(c) Renal clearances is more
(d) Given intravenously

339. Commonest malignant cardiac tumour is

(a) Angiosarcoma
(b) Rhabdomyosarcoma
(c) Fibrosarcoma
(d) Malignant lymphoma

340. Chief composition of heart consist of

(a) Water (b) Fat
(c) Protein (d) Carbohydrate

341. Most common tissue fraction LV is

(a) Cells (b) Interstitium
(c) Capillaries (d) Arteries and veins

342. Which is the largest organ in the body?

(a) Brain (b) Kidney
(c) Spleen (d) Endothelium

343. PCO_2 is decreased in all the following except

(a) Cardiogenic shock
(b) Acute pulmonary embolism
(c) Diabetic ketoacidosis
(d) L–R shunts

344. Which cardiac drug produces osteoporosis with long use?

(a) β-Blockers (b) Aspirin
(c) Dipyridamole (d) Heparin

345. Which cardiac drug produces pulmonary fibrosis?

(a) Phenytion (b) Quinidine
(c) Amiodarone (d) Digoxin

346. Commonest heart disease between 10–30 years is

(a) Congenital heart disease
(b) Rheumatic heart disease
(c) Coronary artery disease
(d) Hypertension

347. Which cardiac disease is rare in females of child bearing Age?

(a) Rheumatic heart disease
(b) Post partum cardiomyopathy
(c) Coronary heart disease
(d) Hypertension

348. Type of surgery which has high risk of cardiovascular events

(a) Thoracic (b) Abdominal
(c) Head and neck (d) Breast

349. Type of surgery which has intermediate risk of cardiovascular events

(a) Vascular (b) Abdominal
(c) Eye (d) Gynecologic

350. Type of surgery which has lowest risk of cardiovascular events

(a) Breast (b) Abdominal
(c) Vascular (d) Head and neck

351. Commonest cause of death at high altitudes

(a) Cold exposure
(b) Fall
(c) High altitude pulmonary edema
(d) High altitude cerebral edema

352. All the following drugs cause pedal edema except

(a) Pioglitazones (b) Calcium blockers
(c) Minoxidil (d) Hydralazine

353. Lithium use during pregnancy may cause which disease?

(a) ASD (b) VSD
(c) PDA (d) Ebsten's disease

354. Which of the following cardiac drug cause fatigue?

(a) α-methyldopa
(b) Ca-blockers
(c) ACE inhibitors
(d) Angiotension receptor blocker

355. All drugs causes autonomic failure except

(a) Phenothiazine (b) Nitrates
(c) Ca-blockers (d) μ-Blockers

356. All of the following metabolic diseases may cause autonomic failure except

(a) DM (b) Porphyria
(c) B12 deficiency (d) Fe deficiency

357. All of the following disease may arise during pregnancy except

(a) Hypertension
(b) Peripartum CMP
(c) Pulmonary embolism
(d) Pericarditis

358. Renovascular murmur is heard at all places except

(a) Beneath costal margins anteriorly
(b) Lateral to aorta
(c) Lumber spine
(d) Epigastrium

359. Which region of heart is most commonly involved by metastasis?

(a) Pericardium
(b) Mural endocarditis
(c) Valvular endocarditis
(d) Myocardium

360. Which is most sensitive ECG finding cardiac amyloidosis?

(a) ST/T changes
(b) High voltages of QRS

(c) QT prolongation
(d) Q waves

361. Most common cardiac involvement in malignant lymphoma is

(a) Pericardial (b) Myocardial
(c) Coronaries (d) Endocardial

362. Which storage disease of myocardium produces valvular calcification?

(a) Gaucher's disease
(b) Horner's syndrome
(c) Fabrys disease
(d) Glycogen storage disease

363. Which storage disease of myocardium produces mitral stenosis?

(a) Fabrys disease
(b) Horner's syndrome
(c) Glycogen storage disease
(d) Gaucher's disease

364. Which storage disease of myocardium produces aortic stenosis?

(a) Fabrys disease
(b) Hurler's syndrome
(c) Glycogen storage disease
(d) Gaucher's disease

365. Pulmonary edema frequently occurs during pregnancy with MS at which Time?

(a) 15 weeks of gestation
(b) 30 weeks of gestation
(c) 25–27 weeks of gestation
(d) > 30 weeks of gestation

366. Human embryonic stem cell have all following properties except

(a) Pluripotant (b) Selforemoval
(c) Rejection occurs (d) Teratirnes occurs

367. Aypical presentation of IDH occurs in all the following except

(a) Elderly (b) Hypertension
(c) Diabetic (d) Young

368. All the following cardiac lesions are associated with blue sclera except

(a) Aortic regurgitaion
(a) Mitral regurgitation
(c) TOF
(d) Aortic stenosis

369. Xanthomas are located all following places except

(a) Eyelids
(b) Planter tendon
(c) Extensor tendons of hand
(d) Palletar tendons

370. Oval hemorrhage near disc with white spotat center on fundus examination indicates

(a) Hypertension
(b) Increased intracranial pressure
(c) Atherosclerosis
(d) Infective endocarditis

371. In Rubella syndrome pulmonary stenosis in at which location?

(a) Valvular (b) Subvalvular
(c) Branch stenosis (d) All of them

372. Which cardiac lesion does not occurs with argyll robert son pupil?

(a) Coronary osteal stenosis
(b) Aortic stenosis
(c) Aortic regurgitation
(d) Aortic aneurysm

373. Eating disorders to loose weight can result in following cardiac changes except

(a) ST/T was changes
(b) Prolonged QT interval
(c) Cardiomyopathy
(d) Coronary artery disease

374. All are major risk factor for non cardiac surgery in cardiac disease except

(a) Severe aortic stenosis
(b) Recent myocardial infarction < 3 month
(c) Decompensated heart failure
(d) Abnormal ECG

375. All are patient related risk factors for venous thromboembolism (VTE) except

(a) Previous VTE (b) Pregnancy
(c) Varicose veins (d) Age < 40 years

376. All are common major risk factor in for VTE except

(a) Malignancy
(b) Major Trauma
(c) Paralysis
(d) Heparin Induced Thrombocytopenia

377. Common major risk factor related to patient is for VTE

(a) Preview VTE (b) Peripartum
(c) Varicose vein (d) Obesity

378. Massive pulmonary embolism causes all following haemodynamic changes except

(a) Right atrial pressure is increased
(b) Right ventricular volume in increased
(c) Systolic vascular resistance is increased
(d) LV volume is increased

379. Hemorrhagic shock causes all the following changes except

(a) RA pressure fall
(b) LA pressure falls
(c) Cardiac output falls
(d) RV volume increase

380. Anaphylactic shock causes all the following haemodynamic changes except

(a) RA pressure decrease
(b) LA pressure increase
(c) LV volume decrease
(d) RV volume decrease

381. Which drug does not decrease preload?

(a) Isosorbid dinitrate (b) Hydralazine
(c) ACE inhibitor (d) Prazosin

382. Use of beta-blocker during pregnancy causes all except

(a) Fetal bradycardia
(b) Fetal hypoglycemia
(c) IUGR
(d) Congenital heart disease

383. Cardiac contractility is increased by which of the following agent?

(a) Halothane (b) Enflurane
(c) Isoflurane (d) Gall amine

384. Coronary blood flow is increased by all except

(a) Enflurane (b) Isoflurane
(c) Thiopental (d) Halothane

385. Heart rate is increased by all following except

(a) Enflurane (b) Isoflurane
(c) Succinyl choline (d) Fentanyl

386. Which is the commonest heart disease in india?

(a) Hypertension (b) IHD
(c) CMP (d) Cor pulmonale

387. Most common cause of death in chronic renal failure is

(a) Heart failure
(b) Myocardial infarction
(c) Sepsis
(d) CVA

ANSWERS

1. (*d*)	2. (*b*)	3. (*c*)	4. (a)	5. (*c*)
6. (*d*)	7. (*c*)	8. (*d*)	9. (*d*)	10. (*a*)
11. (*d*)	12. (*d*)	13. (*d*)	14. (a)	15. (*d*)
16. (*d*)	17. (*a*)	18. (*d*)	19. (*b*)	20. (*b*)
21. (*d*)	22. (*d*)	23. (*b*)	24. (*c*)	25. (*d*)
26. (*b*)	27. (*d*)	28. (*d*)	29. (*d*)	30. (*c*)
31. (*c*)	32. (*c*)	33. (*b*)	34. (*a*)	35. (*c*)
36. (*a*)	37. (*b*)	38. (*c*)	39. (*a*)	40. (*c*)
41. (*a*)	42. (*e*)	43. (*d*)	44. (*c*)	45. (*e*)
46. (*e*)	47. (*a*)	48. (*e*)	49. (*d*)	50. (*d*)
51. (*a*)	52. (*c*)	53. (*a*)	54. (*d*)	55. (*b*)
56. (*b*)	57. (*d*)	58. (*d*)	59. (*d*)	60. (*b*)
61. (*b*)	62. (*b*)	63. (*a*)	64. (*d*)	65. (*d*)
66. (*c*)	67. (*c*)	68. (*c*)	69. (*d*)	70. (*c*)
71. (*b*)	72. (*b*)	73. (*d*)	74. (*c*)	75. (*a*)
76. (*b*)	77. (*d*)	78. (*d*)	79. (*d*)	80. (*d*)
81. (*a*)	82. (*a*)	83. (*d*)	84. (*d*)	85. (*b*)
86. (*c*)	87. (*d*)	88. (*c*)	89. (*d*)	90. (*a*)
91. (*d*)	92. (*d*)	93. (*d*)	94. (*c*)	95. (*b*)
96. (*a*)	97. (*b*)	98. (*d*)	99. (*a*)	100. (*c*)
101. (*d*)	102. (*a*)	103. (*d*)	104. (*c*)	105. (*d*)
106. (*d*)	107. (*d*)	108. (*a*)	109. (*d*)	110. (*d*)
111. (*b*)	112. (*d*)	113. (*d*)	114. (*d*)	115. (*a*)
116. (*a*)	117. (*d*)	118. (*d*)	119. (*d*)	120. (*d*)
121. (*a*)	122. (*c*)	123. (*c*)	124. (*b*)	125. (*c*)
126. (*a*)	127. (*a*)	128. (*d*)	129. (*a*)	130. (*d*)
131. (*d*)	132. (*d*)	133. (*a*)	134. (*d*)	135. (*d*)
136. (*d*)	137. (*d*)	138. (*d*)	139. (*d*)	140. (*c*)
141. (*d*)	142. (*a*)	143. (*d*)	144. (*c*)	145. (*a*)
146. (*a*)	147. (*c*)	148. (*d*)	149. (*d*)	150. (*d*)
151. (*b*)	152. (*d*)	153. (*b*)	154. (*a*)	155. (*a*)
156. (*a*)	157. (*a*)	158. (*b*)	159. (*d*)	160. (*a*)

161. (*d*)	162. (*c*)	163. (*d*)	164. (*d*)	165. (*c*)
166. (*a*)	167. (*d*)	168. (*d*)	169. (*a*)	170. (*d*)
171. (*d*)	172. (*d*)	173. (*a*)	174. (*a*)	175. (*a*)
176. (*d*)	177. (*d*)	178. (*d*)	179. (*c*)	180. (*b*)
181. (*d*)	182. (*d*)	183. (*d*)	184. (*c*)	185. (*b*)
186. (*a*)	187. (*d*)	188. (*a*)	189. (*c*)	190. (*a*)
191. (*d*)	192. (*d*)	193. (*b*)	194. (*d*)	195. (*c*)
196. (*a*)	197. (*d*)	198. (*d*)	199. (*d*)	200. (*d*)
201. (*a*)	202. (*d*)	203. (*b*)	204. (*a*)	205. (*a*)
206. (*d*)	207. (*c*)	208. (*a*)	209. (*c*)	210. (*b*)
211. (*a*)	212. (*d*)	213. (*b*)	214. (*d*)	215. (*d*)
216. (*d*)	217. (*d*)	218. (*d*)	219. (*d*)	220. (*d*)
221. (*d*)	222. (*d*)	223. (*d*)	224. (*b*)	225. (*a*)
226. (*a*)	227. (*d*)	228. (*b*)	229. (*d*)	230. (*d*)
231. (*a*)	232. (*d*)	233. (*d*)	234. (*d*)	235. (*c*)
236. (*b*)	237. (*d*)	238. (*a*)	239. (*d*)	240. (*d*)
241. (*c*)	242. (*d*)	243. (*a*)	244. (*d*)	245. (*b*)
246. (*a*)	247. (*a*)	248. (*c*)	249. (*a*)	250. (*a*)
251. (*c*)	252. (*d*)	253. (*c*)	254. (*a*)	255. (*c*)
256. (*a*)	257. (*b*)	258. (*d*)	259. (*a*)	260. (*d*)
261. (*b*)	262. (*c*)	263. (*d*)	264. (*c*)	265. (*d*)
266. (*d*)	267. (*d*)	268. (*b*)	269. (*d*)	270. (*d*)
271. (*d*)	272. (*c*)	273. (*a*)	274. (*b*)	275. (*c*)
276. (*d*)	277. (*b*)	278. (*c*)	279. (*d*)	280. (*d*)
281. (*a*)	282. (*d*)	283. (*d*)	284. (*d*)	285. (*b*)
286. (*d*)	287. (*b*)	288. (*a*)	289. (*b*)	290. (*a*)
291. (*d*)	292. (*a*)	293. (*d*)	294. (*d*)	295. (*d*)
296. (*d*)	297. (*d*)	298. (*b*)	299. (*a*)	300. (*a*)
301. (*a*)	302. (*d*)	303. (*c*)	304. (*d*)	305. (*d*)
306. (*d*)	307. (*a*)	308. (*c*)	309. (*a*)	310. (*a*)
311. (*d*)	312. (*d*)	313. (*d*)	314. (*d*)	315. (*a*)
316. (*a*)	317. (*a*)	318. (*a*)	319. (*d*)	320. (*a*)
321. (*d*)	322. (*d*)	323. (*d*)	324. (*a*)	325. (*d*)
326. (*d*)	327. (*b*)	328. (*a*)	329. (*d*)	330. (*d*)
331. (*c*)	332. (*a*)	333. (*d*)	334. (*c*)	335. (*d*)

336. (*b*)	337. (*b*)	338. (*c*)	339. (*b*)	340. (*a*)
341. (*a*)	342. (*d*)	343. (*d*)	344. (*d*)	345. (*c*)
346. (*b*)	347. (*c*)	348. (*a*)	349. (*b*)	350. (*a*)
351. (*a*)	352. (*d*)	353. (*d*)	354. (*a*)	355. (*b*)
356. (*d*)	357. (*d*)	358. (*d*)	359. (*d*)	360. (*d*)
361. (*a*)	362. (*a*)	363. (*b*)	364. (*a*)	365. (*c*)
366. (*c*)	367. (*d*)	368. (*d*)	369. (*a*)	370. (*d*)
371. (*c*)	372. (*b*)	373. (*d*)	374. (*d*)	375. (*d*)
376. (*d*)	377. (*a*)	378. (*d*)	379. (*d*)	380. (*b*)
381. (*b*)	382. (*d*)	383. (*d*)	384. (*d*)	385. (*d*)
386. (*a*)	387. (*a*)			

References

1. **Lionel H. Opie Bernard, J. Gersh.** *Drugs for the Heart*, 6th ed., 2005.
2. **Goldman Bennett**. *Cecil Textbook of Medicine*, 21st ed., 2001.
3. **Norman M. Kaplan, MD.** *Kaplan's Clinical Hypertension*, 9th ed., 2006.
4. **David H. Bennett.** *Cardiac Arrhythmias*, 4th ed., 1993.
5. **Muayed AI Zaibag, Carlos M.G. Duran.** *Valvular Heart Disease,* 1994.
6. **James T. Willerson**. **Jay N. Cohn.** *Cardiovascular Medicine,* 1995.
7. **Robert A. O'Rourke, Valentin Fuster R., Wayne Alexander.** *The Heart Manual of Cardiology*, 10th ed., 2001.
8. **Ori Ben- Yehuda.** Cardiology *Clinics Pulmonary Vascular Disease*, Volume 22, Number 3, 2004.
9. **Ezra A. Amsterdam, J. Douglas Kirk.** *Cardiology Clinics Chest Pain Units*, Volume 23, Number 4, 2005.
10. **Michael H. Crawford, Prakash C. Deedwania.** *Cardiology Clinics Therapeutic Strategies in Diabetes and Cardiovascular Disease*, Volume 23, Number 2, 2005.
11. **Otto & Pearlman.** *Textbook of Clinical Echocardiography*, 1995.
12. **Maurice Sokolow, Malcolm B. McIlroy, Melvin D. Cheitlin.** *Clinical Cardiology*, 5th ed., 1990.

13. **Joseph S. Alpert.** *Valvular Heart Disease*, 3rd ed., 2000.
14. **Desmond G. Julian.** *Disease of the Heart*, 1989.
15. **M.J. Gandhi.** *Heart the Best of* 2005 *Edition year Book,* South Asian, 2005.
16. **B. Somaraju.** *Clinical Examination of the Heart*, 1995.
17. **Rajeev Gupta.** *Current Advances in Atherosclerosis Research*, Volume 4, 2001.
18. **Michael H. Crawford.** *Current Diagnosis & Treatment Cardiology*, 2nd ed., 2003.
19. **Roger J. Hajjar, Federica del Monte,** *Heart Failure Clinics Pathogenesis of Heart Failure*, Volume 1, Number 2, 2005.
20. **G. Willam Dee.** *Heart Failure Clinics Myocarditis*, Volume 1, Number 3, 2005.
21. **Gregg C. Fonarow.** *Heart Failure Clinics Neurohumoral Modulators in Heart Failure*, Volume 1, Number 1, 2005.
22. **Lionel H. Opie.** *Angiotensin Converting Enzyme Inhibitors*, 2nd ed., 1994.
23. **I.P. Pina, S. Goldstein, M. Dunlap.** *The Year in Heart Failure*, Volume 1, 2005.
24. **William H. Gaasch, Martin M. Le Winter.** *Left Ventricular Diastolic Dysfunction and Heart Failure.*
25. **Edward A. Gill, John D. Carroll.** *Cardiology Clinics*, Volume 23, Number 1, 2005.
26. **Christopher P. Cannon.** *Management of Acute Coronary Syndromes*, 1999.
27. **Robert C. Schlant.** *The Year Book of Cardiology*, 2002.
28. **H. L. Elliott, J.M.C. Connell & G.T. Mcinnes.** *The Year in Hypertension*, 2000.
29. **Roberto Ferrari, Cristina Opasich, Luigi Tavazzi.** *Heart Failure 181 Questions & Answers*, 2003.
30. **K.M. Fox, W.J. Remme.** *ACE Inhibition and Ischaemic Heart Disease*, 2nd ed., 2004.

31. **James E. Dalen, Joseph S. Alpert.** *Valvular Heart Disease*, 2nd ed., 1987.

32. **Etienne Aliot, Stefan Hohnloser, A. Hohn Camm Bramah N. Singh.** *Atrial Fibrillation Compendium*, 1980.

33. **Amal Mattu, Mark D. Kelemen.** *Cardiology Clinics Emergency Cardiac Care From ED to CCU*, Volume 24, Number 1, 2006.

34. **M. Gabriel Khan.** *Heart Disease Diagnosis and Therapy*, 2nd ed., 2006.

35. **Elliot Chesler.** *Schrire's Clinical Cardiology*, 4th ed., 1981.

36. **Adam D. Timmis, Anthony W. Nathan, Ian D. Sullivan.** *Essential Cardiology*, 3rd ed., 1997.

37. **Paul N. Yu, John F. Goodwin.** *Progress in Cardiology*, Number 4, 1975.

38. **Richard S. Cosby, Michael Bilitch.** *Heart Block*, 1972.

39. **David de Bono, Burton E. Sobel.** *Acute Coronary Syndrome*, 2001.

40. **James T. Willerson, William C. Roberts, Charles E. Rackley, Thomas P. Graham, Dean T. Mason, William W. Parmley.** *Cardiology* 1999.

41. **Roberto Ferrari, Maddalena Lettino, Claudio Ceconi, Luigi Tavazzi.** *Ischemic Heart Disease 130 Questions & Answers*, 2005.

42. **Shilpesh S. Patel, Jay N. Cohn. James T. Willerson.** *Hand Book of Cardiovascular Clinical Trials*, 1997.

43. **Robert A. Kloner, Yochai Birnbaum.** *Cardiovascular Trials Review*, 4th ed., 1999.

44. **Dr. C.R. Maiti.** *Clinical Methods in the Practice of Medicine*, 2nd ed., 2001.

45. **Joseph W. Mason.** *A Heart Attack can Save your Life*, 2006.

46. **Robert C. Schlant, John J. Collins, J.R. Bernard, J. Gersh Thomas, P. Graham**

Norman, M. Kaplan, Albert L. Waldo. *Year Book of Cardiology*, 2001.

47. **Mark Connaughton.** *Evidence-Based Manual of Coronary Care*, 2001.
48. **James T. Willerson.** *Cardiology* 1998.
49. *Nomenclature and Criteria for Diagnosis of Diseases of the Heart and Great Vessels.*, 8th ed., 1973.
50. **Stuart D. Rosen, Sanjay Sharma, Celia M. Oakley,** *Cardiology*, 2nd ed., 2004.
51. **Anthony J. Zollo.** *Medical Secrets*, 4th ed., 2005.
52. **Martin Dolgin.** *Nomenclature and Criteria for Diagnosis of the Heart and Great Vessels*, 9th ed., 1994.
53. **HylaCass.** *St. John's Wort*, 1998.
54. **M. Khalilullah.** *Recent Advances in Cardiology*, 1992.
55. **Jules Constant.** *Bedside Cardiology*, 3rd ed., 1969.
56. **G. Baroldi, F. Camerini, J.F. Goodwin (Eds.).** *Advances in Cardiomyopathies*, 1990.
57. **Joseph K. Perloff.** *The Clinical Recognition of Congenital Heart Disease*, 3rd ed., 1987.
58. **Salim Yusuf, John A. Cairns, A. John Camm, Ernest L. Fallen, Bernard J. Gersh.** *Evidence Based Cardiology*, Volume 1, 1998.
59. **Salim Yusuf, John A. Cairns, A. John Camm, Ernest L. Fallen Bernard, J. Gersh.** *Evidence Based Cardiology*, Volume 2, 1998.
60. **Valentin Fuster R., Wayne Alexander, Robert A. O'Rourke.** *Hurst's the Heart*, Volume 1, 11th ed., 2004.
61. **Valentin Fuster R., Wayne Alexander, Robert A. O'Rourke.** *Hurst's the Heart*, Volume 2, 11th, 2004.
62. **Rakel and Bope.** *Conn's Current Therapy*, 2006.

63. **Tsung O. Cheng.** *The International Textbook of Cardiology*, 1989.

64. **Emilio R. Giuliani, Valentin Fuster, Bernard J. Gersh, Michael D. McGoon, Dwight C. McGoon.** *Cardiology Fundamentals and Practice*, Volume 1, 2nd ed., 1987.

65. **Kanu Chatterjee, Melvin D. Cheitlin, Joel Karliner William W. Parmlry Elliot Rapaport, Melvin Scheinman.** *Cardiology an Illustrated Text Reference*, Volume 1, 1991.

66. **Kanu Chatterjee, Melvin D. Cheitlin, Joel Karliner William W. Parmlry Elliot Rapaport, Melvin Scheinman.** *Cardiology an Illustrated Text Reference*, Volume 2, 1991.

67. **Eric J. Topol.** *Textbook of Interventional Cardiology*, 3rd ed., 1999.

68. **Valentin Fuster R., Wayne Alexander, Robert A. O'Rourke.** *Hurst's the Heart*, 10th ed., 2001.

69. **Kim A. Eagle, Edgar Haber, Roman W. DeSanctic, W. Gerald Austen.** *The Practice of Cardiology*, 2nd ed., Number 1, 1989.

70. **Kim A. Eagle, Edgar Haber, Roman W. DeSanctis, W. Gerald Austen.** *The Practice of Cardiology*, 2nd ed., Number 2, 1989.

71. **Robert A. O'Rourke, Valentin Fuster R., Wayne Alexander.** *The Heart Manual of Cardiology*, 11th ed., 2005.

72. **John D. Rutherford.** *Unstable Angina*, 1992.

73. **Valentin Fuster.** *Assessing and Modifying the Vulnerable Atherosclerotic Plaque*, 2002.

74. **Valentin Fuster.** *Syndromes Atherosclerosis*, 1996.

75. **Anis I. Obeid.** *Echocardiography in Clinical Practice*, 1992.

76. **Michael H. Crawford.** *Current Consult Cardiology*, Part-II 2006.

77. **Isselbacher Braunwald, Wilson Martin Fauci Kasper.** *Harrison's Principles of Internal Medicine*, 13th ed., Volume 1, 1994.

78. **Joseph K. Perloff.** *The Clinical Recognition of Congenital Heart Disease,* 4th ed.

79. **J. Willis Hurst Robert C. Schlant.** *The Heart Arteries and Veins*, 7th ed., 1990.

80. **Dr. S.K. Parashar, Dr. K.K. Aggarwal.** *100 Clinical Questions in Cardiology*, 2006.

81. **J.V. (Ian) Nixon.** *The AHA Clinical Cardiac Consult*, 2nd ed., 2007.

82. **Arati Dave Lalchandani.** *Arati's Textbook of Medicine*, 2007.

83. **Valentin Fuster R., Wayne Alexander, Robert A. O'Rourke.** *Hurst's the Heart*, Volume 1, 2008.

84. **Valentin Fuster R., Wayne Alexander, Robert A. O'Rourke.** *Hurst's the Heart*, Volume 2, 2008.